Self-Care and Stress Management for Academic Well-Being

Karis L. Clarke
Clark Atlanta University, USA

A volume in the Advances in Higher Education and Professional Development (AHEPD) Book Series

IGI Global
PUBLISHER of TIMELY KNOWLEDGE

Published in the United States of America by
IGI Global
Information Science Reference (an imprint of IGI Global)
701 E. Chocolate Avenue
Hershey PA, USA 17033
Tel: 717-533-8845
Fax: 717-533-8661
E-mail: cust@igi-global.com
Web site: http://www.igi-global.com

Library of Congress Cataloging-in-Publication Data

Names: Clarke, Karis, 1979- editor.
Title: Self-care and stress management for academic well-being / Karis Clarke, editor.
Description: Hershey, PA : Information Science Reference, 2022. | Includes bibliographical references and index. | Summary: "Just like educators devote themselves to helping students develop their creativity and their academic voices this book discusses the importance of doing the same for themselves and why self-care for educators is needed to sustain the growth of the students at their institutions"-- Provided by publisher.
Identifiers: LCCN 2022970058 (print) | LCCN 2022970059 (ebook) | ISBN 9781668423349 (hardcover) | ISBN 9781668423356 (paperback) | ISBN 9781668423363 (ebook)
Subjects: LCSH: Teachers--Mental health. | Teachers--Job stress. | Teachers--Job satisfaction. | Self-care, Health. | Stress management.
Classification: LCC LB2840 .S45 2022 (print) | LCC LB2840 (ebook) | DDC 371.1--dc23/eng/20220225
LC record available at https://lccn.loc.gov/2022970058
LC ebook record available at https://lccn.loc.gov/2022970059

This book is published in the IGI Global book series Advances in Higher Education and Professional Development (AHEPD) (ISSN: 2327-6983; eISSN: 2327-6991)

British Cataloguing in Publication Data
A Cataloguing in Publication record for this book is available from the British Library.

Advances in Higher Education and Professional Development (AHEPD) Book Series

Jared Keengwe
University of North Dakota, USA

ISSN:2327-6983
EISSN:2327-6991

Mission

As world economies continue to shift and change in response to global financial situations, job markets have begun to demand a more highly-skilled workforce. In many industries a college degree is the minimum requirement and further educational development is expected to advance. With these current trends in mind, the **Advances in Higher Education & Professional Development (AHEPD) Book Series** provides an outlet for researchers and academics to publish their research in these areas and to distribute these works to practitioners and other researchers.

AHEPD encompasses all research dealing with higher education pedagogy, development, and curriculum design, as well as all areas of professional development, regardless of focus.

Coverage

- Adult Education
- Assessment in Higher Education
- Career Training
- Coaching and Mentoring
- Continuing Professional Development
- Governance in Higher Education
- Higher Education Policy
- Pedagogy of Teaching Higher Education
- Vocational Education

The Advances in Higher Education and Professional Development (AHEPD) Book Series (ISSN 2327-6983) is published by IGI Global, 701 E. Chocolate Avenue, Hershey, PA 17033-1240, USA, www.igi-global.com. This series is composed of titles available for purchase individually; each title is edited to be contextually exclusive from any other title within the series. For pricing and ordering information please visit http://www.igi-global.com/book-series/advances-higher-education-professional-development/73681. Postmaster: Send all address changes to above address.

Titles in this Series

For a list of additional titles in this series, please visit: www.igi-global.com/book-series

Strategy, Policy, Practice, and Governance for AI in Higher Education Institutions
Fernando Almaraz-Menéndez (University of Salamanca, Spain) Alexander Maz-Machado (University of Córdoba, Spain) Carmen López-Esteban (University of Salamanca, Spain) and Cristina Almaraz-López (ArcelorMittal Global R&D, pain)
Information Science Reference • © 2022 • 308pp • H/C (ISBN: 9781799892472) • US $195.00

Dispositional Development and Assessment in Teacher Preparation Programs
Sara Clemm von Hohenberg (Concordia University Ann Arbor USA)
Information Science Reference • © 2022 • 340pp • H/C (ISBN: 9781668440896) • US $195.00

Black Women Navigating Historically White Higher Education Institutions and the Journey Toward Liberation
Stephanie R. Logan (Springfield College, USA) and Tyra Good (Elms College, USA)
Information Science Reference • © 2022 • 330pp • H/C (ISBN: 9781668446263) • US $195.00

Handbook of Research on Teacher Practices for Diverse Writing Instruction
Tracey S. Hodges (The University of Alabama, USA)
Information Science Reference • © 2022 • 425pp • H/C (ISBN: 9781668462133) • US $245.00

Essential Practices for Building STEM Enrichment and College Bridge Programs
Calvin Briggs (Southern Center for Broadening Participation in STEM, USA) and Christopher K. Bass (Clark Atlanta University, USA)
Information Science Reference • © 2022 • 300pp • H/C (ISBN: 9781799871224) • US $195.00

Leadership Wellness and Mental Health Concerns in Higher Education
Cynthia J. Alexander (Acadia University, Canada) and Amy Tureen (University of Nevada, Las Vegas, USA)
Information Science Reference • © 2022 • 365pp • H/C (ISBN: 9781799876939) • US $195.00

Voicing Diverse Teaching Experiences, Approaches, and Perspectives in Higher Education
Wilfredo Alvarez (Utica University, USA) and Patrick S. De Walt (California State University, Fresno, USA)
Information Science Reference • © 2022 • 273pp • H/C (ISBN: 9781799890003) • US $195.00

Preparing Globally Competent Professionals and Leaders for Innovation and Sustainability
Linyuan Guo-Brennan (University of Prince Edward Island, Canada) and Michael J. Guo-Brennan (Troy University, USA)
Information Science Reference • © 2022 • 312pp • H/C (ISBN: 9781668445280) • US $195.00

IGI Global
PUBLISHER of TIMELY KNOWLEDGE

701 East Chocolate Avenue, Hershey, PA 17033, USA
Tel: 717-533-8845 x100 • Fax: 717-533-8661
E-Mail: cust@igi-global.com • www.igi-global.com

Editorial Advisory Board

Table of Contents

Detailed Table of Contents

Human capital is the bundle of information, skills, and talents individuals build for personal well-being and economic productivity. Human capital provides long-term benefits for future generations. It is vital for economic growth, social capital, and the development of networks. Human growth is a challenging and never-ending process. However, the importance of early childhood and youth development is ever crucial. Because youth are susceptible to biological growth, academic and career advancement, and long-term planning, stress can come to them in various forms and sources. Stress represents an undeniable reality of life, particularly in youth concerning the academic sphere. Taking care of oneself represents a regularly practiced concept to relieve stress. Learning about self-care helps carefully maintain and improve short and long-term health and well-being. Its cohorts to improve overall health and well-being thus required scholarly attention to find the new way to benefit children and youth development.

This chapter focuses on how the stress of teaching can lead to compassion fatigue. It will examine the general stressors of teaching which have led to the current teacher shortage with a special focus on the unique stress of teaching students who have experienced trauma. In addition, it will offer a snapshot of how trauma presents itself in the classroom and some of the challenges that educators experience. This chapter will share one school's experience with helping their teachers cope with compassion fatigue through a professional development series covering these topics: defining compassion fatigue and its impact, coping strategies, and the importance of self-care. Data will be presented to show the effectiveness of this intervention at this author's school.

The global COVID-19 pandemic has dramatically changed the scope of teaching and leading and has had negative effects on the academic outcomes for students. As a result of stress-induced demands provoked by this pandemic, school leaders are at an increased risk for physical, emotional, and mental health challenges. Recent studies about the pandemic's psychological impact on the general population reveal increased depression and stress levels. This chapter discusses ways university educational leadership programs can integrate self-care using mindfulness practice to effectively prepare aspiring school leaders. Practical approaches and resources for university programs are provided. In addition to suggestions for practical application, this chapter also discusses recommendations for universities and school districts regarding self-care for school leaders.

Educators have the best job in the world. They have the responsibility of helping others find their purpose in life. Every profession there is depends on them. Why is it that people with the greatest responsibility tend to not make time to care for themselves? We have often heard you cannot pour from an empty cup. In order for you to be effective and make a difference in the lives of others, you must be certain you are up for the task. The responsibility of helping others achieve their goals sometimes means putting yours on the back burner. This can lead to burnout. Educators must be better to themselves so they can be good to their students.

Preface

Anyone who's interested in making change in the world, also has to learn how to take care of herself, himself, theirselves. – Angela Davis (1981)

As an educator in p-12 and higher education settings, I have found that educators do not do a great job of taking care of ourselves. We work too many hours, do not get enough sleep or exercise, eat too many unhealthy foods, and do not spend enough time doing things that refresh and energize us.

This book is an effort to begin a necessary conversation. Too many educators have reached the conclusion that this lifestyle is just part of the job. One simply cannot be a good educator and take care of oneself (Cachero, 2019). Self-care is merely something that is done during breaks from work.

The Covid-19 pandemic really put things into perspective for me. I was beginning to question if I even needed to remain in the profession. I have devoted so many years to educating others and was not doing a good job of taking care of myself. I found myself exhausted. I thought this meant that I needed to leave the profession. What it really meant was that I was in the beginning stages of burnout. I also noticed the same was happening to my colleagues. Self-care for academic well-being has never been more important!

Educators are amazing individuals. It is our job to help our students along the journey of them becoming who they are meant to be. For people charged with such an important task, it seems important for us to take care of ourselves. This could never be truer than it is in the current times in which we live. Many of us saw the Covid-19 pandemic as a much-needed wake up call. Work was a constant. As we worked from home the boundary of workplace and time did not exist. At times, our loved ones were additional obstacles to our workload. For some, remembering to exercise, healthy eating, adequate rest, and other recommended self-care practices seemed to be only a pipe dream.

This book is a love letter to my colleagues in P-12 and Higher Education settings. We must make self-care a priority. How can we be the best versions of ourselves for our students and in our personal lives if we are exhausted (Hart et.al, 2019)? My goal with this book is to remind educators that we cannot achieve teaching excellence without first having healthy mental, physical, and psychological well-being.

We must determine comfortable boundaries such as:

Consider setting specific hours for answering students emails every day and communicating that to students.

For office hours, consider holding these hours at the same time every week and/or by appointment. As much as possible, try to be consistent about when you will hold them and communicate to students that you encourage them to utilize this option, whether they have specific questions to ask.

Setting clear boundaries with students is key! While you should communicate that you care for their wellbeing and success, boundaries help indicate to them when you are and are not available to support them (Konen, 2017).

When assigning students work, consider the time it will take you to provide feedback:

If a particular assignment will take you longer to provide feedback and students will not be able to use it for their next assignment, consider shortening the assignment, scaffolding the assignment into smaller component parts, or combining a few options together so that students have choices, and you have enough time to support their progress.

Consider other ways to provide feedback, such as voice or video feedback, check marks with longer comments, or a rubric in combination with written feedback, which can often be faster than only written feedback.

Take breaks every day for yourself.

Dedicate time every day for your other work obligations such as research or writing, family, and other life obligations, checking in on loved ones, and for moments to relax, even if only for a few minutes.

Taking short breaks throughout the day to look out the window, go for a (socially distant) walk, or participating in other relaxing activities, will provide a much-needed break from the computer screen and help keep you centered on your own needs.

Self-Care and Stress Management for Academic Well-Being discusses why self-care for educators is needed for them to sustain the growth of the students at their institutions. It explores the ways in which educators devote themselves to helping students develop their creativity and their academic voices but do not always give themselves the same permission.

WHERE DOES THIS TOPIC FIT INTO THE WORLD TODAY?

This topic fits into the world today because faculty members need to remember that our time is always a gift. Daily, those of us who work in higher education should purposefully attend to our important needs, even if only for a short time each day (Maslach & Leiter, 2016). We need to schedule wisely and carve out regular time to unplug and recharge.

Self-care can help educators prevent burnout, interact more effectively with students, and can even create climates more conducive to learning. Educators have faced so many challenges this year as they straddled in-person and remote learning, and many who dealt with personal losses.

This can be difficult for educators because many of us who do into helping professions may tend to focus more on others, sometimes at the expense of ourselves. It can be a difficult shift for some people for a variety of different reasons, to include upbringing or the way in which we practice (Patteron et. al, 2014). We simply do not prioritize self-care as something important to do.

Burnout is not a new challenge in the field of education (Darling-Hammond, 2001); however, the pandemic has presented some unique challenges. People are coping with loss of loved ones, concern for loved ones who are at increased risk, loss of jobs, loss of many of our daily routines that fuel us and connected us that are no longer in place at this time. All the while, educators are trying to support students who are often experiencing similar concerns in addition to other challenges, some that have been standing before the pandemic and some that have been exacerbated during this time and others that have presented new challenges because of the current time we are in.

One new challenge is the increased awareness about advocating for equity, which is so important. To do so effectively, requires a great deal of self-reflection and often challenging conversations. Self-care in important to sustain educators who are advocating with students and their families for social justice (Phoenix, 2017). This is a time where many educators are navigating remote schooling as teachers, while also trying to balance their personal responsibilities, which can often include remote schooling their own children. This remote schooling has required all of us as educators to be nimble and adapt to new technologies and methods of teaching in really a relatively short period of time. While I think educators understand the need for remote schooling, at the same time, some are really missing the in-person interactions with students, some of the hands-on and play-based work they were able to do before, as well as just the sense of community that they felt when they were walking through the hallways of their school building.

THE TARGET AUDIENCE

The target audience of this manuscript are educators in P-12 and higher education settings. This text is ideal for researchers, academicians, practitioners, scholars, administrators, instructors, and students.

ORGANIZATION OF THE BOOK

Chapter 1 talks about well-being, a relatively new research area in relation to teachers, being at the heart of the issue of teacher retention. This chapter provides background information on teacher retention, an overview of self-care and self-advocacy for teachers, and strategies for teachers and administrators to implement for teachers' overall well-being. Teachers who work in supportive environments that allow for innovation, authentic collaboration, and leadership opportunities often have higher job satisfaction and perceptions of self-efficacy. Additionally, teachers whose well-being is cared for are better teachers, and student outcomes are positively correlated to increased teacher satisfaction, self-efficacy, and empowerment.

Chapter 2 is designed to speak to those educators in the field that can relate to functioning on a mental, emotional, and physical low frequency based on the challenges of the workplace. The author unravels how he, as an educator, struggled to find balance in his own self-care practices while simultaneously devoting himself to helping students, and a school community flourish. This work will unpack some actional strategies that have been helpful by being proactive, rather than reactive, in coping with the challenges that educators face.

Chapter 3 is a reflection of two public school teachers and recent doctoral graduates' account of the ways in which their critical dialogues inform their rendering of the stressors weighing on educators since the onset of the COVID-19 pandemic in early 2020. The teachers-one, a Black woman in Texas, the other, a White man in New Jersey-explore how their shared, liberatory, educational goals are compromised by institutional pressures, economic uncertainties, uneven enforcement of localized curricular policies, and ongoing resistance to healthcare initiatives instituted to combat the spread of COVID-19. To accomplish this, the authors highlight how race, identity, and pedagogy are disparately addressed in their respective workplaces.

Chapter 4 identifies the predominant sources of stress and declined well-being of teachers. This chapter proposes the 'Me Within We' model of social self-care to enable teachers to experience a high level of well-being by fostering belongingness through emphatic relationships and the establishment of group identity. Future researchers are urged to empirically investigate the holistic efficacy of various dimensions of educator self-care-including social, physical, emotional, and spiritual.

Chapter 5 is about the nature of Covid-19 recovery and what teachers can do to support themselves and their students through these challenging times. This chapter provides a wide variety of research-based approaches for teachers to implement that take into account the mind, body and spirit. Recommendations, considerations, and tips for going back to the classroom, whether virtual or online, are also addressed.

Chapter 6 discusses the importance of understanding the impact stress can have on biological growth, academic and career advancement, and long-term planning. Taking care of oneself represents a regularly practiced concept to relieve stress. Learning about self-care helps carefully maintain and improve short and long-term health and well-being.

Chapter 7 focuses on how the stress of teaching can lead to compassion fatigue. The chapter will share one school's experience with helping their teachers cope with compassion fatigue through a professional development series covering these topics: defining compassion fatigue and its impact, coping strategies, and the importance of self-care. Data will be presented to show the effectiveness of this intervention at the author's school.

Chapter 8 discusses how the global COVID-19 pandemic has dramatically changed the scope of teaching and learning, as well as the negative effects on the academic outcomes for students (Kuhfeld et al., 2020). ways university educational leadership programs can integrate self-care using mindfulness practice to effectively prepare aspiring school leaders. Practical approaches and resources for university programs are provided.

Chapter 9 considers one can have success, but solace and satisfaction would only come if that success is attained through hard work by a pure mind. The chapter discusses science teaches us physical laws that govern the material world but knowledge of absolute or true understanding comes through discrimination which is a byproduct of leading a spiritual life. Also, it stresses the need for yoga of synthesis in our thoughts, beliefs and actions as being the key for one to practice enjoying holistic development for a bright career and peaceful life.

Chapter 10 examines the lack of awareness to take care of emotional aspects can lead to high levels of stress that affect educators' health and well-being, causing burnout, lack of engagement, job dissatisfaction and poor performance. The fact that having good self-care and effective stress management may result in excellent work performance and increases motivation in teaching and learning. The chapter demonstrates the need for educators to understand the stress phenomenon to include the causes and effects as well as the coping strategy.

Chapter 11 presents an overview of occupational health in remote work from the self-care perspective. A literature review regarding remote working conditions and their effects on health and well-being is included, along with an analysis of the most relevant self-care and practices that have been developed for working at the distance. The concept of health circles is introduced to help explain specific actions taken to promote self-care and group care.

Chapter 12 presents a reflection on how self-care strategies and techniques can be used to combat compassion fatigue among psychologists/psychology professionals when dealing with different stressors at the workplace front. The first section of this chapter discusses compassion fatigue, including its causes, symptoms, and progression. It entails the creative of the notion of compassion fatigue, as well as how it is stated in the literature and comprehended by psychologists. The second part explores the resilience skills of the psychology professionals to mitigate distress, discomfort, and anxiety caused due to compassion fatigue. Implications for practice as well as future research would be discussed in the chapter further.

Chapter 13 informs us to be well, our self-care cannot happen only at a micro-level. The chapter examines educator wellness from the perspective of the ecological model. It is important to examine all the impacts on our wellness and understand the control we can have over our systems. This chapter will look at the impacts of wellness and how to implement self-care strategies both at a personal and university level to reduce the impact of burnout.

Chapter 14 will explore the experiences of a Black male, full-time tenure track faculty member at a Community College. It will delve into the experiences of a Black faculty member in part-time (adjunct positions) and full-time tenure-track positions. Additionally, the author will share the importance of protecting space and time as a Black academic to prevent burnout. Lastly, the chapter will provide strategies that would be helpful to Black academics and administration that can help one to cope with challenges before situations occur.

Chapter 15 examines that while higher education seeks to foster knowledge advancement and human development through research communities, stress is alarmingly on the rise. This chapter is an acknowledgment of the trails of faculty in higher education and the importance of making self-care a priority. The author seeks to assist educators in the profession prevent burnout. The chapter addresses the need for educators to prioritize self-care to successfully educate students.

CONCLUSION

Faculty members devote themselves to helping students develop their creativity and their academic voices; however, faculty members do not always give themselves the same permission (Sinclair, 2018). This publication is a way of allowing time and space to do the same things we encourage our students to do. Administrators do not always encourage and support these efforts. This publication could be a way to education administrations on the reasons self-care for faculty members is important; self-care is needed for educators to sustain the growth of the students at their institutions of higher learning.

This publication allows me to reflect on my own experiences in this area and allow my colleagues in P-12 and higher education settings to do the same. I have spent my career supporting educators. Self-care is an area that is not discussed enough in education profession (Will, 2018). It is my sincere desire my colleagues will begin to implement strategies such as the following: insisting that your students take responsibility for their actions; learn to say no; learning to identify burnout in your yourself and/or colleagues; establishing a network of family and friends; schedule breaks; do things you enjoy; take care of yourself; and stop trying to be a perfectionist.

Educators are required to learn to teach, advise, and cope with organizational change. They must learn to insist their students take responsibility for their actions, say no, identify burnout, establish a network of family and friends, schedule breaks, do things you enjoy, and take care of themselves physically (Rimm-Kaufman & Sandilos, n.d.). The aim of this book is for readers to understand more comprehensively some of the challenges of educators and to acquire some strategies that can help one to cope with these challenges before situations occur.

This edited volume promotes voices that can be triangulated with the intentionality of the reminder that self-care has dimensions. Moreover, the final chapter of this volumes posits that recent works such as (Johnson-Arnold, 2020), which promotes the need for Self-care among educational leadership candidates at the masters degree and doctoral degree levels, should be promoted by colleagues in P12 and higher education instructional roles, leadership roles and governance roles in the policy venues of education at every level. The manifestation of change in educational leadership with an inventory of holistic health through models developed by the AERA Distinguished Research Award Winning Dissertation by Johnson-Arnold (2020) captured perspectives of those seeking and holding educational leadership roles. Nevertheless, the concept of Educare as a construct that has operational significance on the teaching and learning process should be visited as much as strategic planning is used to move the organizational ethos in the academic enterprise.

It is my hope readers will understand taking time for oneself is vital for making our classrooms reach the level that our students deserve. We can only perform excellently if we unplug and recharge. Our loved ones and students are well worth the investment.

Karis L. Clarke
Clark Atlanta University, USA

REFERENCES

Cachero, P. (2019, October 1). *Depression, anxiety, and suicidal thoughts: How teachers' stress affects their mental health*. Retrieved from https://www.yahoo.com/lifestyle/treating-the-new-ptsd-postteaching-stress-disorder-were-trying-to-survive-a-career-thats-destroying-us-155043903.html

Darling-Hammond, L. (2001). The challenge of staffing our schools. *Educational Leadership*, *58*(8), 12–17. http://www.ascd.org/publications/educational-leadership/may01/vol58/num08/The-Challenge-of-Staffing-Our-Schools

Hart, D., Paetow, G., & Zarzar, R. (2019). Does implementation of a corporate wellness initiative improve burnout? *The Western Journal of Emergency Medicine*, *20*(1), 138–144. doi:10.5811/westjem.2018.10.39677 PMID:30643617

Johnson-Arnold. (2020). Self-Care Practices and Perceptions of Holistic Health Among Selected Educational Leadership Graduate Students Attending Historically Black Colleges and Universities or Minority Serving Institutions. Academic Press.

Johnson-Arnold, L. P. (2020). Practicing Holistic Health and Self-Care Throughout the Dissertation Journey: Practical Applications and Self-Reflections for Doctoral Students. In *Creating a Framework for Dissertation Preparation: Emerging Research and Opportunities* (pp. 1-22). IGI Global. doi:10.4018/978-1-5225-9707-0.ch001

Konen, J. (2017, April). *Managing classroom procedures*. Retrieved from https://www.teacher.org/daily/managing-classroom-procedures/

Kuhfeld, M., Soland, J., Tarasawa, B., Johnson, A., Ruzek, E., & Liu, J. (2020, June 13). *Projecting the potential impacts of COVID-19 school closures on academic achievement*. Annenberg Institute at Brown University. doi:10.26300/cdrv-yw05

Maslach, C., & Leiter, M. P. (2016). Understanding the burnout experience: Recent research and its implications for psychiatry. *World Psychiatry; Official Journal of the World Psychiatric Association (WPA)*, *15*(2), 103–111. doi:10.1002/wps.20311 PMID:27265691

Morgan, M. (2018, December 17). Angela Davis on radical self-care. *Afropunk*. https://www.youtube.com/watch?v=Q1cHoL4vaBs

Patteron, J. H., Collins, L., & Abbott, G. (2014). A study of teacher resilience in urban schools. *Journal of Instructional Psychology*, *31*(1), 3–11. https://eric.ed.gov/?id=EJ774036

Phoenix, S. M. (2017, November 12). *The challenges of mental/emotional health for teachers*. Retrieved from https://theeducatorsroom.com/stress-management-challenges-mentalemotional-health-teachers-public-education/

Rimm-Kaufman, S. & Sandilos, L. (n.d.). *Improving students' relationships with teachers to provide essential supports for learning*. PsycEXTRA Dataset. doi:10.1037/e501992017-001

Sinclair, A. L. (2018, February 22). Teaching while afraid. *The Atlantic*. Retrieved from www.theatlantic.com

Will, M. (2018, October 16). *Educators are more stressed at work than average people, survey finds*. Retrieved from https://blogs.edweek.org/teachers/teaching_now/2017/10/educator_stress_aft_bat.htm

Acknowledgment

I would like to thank my family and friends for their love and support during this project.

To my parents, John and Bessie, I thank you for your spiritual guidance. None of this would have been possible without you.

To my sister, Dayna, thank you for showing me how to leave work at work and reminding me to always make time for the people you love.

To my mentor, Noran, thank you for your friendship when it mattered most. Thank you for teaching me about radical self-care.

To my colleague, Annette, thank you for your wise counsel. You have proven to be a true friend.

To the authors and reviewers, thank you for being involved in this project. You made this book at reality.

Chapter 1
Self-Care and Self-Advocacy for Improved Educator Engagement and Satisfaction:
A Guide for Teachers and Administrators

Brennan Davis
Columbia College, USA

Whitney Chick
Columbia College, USA

ABSTRACT

Teachers are leaving the profession at high rates for myriad reasons, including heavy workloads, too little time to complete tasks, lack of administrative support, inadequate professional development, and insufficient collaborative support. Well-being, a relatively new research area in relation to teachers, is at the heart of the issue of teacher retention. This chapter provides background information on teacher retention, an overview of self-care and self-advocacy for teachers, and strategies for teachers and administrators to implement for teachers' overall well-being. Teachers who work in supportive environments that allow for innovation, authentic collaboration, and leadership opportunities often have higher job satisfaction and perceptions of self-efficacy. Additionally, teachers whose well-being is cared for are better teachers, and student outcomes are positively correlated to increased teacher satisfaction, self-efficacy, and empowerment.

INTRODUCTION

Teacher retention is a well-documented issue in the United States. Sutcher et al. (2016) note that new teachers leave the profession at rates between 19 and 30% during their first five years of teaching, but this can be reduced by more than half if teachers are provided with mentoring, collaboration, and resources.

DOI: 10.4018/978-1-6684-2334-9.ch001

With so many teachers working in environments that do not provide this comprehensive support, it is no surprise that recent studies have highlighted that "half (51%) of teachers report feeling under great stress several days a week, an increase of 15 percentage points over 36% of teachers reporting that level in 1985" (MetLife, 2013, p. 6) and that 69% of teachers are either not engaged or are actively disengaged at work (Gallup, 2014). Educators in general, and beginning teachers in particular, are struggling to remain engaged and satisfied in schools across the United States. Considering this information, educators must look within to prepare themselves to thrive in academic environments and to advocate for changes that will improve the current and long-term practices within the education profession. This chapter aims to inform teachers and school administrators about the importance of self-care and self-advocacy in teacher retention and well-being as well as to provide a myriad of strategies for both groups to work toward these goals.

LITERATURE REVIEW

Teacher Retention

In a study of hundreds of first-year teachers, researchers found that teachers reported several stressors that lead to teacher attrition:

They are asked to do too much with too little time; they are compensated so poorly they cannot pay for living expenses and health care and keep up with student loan payments; they lack opportunities for collaborative support; they are overwhelmed by the state's relentless focus on data at the expense of the whole child; and they are acutely aware of their starring role in dominant political narratives as scapegoats for conditions well outside of their realm of control. (Educator Policy Information Center [EPIC], 2016, p. 28)

In addition to these factors, Holmes et al. (2019) note the following:

Teachers are exiled by fractious decision-making systems, lack of support by school leaders and by policy priorities that do not focus on student learning and developing professional learning communities. It is also postulated that good teachers leave because no one asks them to stay. Teachers also leave because of lack of respect. (p. 27)

Holmes et al. also concluded that "structural framing of the educational environment, student behaviors, school district demands for improvement, and teacher perspectives on administrative support" had significant impacts on teacher retention (p. 27). According to these studies, teachers are leaving the profession for a wide range of issues, including several factors that can be addressed within a school, such as collaboration, professional development, and school administration support. Furthermore, student outcomes are negatively affected by high teacher attrition rates across the United States (EPIC, 2016; Holmes et al., 2019; Kaynak, 2020; Kiral, 2020; Pearman et al., 2021; Robertson et al., 2020).

Teacher attrition has been linked to a variety of factors, but Carver-Thomas and Darling-Hammond (2019) found the following:

Teachers are more likely to leave schools where there are more students of color and more low-income students, where salaries are lower, and where working conditions are worse. These are frequently conditions that coexist. In schools with a majority of low-income students and students of color, turnover rates can be double the rates in schools with more White students and fewer low-income students. These schools wind up with teachers who have fewer years of experience and, often, significantly less training to teach. (p. 16–17)

This finding supports the idea that professional development is essential to better preparing teachers to support and respond to the needs of students of color and students living in poverty to build competence and self-efficacy in teachers.

School districts and governing boards must find ways to meet the needs of teachers to retain them year after year. In a recent study by Hasselquist and Graves (2020), participants "discussed the benefits of having a positive role model and mentor as part of one's professional network...The need to have peers to confide in and seek advice from came up often within the focus group" (p. 9). They also found that "programming for preservice and early career teachers should help them identify factors they can control and ways to improve job satisfaction through adjusting those factors over which they do have control" (Hasselquist & Graves, 2020, p. 10). Furthermore, Holmes et al. (2019) found that several administrative factors affected teacher retention: "supporting teacher professional development, and providing opportunities for sharing expert knowledge, professional learning outcomes" (p. 29). Therefore, more professional development is needed to provide teachers with supportive networks and empower them to use innovative and responsive practices to improve student performance.

In a study of teacher morale in a turnaround school, "interview results produced 6 themes relating to factors that influence teachers' perspectives of morale: (a) powerlessness, (b) excessive visitations, (c) loss of confidence, (d) ineffective instructional practices, (e) stress and burnout, and (f) ineffective professional development opportunities" (Lane et al., 2019, p. 1). Hasselquist and Graves (2020) also found that innovative teaching practices are key elements in teacher confidence and retention, as "improving existing lessons, incorporating new technology, adding new units, and trying new teaching techniques all received mention as important ways to stay invigorated in the classroom" (p. 12). Furthermore, Holmes et al. (2019) found that "hostile behavior exhibited by students comprise school culture and raise the stress levels of teachers throughout the day...minimizing undesired student behaviors provides opportunities for students to gain better understanding and adds to teacher longevity within schools" (p. 28). Professional development, collaboration, and innovative practices can provide teachers with strategies to mitigate undesired student behaviors and manage the stress they cause. As "specific school characteristics are highly predictive of teacher attrition rates" (EPIC, 2016, p. 28), the following strategies are recommended for teacher retention:

- Provide the resources to allow educators and administrators to build collaborative working environments;
- Increase support for teacher agency, which means granting autonomy to teachers as they respond to student needs and involving teachers in the schoolwide decision-making process;
- Provide a stronger menu of financial benefits for all educators;
- Invest in quality professional development for all educators;

- Invest boldly in new strategies that help retain teachers of color, including creating avenues for teacher autonomy, diversifying curriculum, reducing financial barriers, and providing meaningful, ongoing professional development and induction;
- Decrease the professional demands and work stressors placed on special educators; and
- Give more attention to the mental health and well-being of all educators. (EPIC, 2016, p. 28–29)

Professional Development and Administrative Support

Professional development can have positive or negative effects on teachers. Wang et al. (2020) found that teachers were "frustrated at the variability in the quality of their professional development and the lack of administrative support they received" and that, "while some teachers found their administrators to be effective in supporting their instruction, others found their school leaders to be uninterested or too busy" (p. 9–10). In another study by Lane et al. (2019), teachers reported that

Repetitive and ineffective professional development sessions had a negative influence on their perceived levels of morale. Teachers reported that there were too many professional development meetings, and that these were delivered in a regimented style of direct instruction without opportunities for discussion or participation. Most sessions focused overly simply on basic instructional practices. Other professional development sessions were either only partly useful or not helpful to veteran teachers. (p. 6)

Professional development should be collaborative and engaging, and it should provide opportunities for teachers to improve their practices in meaningful ways (Lane et al., 2019; Wang et al., 2020). Furthermore, Lane et al. (2019) found that schools should "provide participative professional development training that is appropriate to the needs of both beginning and veteran teachers and that is delivered in a way that reflects principles of andragogy and constructivism" (Lane et al., 2019, p. 6). Professional development can positively impact teachers when it serves teachers at all levels and provides opportunities for teachers to make meaning through exploration and collaboration.

Autocratic Leadership

According to Gallup (2015), 75% of people who quit their jobs do so because of a bad manager. Harsh leadership can drive employees toward a feeling of powerlessness. In education, teachers who work for poor leaders are more likely to change jobs and leave the profession (Wang, et al., 2020). In general, "autocratic leadership might not be the ideal style to lead a company that needs more innovation or better employee morale" as "autocracy is likely to decrease, not increase, employee engagement" (Murphy, 2019, para. 35). According to the same study, Murphy found that only about 11% of people prefer a leader who tells them precisely what to do and how to do it. Autocratic leaders tend to make decisions in the workplace without gathering input from others, and they frequently make all decisions regarding individuals' work assignments and processes. Failing to recognize the expertise of their employees and excluding them from decision making inevitably leads to employment dissatisfaction and damages the overall success of the group (Cherry & Susman, 2020). According to Maxwell's (2016) five levels of leadership, the second-highest level of leadership is in people development. When leaders invest in others, they can "reproduce" themselves and improve the work lives of their employees; "the more you raise up new leaders, the more you will change the lives of all members of the team. As a result, people will follow you because of what you've done for them personally" (Maxwell, 2016, para. 12).

As school administrators develop their leadership styles, it is important to emphasize that teachers are leaders and that their agency is important. Effective principals embrace the expertise of their teachers, delegate responsibilities, and develop leadership skills in stakeholders to ensure student and school success (Regional Educational Laboratory, 2019). Simply put, teachers want to be given opportunities to participate in decision making, take on leadership roles among the faculty, and lead professional development and collaboration opportunities within the school. Administrators who tap into this desire will support their teachers' development, enhance teachers' sense of empowerment and agency, and increase their likelihood of remaining in that school and in the profession overall. School administrators who increase teacher engagement and well-being will likely also see improvements in school performance in addition to improvements in teachers' adaptability, health, retention, and productivity (Witters & Agrawal, 2015).

Teacher Well-Being

According to Sharrocks (2014), "happiness and feelings of achievement are likely to be impacted on by skills possessed in interacting with others, and also by the internal thought processes in which responsibility for positive and negative experiences are ascribed internally, and hence more within one's control, or externally, and therefore less within the scope of one's control" (p. 20). Teaching is a stressful profession that many educators choose for altruistic reasons, so "maintaining a belief in a long-term aim, together with one's efficacy to attain it, is of great importance to well-being" (Sharrocks, 2014, p. 20). De Stasio et al. (2017) define work-related burnout as "the degree of physical and psychological fatigue and exhaustion perceived by the teacher specifically in relation to his/her work" (p. 473). Burnout is common within the teaching field and is often a contributing factor in teacher attrition (De Stasio et al., 2017; EPIC, 2016; Kaynak, 2020; Sharrocks, 2014; Soulen, 2020).

One of the key strategies recommended for combating teacher attrition is paying more attention to the overall health and well-being of teachers (EPIC, 2016; Kaynak, 2020; Soulen, 2020). While new teachers enter the profession engaged and enthusiastic, research has shown that their engagement begins to wane within six months, as "teachers are overworked and face enormous pressures. Occupational stressors are leading to burnout, and they are causing many educators to leave the classroom" (EPIC, 2016, p. 51). To build capacity and resilience, school administrators and veteran educators are encouraged to implement a structured system of support, which provides a variety of interventions and support across the school year or a continuum of care (Soulen, 2020).

In a study of well-being in elementary teachers, Kaynak (2020) found that teachers' well-being is attached to their sense of self-efficacy, autonomy, and empowerment, their job satisfaction in relation to a sense of achievement, engagement, and pleasure, as well as their experiences with a supportive school culture that provides sufficient time to complete their tasks. Teaching contexts must be restructured to make space for teacher well-being. Kaynak states that, "when schools are places in which teachers feel valued, respected, empowered and involved in decision-making processes, they are likely to have a better sense of well-being" (p. 32), which will improve student outcomes.

Early Career Teacher Study

This chapter is also informed by the authors' current longitudinal study of 20 beginning P-12 teachers (years 1–3) who were identified using convenience sampling. Teachers were invited to join the five-year study of beginning teachers just after their graduation from EPPs in the Southeastern region of the US. The participants are currently first- through third-year teachers, female, and in the age range of 21-46. There is a representative sample of White, African American, and Latinx teachers. A new cohort has been recruited each year since the study began in 2019. Three cohorts are currently active: Cohort 1 includes seven third-year teachers, Cohort 2 includes 5 second-year teachers, and Cohort three includes 8 first-year teachers. The authors believe it is important to note, however, that while these teachers are in their first through third years of teaching, participants in Cohorts 1 and 2 have had the first year(s) of their teaching experience altered by the onset of the COVID-19 pandemic, which has caused many of them to feel as though they are in a perpetual first-year experience.

The purposes of the study are to describe how teachers experience the transition from student to beginning teacher and to identify support interventions to enhance their experiences in the classroom. The overall aim is to better understand low first- to fifth-year teacher retention rates and to explore interventions to improve the current outcomes.

Data collection is conducted through a variety of methods. Participants complete an entrance survey during the summer prior to their first year of teaching, followed by an annual written reflection after the first two weeks of school and annual focus group interviews (audio recording) after one-month, second quarter, third quarter, and the final month of school. While all focus groups were held in person during 2019 and early 2020, all meetings since March 2020 have been held using Zoom. The authors will refer to participants throughout this paper as numbered participants (e.g., Participant 1) or cohorts (e.g., Cohort 1) for clarity.

Preliminary findings reveal that beginning teachers are impacted by their relationships with mentors in both positive and negative ways, with many of the participants noting that their mentors are not carefully selected. Participants with positive experiences are mentored by teachers on their team or in their content area. Communication is essential to new teachers' success, and they need more specific feedback from observations at school and district levels. Further, these teachers also found that expectations for their teaching positions were not clear and accessible (i.e., manuals, lists, protocols). Two-thirds of the participants would welcome classroom management mentorship and feel that self-care support is needed.

Participants also report that school-based supports could be extremely helpful to new teachers: anticipate the needs of first-year teachers through communication, train faculty to address the needs of first-year teachers, clarify the roles of teachers and administration regarding mentorship and first-year teacher support, create a "look book" of the school's who's who that includes pictures, locations, titles, and responsibilities of faculty and staff members.

The authors believe that it is essential that schools and administrators encourage and provide opportunities for self-care and self-advocacy for teachers and that it is the only way that administrators can hope to retain their teachers and maintain the quality of education in their schools.

SELF-CARE AND SELF-ADVOCACY FOR TEACHERS

Self-Care

When referring to self-care, it is important not to generalize that self-care is associated with merely a lack of sleep, too many working hours, etc. In practicing self-care, social, emotional, physical, and psychological care should each be considered independently of each other, although there are some overlapping elements. Preservice educators anticipate having their own classrooms where they will nurture students' social skills and facilitate their academic and emotional growth, but they have little preparation for supporting their own well-being once they are in the field. In addition to a lack of preparation for professional self-care, beginning teachers in their 20s often struggle with their roles. These teachers are managing their transition from student to teacher while also navigating their perceptions and perceived roles as emerging adults, which can compound struggles with self-efficacy and classroom management (Dugas, 2017). In general, teachers are conditioned to support positive attitudes and practices around well-being in students, but they do not always do the same for themselves (Sharrocks, 2014).

According to Martin et al. (2020), "professional self-care is the process of purposefully engaging with practices that promote an effective professional self, which may involve attention to workload, professional development, and time management" (p. 75). Barriers to self-care are bountiful, and a "lack of self-care leads to greater risks of burnout, compassion fatigue, vicarious trauma, and other workplace hazards" (Martin et al., 2020, p. 74). The concept of self-care is related to well-being, which is often presented through two perspectives: "the subjective experience of happiness (affect) and life satisfaction (the hedonic perspective) and positive psychological functioning, good relationships with others and self-realization (the eudemonic perspective)" (Sharrocks, 2014, p. 19–20). Prioritizing well-being within human service fields can help sustain teachers (Martin et al., 2020). Teachers must actively address their social, emotional, physical, and psychological well-being throughout their careers.

What Teachers Need

While research has shown that teaching is among the most stressful professions, "there has been a failure to recognize the critical role that teacher stress and social-emotional well-being plays in this process" (Cook et al., 2017, p. 14). In fact, teachers frequently experience a decline in their mental health as early as their first year of teaching (McLean et al., 2017). To support teacher well-being, "self-care can be framed as a critical practice with pragmatic and ethical aspects, also serving as a launching point for meaningful critical engagement" (Lee et al., 2020, p. 26). Teachers have reported several barriers to self-care, including "personal/family, not enough time/too many demands, and work-related issues and money" (Martin et al., 2020, p. 78). In this sense, teacher self-care is negatively impacted by professional demands, isolation, and negative environments. In addition to these factors, teachers are also concerned about the implications of appearing unwell:

Although staff clearly valued promoting their well-being out of school, it did not appear to be valued or permitted overtly in the school culture... Well-being in school appeared to be the responsibility of the member of staff who "learned" the required skills to cope and carry out both specific and perceived duties. Failure to acquire these skills was perceived to indicate that staff were not "good enough." Not coping or being seen to be mentally unhealthy was described in weighty and emotive terms and staff referred to "admitting" poor mental health and poor well-being conferring a "death penalty" from which "you can never come back. (Sharrocks, 2014, p. 28)

Furthermore, Cook et al. (2017) found that "the well-being of teachers is ignored, and the results are that teachers who are stressed and overwhelmed leave the profession" (p. 24).

Teachers need safe professional spaces to work on self-care and well-being. McLean et al. (2017) found that "in-school features, especially those concerning the relations among colleagues and with superiors (principals), tend to be the most salient when teachers are assessing their school's climate and hold the most sway when predicting teachers' mobility" (p. 232). Principals should work to establish environments in which well-being is promoted through breaks from work and social supports, and individual needs are honored (McLean et al., 2017). Educator preparation programs (EPPs) should provide curriculum on teacher well-being (Cancio et al., 2018; Cook et al., 2017), and school administrators "need to adopt a balanced perspective that values teacher well-being as an essential piece to creating high-quality learning environments in which students thrive" (Cook et al., 2017, p. 24). Well-being should become a part of everyday school life, and principals should create supportive work environments, provide spaces for conversations around well-being and self-care, and time to practice them (Martin et al., 2020). Principals can further support teachers' well-being by providing PD on the topic (Cancio et al., 2018).

Teacher Well-Being Affects Students

When teachers practice self-care and attend to their well-being, their ability to work with students successfully increases (Cancio, 2018; De Stasio, 2017; Sharrocks, 2014). Teachers who are satisfied in their jobs often perform better or more consistently (De Stasio, 2017). According to Cancio et al. (2018), educators who "view themselves as stress-free are more likely to engage in effective classroom practices, experience greater job satisfaction, improve their instructional capacity, and positively impact student achievement" (p. 476). However, low self-efficacy often reduces motivation (De Stasio et al., 2017). In addition to aiding in more effective instruction, teachers who practice self-care also report more positive relationships with students. As Sharrocks (2014) found, "after focusing on their own well-being, they [teachers] managed incidents relating to children's emotions in class better, perhaps highlighting that those who are involved in supporting the well-being of others should themselves have access to support" (p. 32).

Self-Advocacy

While self-advocacy is frequently discussed within other professions, it is rarely a topic among educators except in terms of developing self-advocacy in students. According to Abrell (2020), self-advocacy is necessary for all professionals, and it should be accessed through an individual's entitlement, confidence, comfort with discomfort, and knowledge of one's worth. Abrell (2020) goes on to encourage professionals to "understand and justify your place in the organization. You have a responsibility to yourself and your family to make sure that your value is recognized and rewarded appropriately" (para. 4). While it is not often discussed, the same is true for teachers. Participants in the current teacher study reported that they struggle with this due to concerns that they will not be heard. However, self-advocacy is an important element of every professional's work, and educators must advocate for changes in their schools to improve current systems and innovate new, more effective processes. Teachers must advocate for the roles and reforms they believe will improve academic environments. According to participants in the current beginning teacher study, examples of these reforms include improved communication systems, more time dedicated to planning and student feedback, and more teacher voice and choice in PD.

What Teachers Need

Additional research has indicated that teachers need to develop several skills and receive support to help them stay in the profession long term. According to Kaynak (2020), the aspects of teacher well-being include a reasonable workload, supportive school culture, job satisfaction, a sense of autonomy, and a sense of efficacy. In addition, teachers are more motivated and satisfied when they are "entrusted with more autonomy and decision-making power, resulting in increased teacher authority" (Kaynak, 2020, p. 22). Fix et al. (2021) further posit that self-determination theory "implies that teachers' learning is stimulated by support of teachers' perceived autonomy, which applies to opportunities to bring in their own ideas, opinions and personal experiences" (p. 9). Kiral (2020) also found that "involving teachers in the decisions regarding the school by administrators is one of the most significant components of empowerment" (p. 250).

Additional factors that significantly impact teacher empowerment are teamwork and effective communication with administrators (Kiral, 2020). Collectively, these studies support the idea that teachers' self-efficacy is tied to many factors, including confidence, collaboration, voice, and a variety of support from administrators. Finally, in their study, Pearman et al. (2021) found that the characteristics of teacher self-efficacy include "confidence/self-empowerment, commitment, ability to meet challenges, innovative thinking, and facilitation" (p. 84). Teachers who develop a strong sense of self-efficacy "possess characteristics of resiliency, perseverance, and motivation. They demonstrate creativity and curiosity when faced with challenges and believe failure can be surmounted by skill-acquisition or further investigation to increase their knowledge base" rather than blaming others for their circumstances or feeling powerless in difficult situations (Pearman et al., 2021, p. 81).

Teacher Empowerment Affects Students

Teacher empowerment and self-advocacy result in improved outcomes for students (EPIC, 2016; Holmes et al., 2019; Kaynak, 2020; Kiral, 2020; Pearman et al., 2021; Robertson et al., 2020). Wellness is a benefit that extends beyond the individual teacher, as "the wellness of teachers directly influences the wellness and performance of students. Teachers will be able to perform better in their classrooms if they have the occupational resources needed to sustain their work" (EPIC, 2016, p. 56). When teachers have self-efficacy, they are better able to demonstrate their competence, and teachers who experience autonomy and empowerment will more freely apply their best teaching methods. Likewise, when teachers have access to agentive professional development, they are more likely to transfer this agency to their work with students, thus increasing student motivation (Robertson et al., 2020). A significant relationship is found "between teachers' empowerment perception levels and their organizational-professional commitment and organizational citizenship behavior" (Kiral, 2020, p. 258). Furthermore, "as a teacher's self-efficacy increases, their belief in their students' abilities and confidence in their own teaching practices also increases" (Pearman et al., 2021, p. 82).

SOLUTIONS AND RECOMMENDATIONS

Self-Care and Self-Advocacy Implementation

Teachers must take actions to secure self-care and self-advocacy practices that will sustain them through the challenges of teaching and provide them with improved engagement and satisfaction with the profession. Likewise, administrators must encourage, support, and provide access to the self-care and empowerment of teachers.

Self-Care

Across more than two years of focus group meetings with beginning teachers, participants in the current study consistently demonstrated their excitement and enthusiasm as they entered the classroom for their first year of teaching. After their first month of teaching, participants said they were prepared and committed to facilitating student growth. They were very hopeful about the work they would do with their students:

I love my job despite the challenges...The reward of reaching difficult students and building close bonds with my students makes it so worth it. I love how no day is the same and I am always on my toes. I have also found a confidence in myself that I never had before. (Participant 6, October 4, 2019)

Quickly, however, their excitement turned to frustration, disappointment, and even anger. Beginning teachers shared that they have struggled with the realities of teaching: "I'm feeling overwhelmed in juggling the amount of paperwork and organization that goes into it. I was told to expect it, but I never understood how challenging it is until I had to do it myself" (Participant 6, September 24, 2019). They noted repeatedly that ineffective communication, unclear expectations, lack of mentoring, and insufficient professional development specifically designed for beginning teachers have contributed to this shift in their perception of the profession.

The participants also struggled to maintain work–life balance, and they indicated that they frequently work all weekend and late in the evenings. These teachers also shared that they struggle to maintain relationships with friends and family and that they are often too tired after work to engage in social activities. Participants have used self-care strategies, such as shopping, setting work cut-off times, putting their phones away for established times, yoga, meditation (Cohort 1, October 25, 2021), not taking work home, making Saturdays a dedicated day off, and taking day trips with friends (Cohorts 2 & 3, October 28, 2021).

Knowing that self-care is multifaceted, educators and individuals alike must consider social, emotional, psychological, and physical aspects of their self to adopt better self-care practices. Because the profession of education has many practices that align with the field of social work, practices supporting these professionals can be used to benefit educators. Literature from the field of social work supports the efficacy of self-care practices, which can be practiced by educators for the improvement of professional well-being and overall health (Lee et al., 2020; Martin et al., 2020). The practice of "self-care enhances well-being and involves purposeful and continuous efforts that are undertaken to ensure that all dimensions of the self receive the attention that is needed to make the person fit to assist others" (Moore et al., 2011, p. 1). Individual educators hold a great responsibility in implementing strategies to improve personal self-care practices; however, administrators have an opportunity to support the overall mental health of teachers. Through a school's culture, climate, and supportive initiatives, administrators can implement practices (Table 1) to address the need for self-care to reduce stress.

Social Well-Being

Social well-being refers to "positive functioning and involves having something to contribute to society (social contribution), feeling part of a community (social integration), believing that society is becoming a better place for all people (social actualization), and that the way society works makes sense to them (social coherence)" (Galderisi, 2015, p. 231). Participants in the current study have noted that their social well-being is at risk. While first-year teachers report inordinate hours of work that keep them from enjoying valuable down time and time with friends and family, participants in Cohorts 1 and 2 have shared in the past year that they are utilizing a variety of self-care measures for their social well-being: setting boundaries with work hours, reflecting on their work, taking Saturday trips with friends, reserving particular nights during the week to do something by themselves or with others, and shopping (Cohort 1, October 25, 2021).

To build social well-being, self-care practices for educators include finding time to be alone, completing an activity with others, and spending time with friends and family. Part of developing social well-being includes professional awareness of who you are in relation to your work. Vekeman et al. (2017) posit that job fit (or person–organization [PO] fit) is an essential part of a teacher's job satisfaction. Therefore, teachers should take time to identify, clarify, and commit to personal values related to education that will aid them in selecting the best job fit for their satisfaction and will provide them with a framework for acting according to their values when confronted with stressful situations at work (Cook et al., 2017). Teachers should be aware of their own values so they can determine which working environments will most closely align with their values and, therefore, provide them with a sense of community and belonging.

In addition to establishing a set of values to sustain teachers through challenging moments, educators should also seek supportive networks, whether they are local school networks or professional networks through membership (Cancio et al., 2018). Teachers are best served in their "overall personal and professional wellness" by developing social support, which "includes time with family, friends, and significant others"; collegial support, which involves "processing stress as a professional team and raising morale in the work environment"; and professional support, which refers to counseling (Martin et al., 2020, p. 77). Administrators should work with teachers to create supportive, encouraging environments (Martin et al., 2020).

Emotional Well-Being

Emotional well-being is characterized as "happiness, interest in life, and satisfaction" (Galderisi, 2015, p. 231). In the current study, Participants 7 and 13 shared that it is "hard to be happy about anything at all" because of stressors at work (October 29, 2020).

Self-care strategies to support emotional well-being and self-care require personal reflection and changes to one's lifestyle. At the beginning of the 2020-2021 school year, participants in Cohort 1 shared that they were experiencing stressors that were affecting their mental health; one participant's main concerns included the "health and safety for my family/students. I am currently at home sick, waiting for test results to be able to go back to work. I'm worried about missing valuable face-to-face instruction time" (Participant 10, September 24, 2020).

Taking time away from work to spend time in nature or visit with friends allows for a balance of personal enjoyment with work life, or work–life balance. According to Taylor (2018), "the experience of social and emotional well-being is a precursor to good mental health and provides a barrier to the normal stresses of everyday life" (p. 243). Furthermore, "past studies have shown that school-based implementation of mental health training and support for teachers can lead to positive outcomes for both teachers and their students through improvements in classroom climate, teacher sensitivity to student needs and behavior management, as well as diminished teacher burnout, anxiety, and depression" (McLean et al., 2017, p. 232). Cook et al. (2017) suggest that teachers integrate the following resilience practices:

1. Awareness and empowerment through mindfulness-based practices;
2. Choosing to pay attention to the positive and practicing gratitude;
3. Helping and doing good deeds for others;
4. Identifying unhelpful thoughts and altering them to be more helpful;
5. Engaging in good sleep, exercising regularly, and eating well;
6. Clarifying values and making commitments;
7. Establishing good social support, role model(s), and a mentor (relationships); and
8. Rewarding yourself through relaxation and recreation. (p. 18)

Several of these recommended practices focus on emotional well-being, such as mindfulness, practicing gratitude, monitoring unhelpful thoughts, and doing good deeds for others. In addition to these actions, teachers can learn to deal with their automatic thoughts and learn to resolve conflict to reduce stress (Taylor, 2018). In terms of resilience, it is important to note that "people can alter their physical and mental states through proactive behaviors, even if the actual work environment does not alter," so teachers can work toward happiness even if their work environments are not ideal (Taylor, 2018, p. 255). However, administrators have an opportunity to greatly improve work environments by supporting teachers and providing opportunities for reducing stress, practicing mindfulness, and creating spaces for teachers to relax and think in the school building. According to McLean et al. (2017), "understanding teachers' mental health is important not only for the objective of supporting teachers, but also because these symptoms have implications for students" (p. 231). School administrators should move beyond an acknowledgement of the role of emotional well-being in teacher satisfaction and performance by providing supports for teachers (Cook et al., 2017).

Physical Well-Being

In a focus meeting with Cohort 1, participants reported that they were increasingly worried about their physical health, which had been in decline due to long hours of working and isolation because of the pandemic. This feeling is exacerbated by the feeling that teachers are "playing a never-ending game of catch-up that seems impossible" (Participant 8, September 24, 2020).

While mental and social self-care practices contribute to an overall positive outlook and interactions with others, physical self-care also plays a critical role. Physical self-care practices include creating exercise regimens that begin with a tangible goal that can be increased over time, focusing on hydration, and eating a healthier diet (Moore et al., 2011).

Relaxation can also be a critical element of physical well-being and can include various practices, such as deep-breathing exercises and progressive muscle relaxation, which involves the systematic tensing and relaxing of all body parts (Taylor, 2018). Sleep also plays a major role in physical well-being. According to Taylor (2018), "sleep deprivation appears to be affecting a significant proportion of the population, in part due to the widespread use of technology" (p. 261), and therefore, teachers are encouraged to consider their sleep habits and identify practices that might improve their quality of sleep.

Finally, teachers can make room for additional coping strategies, such as listening to music and dancing, which have been linked to lower stress levels (Cancio et al., 2018). Administrators can assist teachers in the development of physical well-being by providing access to fitness rooms on school grounds and incorporating physical activities, such as yoga, into professional development opportunities.

Psychological Well-Being

Participants in the authors' study consistently report that a lack of time to complete their work and communication challenges with administrators have impeded their productivity. Teachers shared that time is one of their "lows"; Participant 1 shared that she "[gets] to school around 6:30 a.m. to get a head start on my day...planning lessons is taking up the majority of my weekends—roughly 10 hours total" (September 24, 2019).

According to Galderisi (2015), "psychological well-being includes liking most parts of one's own personality, being good at managing the responsibilities of daily life, having good relationships with others, and being satisfied with one's own life" (p. 231). Organizational tools, such as planners and visual schedules, help develop structured routines to support time assessments and management, and teachers can use daily, weekly, monthly, and yearly calendars to organize their responsibilities and prioritize tasks. In addition to organizational tools, teachers can employ coping strategies to develop psychological well-being, as "capacity can be increased by effective coping resources in a supportive environment that contributes to professional growth" (Cancio et al., 2018, p. 461).

Coping mechanisms, such as mindfulness, can help teachers manage stress and become more accepting of themselves and their feelings. Martin et al. (2020) suggest that self-preservation should begin early in one's teaching career and that practicing self-awareness, self-compassion, and work–life balance mitigates stressful work factors. Finally, the implementation of positive psychology aims "to increase the degree to which people experience positive emotion while at the same time, decrease the degree of negative emotion" (Taylor, 2018, p. 249). Teachers could implement positive psychology practices, such as expressing gratitude to others or journaling positive events in their lives daily.

The "vital intersection of psychological and organizational self-care" provides administrators with the opportunity to model and facilitate positive practices in each area (Martin et al., 2020). Cancio et al. (2018) suggest that administrators should actively search for activities that relieve stressors and provide teachers with opportunities to participate in them, constantly evaluate teachers' job satisfaction and provide support, and provide professional development on dealing with stress.

Self-Advocacy

Self-advocacy, or representing oneself or ideas (Oxford, 2021), is essential to the long-term success of teachers. Developing and implementing self-advocacy is necessary, but often difficult, work that should be supported and encouraged by school administrators and EPPs alike.

Table 1. Self-care implementation practices

Domain	Self-Care Practices
Social	• Evaluate job fit/satisfaction • Identify values and commit to them • Engage with family, friends, and neighbors • Seek out social, collegial, and professional support
Emotional	• Spend time alone • Practice mindfulness • Do good deeds for others • Practice gratefulness • Journal your thoughts and feelings • Find something positive to share about your day with someone who cares
Physical	• Develop a realistic exercise regimen • Maintain a regular sleep schedule • Practice intentional relaxation • Listen to music • Dance • Stay hydrated • Develop a healthy eating plan
Psychological	• Practice mindfulness • Employ time management strategies • Take breaks from work and the demands of the tasks at hand • Embrace your agency • Practice self-awareness/compassion

Participants across all cohorts in the current study have noted repeatedly that ineffective communication, unclear expectations, lack of mentoring, and insufficient professional development specifically designed for beginning teachers have contributed to a shift in their perceptions of the profession. Teachers in this study noted that "college me and first-year me would hate each other" and "I thought student teaching was hard...first year is hard" (Participant 7, October 29, 2020). The daily frustrations of not knowing who to go to for information or tasks, having little-to-no time with their mentors or for planning, and adjusting to the demands of planning, teaching, grading, classroom management, etc. worked quickly to change their perspectives.

As these teachers unpacked their experiences over the first year of teaching, they suggested several ideas for improving the experience for future teachers: intentional mentoring, clear communication about responsibilities, expectations and processes, and more training designed specifically for beginning teachers to support their growth and development over the first years of teaching. Specific actions for teachers and administrators toward this goal include communication, collaboration, professional development, innovation, and leadership (Table 2).

These teachers have also started to explore self-advocacy to varying degrees as a coping strategy. One third-year teacher shared that she is comfortable with self-advocacy but that, after using the chat feature to advocate for herself and others during a virtual faculty meeting, "administration did not appreciate it and turned the chat feature off in subsequent faculty meetings" (personal communication, October 28, 2021). First- and second-year teachers shared that they are also somewhat comfortable with self-advocacy: "I'm new but I'm not stupid...you can only advocate for what you know" (Cohorts 2 & 3, October 25, 2021).

Communication

Challenges with school administrators were prevalent among participants in the current study who shared that they are overwhelmed by excessive and conflicting communication from administrators; participants believe that more support is needed from administrators in the areas of student behavior and performance (Cohort 1, February 12, 2020). Participant 12 shared that "there is a high expectation that we openly and consistently communicate with administration, but that isn't modeled or received" (September 15, 2021). Communication is essential in any relationship, and this is especially true in schools where teachers are often micromanaged and infrequently given voice in decision making (EPIC, 2016).

Teachers should be vocal about their concerns and beliefs, and administrators must listen to teachers' voices and take heed of the challenges teachers are facing, such as insufficient time to complete work, ineffective administrator communication, and too many school and district initiatives. Ultimately, to retain and grow effective teachers, "they need to be in a safe learning environment that support[s] risk to remove the affective filter and allow optimal learning to occur. They must feel free to admit when they don't know something, and they have to feel that their ideas will be listened to and taken seriously" (Martin, 2020, p. 37). Lack of effective communication often leads to a decreased sense of self-efficacy and, therefore, a diminished sense of job satisfaction. Radical candor based on caring personally and challenging directly is one way that teachers and administrators can develop more effective communication and support each other's growth (Martin, 2020). Kiral (2020) also found that "by enhancing their communication with teachers, school administrators can help teachers increase their school commitment levels" (p. 259), which can improve efficacy, job satisfaction, and student outcomes. Finally, it is important for both teachers and administrators to remember to reflect rather than react. Reflection is looking back "to experiences a teacher has had and being able to step away and look at the evidence to enhance future practices" (Reitman & Karge, 2019, p. 16). As issues occur, teachers and administrators should reflect and respond constructively rather than simply reacting to the situation. This reflection is imperative in effective communication within school settings.

Collaboration

Collaboration is a natural part of schooling, especially for students. Teachers, however, rarely have the time for or access to meaningful collaboration with peers or school administrators. Participants in the current teacher study shared that they have very little time with mentors, teams, and administrators, but that they do benefit from authentic collaboration when it is accessible. One participant shared that mentoring at the teacher, school, and district levels are a "great concept, [but a] challenging expectation" (Participant 8, February 12, 2020). Another teacher shared that "I wish I had collaborating teammates with a positive mentality and a drive to help students learn. I also wish I had more support from administration especially in circumstances in which kids are disrespectful and do not want to do their work" (Participant 9, February 18, 2020).

Collaboration must move beyond surface-level interactions. As an EPIC (2016) report notes, "to retain teachers, it is vital that schools be collaborative environments. Policies that inspire and nurture authentic collaboration—between teachers and administrators, between teachers and paraprofessionals, between teachers and parents, and among teachers themselves" are needed (p. 29). Furthermore, EPIC (2016) also found that "when teachers and administrators work collaboratively on student behavior policies and procedures, attrition rates drop" and that teachers "cite collaborative relationships as important factors when asked about their desire to stay in or leave teaching" (p. 30). These types of relationships, specifically for beginning teachers, can also be connected to the school culture and the type of interactions between colleagues within the school. McLean et al. (2017) report that "there is evidence to suggest that within-school/program supports such as guidance and mentoring from colleagues and superiors and a cohesive work environment may be related to more positive mental health among beginning teachers." To establish effective collaborative environments, teachers and administrators must achieve psychological safety, a state of comfort with being oneself, through radical candor, normalizing failure, and welcoming direct feedback (Martin, 2020). Teachers must advocate for collaborative time with peers and administrators and be willing to lead these opportunities when they are allowed. Administrators should be active participants and supporters of authentic collaborations. Robertson et al. (2020) found that agentic professional development works "in iterative and interdependent ways to foster collective agency…Thus, the social and contextual factors in which the groups are interacting facilitate intrinsic motivation through increased autonomy and self-efficacy" (p. 193). Authentic collaborative relationships among school faculty and staff support the long-term retention of teachers by increasing their knowledge and efficacy.

Professional Development

Participants in the current study have called for professional development that is designed specifically for beginning teachers. Further, participants have suggested that administrators spend time with them as a group to discuss what they need and provide it personally, if possible, to develop a more collaborative PD model. Additional individualized PD on classroom management and instructional strategies would be welcomed.

Traditional professional development, though common, "rarely leads to meaningful change in teachers' practice or student achievement"; thus, an agentive approach to professional development "where all educators act individually and intentionally to promote student learning" is recommended (Robertson et al., 2020, p. 192). This approach to professional development includes four elements: "leadership that privileges teachers' co-construction and application of new knowledge from the outset, autonomy in designing PD reciprocally with teachers and situating learning in teachers' actual classrooms, intentionality and coherence across multiple PD sessions, and reflectivity that is consistently focused on student learning of context-embedded curriculum goals" (Robertson et al., 2020, p. 195).

Professional development that is designed for specific schools, teachers, and classrooms has a positive effect on teacher retention (EPIC, 2016). In fact, "many young teachers report feeling unsupported and unprepared for the classroom, and a large number of the new teachers who leave the profession cite lack of training as a primary reason" (EPIC, 2016, p. 40). Teachers should advocate for the professional development they need to be successful, and administrators should provide professional development opportunities that focus on the authentic questions, experiences, and problems that teachers face over time (EPIC, 2016). Ultimately, administrators must understand that teacher retention requires that they "put time and effort into planned professional learning, based on solid research and individualized support, for teachers during the first five years of their careers" (Reitman & Karge, 2019, p. 17).

In addition to self-advocacy for responsive professional development sessions, teachers should also practice self-advocacy by pursuing their own professional learning in the form of professional organization membership, conference attendance, and professional reading. These professional communities can provide resources, pedagogical knowledge, and relationships that can sustain teachers through their first years of teaching.

Innovation

Teachers are frequently micromanaged, which often leads to teacher burnout (EPIC, 2016). Teachers must advocate for their own innovation in school settings. According to Fix et al. (2021), "Teachers' perceived autonomy in innovation leaves an important role for school leaders, for example, as they make sure teachers feel safe to change their individual ideas and respect the identities of individual teachers" (p. 9). One teacher in the current study shared her belief that teachers deserve more respect and acknowledgement because they "are innovators, we adapted to any and everything" (Participant 11, October 2, 2020).

When teachers advocate for safe spaces to innovate and administrators support them, teachers improve their sense of competence. As teachers develop the "ability to view difficulties as growth opportunities… they utilize creativity in their ability to apply knowledge and make professional decisions" (Pearman et al., 2021, p. 86). Teachers need to feel ownership of their work, and administrators must foster this feeling in schools. Through professional learning and reflection, teachers can develop the knowledge to support and advocate for their innovations.

Leadership

Teachers are often interested in leadership roles outside of the classroom (MetLife, 2013), but leadership roles are frequently reserved for administrators. Participants in the current study have reported no leadership opportunities over the previous three years, and they believe that this is, in part, because administrators do not see them as leaders in their first three years of teaching.

Teachers should identify and advocate for the leadership roles they believe would improve school culture and student outcomes. Teachers could serve as leaders in a myriad of formal ways, including assigned mentorship, team leaders, department leaders, professional development leaders, and professional learning community leaders, and in many informal ways, such as unofficial mentoring, modeling professionalism, advocating for teacher agency, and providing feedback to peers and administrators.

Administrators can support teachers in their development of leadership through coaching (Mayer, 2013) and a continuum of care (Soulen, 2020). The role of teacher leaders "differs from that of other school leaders…The clarification of roles is best established through collaboration with administrators" (Mayer, 2013, p. 32). Administrators should identify emerging teacher leaders and provide them with opportunities and feedback to facilitate their growth. A continuum of care model can be utilized to develop "resilient faculty who contribute positively to the school ecology" (Soulen, 2020, p. 38). In this model, beginning teachers are provided with structured support that includes intentional mentoring, collaboration, and reflection to "build resilience of new teachers, reduce burnout, and increase the commitment and effectiveness of new teachers" (Soulen, 2020, p. 42). Administrators should engage in a leadership approach in which "power is distributed across principal and teachers, facilitating a sense of collective agency that facilitates the process of teachers working toward a common goal" (Robertson et al., 2020, p. 195). This distributed leadership approach allows administrators to model effective leadership while fostering the growth of leadership skills in teachers. Furthermore, Fix et al. (2021) found that "distributed leadership contributed to the quality of the innovation" and that school leaders "posited that freedom for teachers' expertise led to an innovation that was very well adapted for students" (p. 19). Teachers who are interested in leadership roles should identify opportunities for assuming these roles and advocate for themselves with school administrators. Administrators can encourage teacher leaders by identifying emerging leaders, modeling a distributed leadership approach, and fostering the development of leadership skills.

Table 2. Self-advocacy implementation practices

Implementation Practice	Teacher Strategies	Administrator Strategies
Communication	• Identify communication needs and articulate them to administrators • Share concerns and beliefs • Admit when you do not know something • Ask for help • Reflect and respond; do not react	• Cultivate a supportive environment in which teachers feel free to be themselves (psychological freedom) • Embrace and value radical candor • Be responsive to teachers' needs • Reflect and respond; do not react
Collaboration	• Advocate for authentic collaborative opportunities with teachers and administrators • Be prepared to lead collaborative activities	• Provide opportunities for meaningful collaboration • Develop intentional, collaborative relationships with teachers to develop agency in daily decision making
Professional Development	• Advocate for specific professional development opportunities/topics • Engage in self-directed professional learning	• Design professional development that is school, teacher, and classroom centered • Provide responsive professional development opportunities
Innovation	• Advocate for your agency as a professional • Prepare to defend innovations by doing the research/professional learning necessary	• Provide teachers with a low-risk environment for innovation • Embrace teacher voice and include them in decision making • Develop teacher autonomy; do not micromanage them
Leadership	• Identify needed teacher leadership roles and responsibilities • Advocate for your desired leadership development/role • Take on formal and/or informal leadership roles	• Identify emerging leaders and foster their development of leadership skills • Model a distributed leadership approach

FUTURE RESEARCH DIRECTIONS

While self-care and well-being are well-established areas of study in psychology and health care, they are relatively new research areas within the field of education. Educators often enter the field with altruistic aims and the hopes of encouraging and supporting student growth, well-being, and achievement. However, space for teachers to nurture their own well-being is often limited or nonexistent. Some progress has been made toward more awareness around these issues in education, but there is still a long way to go in the restructuring of teaching environments to better support and serve teachers and students. As EPPs seek to build programs that prepare teachers to teach students who experience challenges such as poverty and trauma, more attention should be given to building a curriculum around teacher self-care and self-advocacy to best prepare teachers to care for themselves along with their students. More research is needed in this area to determine which strategies are the best practices for the overall health and persistence of educators. Future research should focus on how teachers process job stressors, when support is needed, and how administrators can best support self-care and self-advocacy among teachers. Additionally, more research investigating the connection between teacher perceptions of self-care and self-advocacy, administrator attitudes and practices, and teacher retention is needed.

CONCLUSION

Educators must develop effective self-care and self-advocacy practices to thrive in academic environments in which time constraints and increasing demands create stressful working conditions. Educators who develop practices that allow them to use their time and energy most effectively while at work will improve their job satisfaction and work–life balance. As educators take a more proactive role in schools through self-advocacy, they will also develop a deeper engagement and satisfaction in their work. Likewise, when teachers feel more in control of their work and become more engaged and satisfied in their academic environments, they will be more inclined to persist in the education profession.

Administrators play an essential role in this process. While teachers cite heavy workloads, too little time, lack of administrative support, a need for more collaborative support, and many more reasons for leaving the education field, administrators can implement practices to ease these challenges. Administrators should create an environment in which teachers are encouraged and given time to collaborate in meaningful ways, listen and respond constructively to teacher feedback about their needs, and identify and support teachers as leaders in schools.

As education deals with the ongoing demands of the pandemic, remote learning, and public opinion, it is essential that teachers and administrators work together to develop strategies for self-care and self-advocacy among teachers. These strategies, such as time management, collaboration, innovation, and leadership, will enhance teachers' job satisfaction, sense of efficacy, and persistence in the profession.

REFERENCES

Abrell, T. (2020, September 12). A year-round guide to self-advocacy. *Forbes*. https://www.forbes.com/sites/ellevate/2020/10/01/a-year-round-guide-to-self-advocacy/

Bradberry, T. (2021, June 24). *70% of Employees Say They Are Disengaged at Work. Here's How to Motivate Them.* World Economic Forum. https://www.weforum.org/agenda/2016/11/70-of-employees-say-they-are-disengaged-at-work-heres-how-to-motivate-them/#:%7E:text=The%20scariest%20thing%20is%20how%20prevalent%20this%20lack,happen.%20When%20they%20don%E2%80%99t%2C%20the%20bottom%20line%20suffers

Cancio, E. J., Larsen, R., Mathur, S. R., Estes, M. B., Johns, B., & Chang, M. (2018). Special education teacher stress: Coping strategies. *Education & Treatment of Children, 41*(4), 457–482. doi:10.1353/etc.2018.0025

Carver-Thomas, D., & Darling-Hammond, L. (2019). The trouble with teacher turnover: How teacher attrition affects students and schools. *Education Policy Analysis Archives, 27*(36), 1–28. doi:10.14507/epaa.27.3699

Cherry, K., & Susman, D. (2020, June 10). *What Are the Pros and Cons of Autocratic Leadership?* Verywell Mind. https://www.verywellmind.com/what-is-autocratic-leadership-2795314#:%7E:text=Because%20autocratic%20leaders%20make%20decisions,hurt%20the%20group%20from%20performing

Cook, C., Miller, F., Fiat, A., Renshaw, T., Frye, M., Joseph, G., & Decano, P. (2017). Promoting secondary teachers' well-being and intentions to implement evidence-based practices: Randomized evaluation of the achiever resilience curriculum. *Psychology in the Schools*, *54*(1), 13–28. doi:10.1002/pits.21980

De Stasio, S., Fiorilli, C., Benevene, P., Uusitalo-Malmivaara, L., & Di Chiacchio, C. (2017). Burnout in special needs teachers at kindergarten and primary school: Investigating the role of personal resources and work wellbeing. *Psychology in the Schools*, *54*(5), 472–486. doi:10.1002/pits.22013

Dugas, D. (2017). The perils of feeling in-between: The experiences of emerging adult novice teachers. *Journal of Adult Development*, *24*(3), 189–198. doi:10.100710804-016-9257-2

Educator Policy Innovation Center. (2016). *Smart solutions to Minnesota's teacher shortage: Developing and sustaining a diverse and valued educator workforce.* EPIC. https://educationminnesota.org/wp-content/uploads/2021/08/EPIC-Recruitment-Retention-Report.pdf

Fix, G. M., Rikkerink, M., Ritzen, H. T. M., Pieters, J. M., & Kuiper, W. A. J. M. (2021). Learning within sustainable educational innovation: An analysis of teachers' perceptions and leadership practices. *Journal of Educational Change*, *22*(1), 131–145. doi:10.100710833-020-09410-2

Galderisi, S., Heinz, A., Kastrup, M., Beezhold, J., & Sartorius, N. (2015). Toward a new definition of mental health. *World Psychiatry; Official Journal of the World Psychiatric Association (WPA)*, *14*(2), 213–233. doi:10.1002/wps.20231 PMID:26043341

Gallup. (2014). *State of America's schools report.* https://www.gallup.com/education/269648/state-america-schools-report.aspx

Hasselquist, L., & Graves, N. A. (2020). CTE teacher retention: Lessons learned from mid-career teachers. *Career and Technical Education Research*, *45*(1), 3–16. doi:10.5328/cter45.1.3

Holmes, B., Parker, D., & Gibson, J. (2019). Rethinking teacher retention in hard-to-staff schools. *Contemporary Issues in Education Research*, *12*(1), 27–33. doi:10.19030/cier.v12i1.10260

Kaynak, N. E. (2020). A close look at teachers' lives: Caring for the well-being of elementary teachers in the US. *The International Journal of Emotional Education*, *12*(1), 19–34.

Kiral, B. (2020). The relationship between the empowerment of teachers by school administrators and organizational commitments of teachers. *International Online Journal of Education & Teaching*, *7*(1), 248–265.

Lane, L., Jones, D., & Penny, G. E. (2019). Qualitative case study of teachers' morale in a turnaround school. *Research in Higher Education*, *37*(Nov), 1–12.

Lee, J. J., Miller, S. E., & Bride, B. (2020). Development and initial validation of the self-care practices scale. *Social Work*, *65*(1), 21–28. doi:10.1093wwz045 PMID:31846041

Martin, E. M., Myers, K., & Brickman, K. (2020). Self-preservation in the workplace: The importance of well-being for social work practitioners and field supervisors. *Social Work*, *65*(1), 74–81. doi:10.1093wwz040 PMID:31846026

Martin, J. (2020). Teaching without fear: Psychology safety can alter the professional learning landscape. *The Learning Professional*, *41*(2), 36–38.

Maxwell, J. (2016, August 30). *The 5 Levels of Leadership.* John Maxwell. https://www.johnmaxwell.com/blog/the-5-levels-of-leadership1/

Mayer, L. (2013). Empowerment zone: Coaching academy primes teachers to become instructional leaders. *Journal of Staff Development*, *34*(6), 30–33.

McLean, L., Abry, T., Taylor, M., Jimenez, M., & Granger, K. (2017). Teachers' mental health and perceptions of school climate across the transition from training to teaching. *Teaching and Teacher Education*, *65*, 230–240. doi:10.1016/j.tate.2017.03.018

MetLife. (2013). *The MetLife Survey of the American Teacher: Challenges for School Leadership.* https://www.metlife.com/content/dam/microsites/about/corporate-profile/MetLife-Teacher-Survey-2012.pdf

Moore, S. E., Bledsoe, L. K., Perry, A., & Robinson, M. A. (2011). Social work students and self-care: A model assignment for teaching. *Journal of Social Work Education*, *47*(3), 545–553. doi:10.5175/JSWE.2011.201000004

Murphy, M. (2019, November 25). Does Anyone Actually Like Autocratic Leaders? New Data Says Yes. *Forbes*. https://www.forbes.com/sites/markmurphy/2019/11/24/does-anyone-actually-like-autocratic-leaders-new-data-says-yes/?sh=5697cbc610de

Pearman, C., Bowles, F., & Polka, W. (2021). Teacher educator perceptions of characteristics of self-efficacy. *Critical Questions in Education*, *12*(1), 81–99.

Regional Educational Laboratory at Mathematica Policy Research. (2019, March). *What are effective school leaders, and how can states and districts develop them?* REL Mid-Atlantic. https://ies.ed.gov/ncee/edlabs/regions/midatlantic/pdf/RELMA_Characteristics_effective_school_leaders_fact_sheet.pdf

Rietman, G. C., & Karge, B. D. (2019). Investing in teacher support leads to teacher retention: Six supports administrators should consider for new teachers. *School Administration, Multicultural Education, and Inclusion*, *27*(1), 7–18.

Robertson, D. A., Padesky, L. R., & Brock, C. H. (2020). Cultivating student agency through teachers' professional learning. *Theory into Practice*, *59*(2), 192–201. doi:10.1080/00405841.2019.1705090

Sharrocks, L. (2014). School staff perceptions of well-being and experience of an intervention to promote well-being. *Educational Psychology in Practice*, *30*(1), 19–36. doi:10.1080/02667363.2013.868787

Soulen, R. R. (2020). The continuum of care: A model of collaboration with new teachers. *Knowledge Quest*, *48*(4), 36–42.

Sutcher, L., Darling-Hammond, L., & Carver-Thomas, D. (2016). *A coming crisis in teaching? Teacher supply, demand, and shortages in the U.S. Learning Policy Institute.* Learning Policy Institute. https://learningpolicyinstitute.org/

Taylor, M. (2018). Using CALMERSS to enhance teacher well-being: A pilot study. *International Journal of Disability Development and Education*, *65*(3), 243–261. doi:10.1080/1034912X.2017.1394985

Vekeman, E., Devos, G., Valcke, M., & Rosseel, Y. (2017). Do teachers leave the profession or move to another school when they don't fit? *Educational Review*, *69*(4), 411–434. doi:10.1080/00131911.2016.1228610

Wang, J., Straubhaar, R., & Ong, C. (2020). Teacher and administrator experiences with teacher recruitment, retention, and support in a California charter-led turnaround school. *Inquiry in Education*, *12*(1), 1–17.

Witters, D., & Agrawal, S. (2021, December 6). *Well-Being Enhances Benefits of Employee Engagement.* Gallup.com. https://www.gallup.com/workplace/236483/enhances-benefits-employee-engagement.aspx

ADDITIONAL READING

Aragon, S. (2016). *Teacher shortages: What we know*. Education Commission of the States. https://files.eric.ed.gov/fulltext/ED565893.pdf

Berry, B., & Shields, P. M. (2017). Solving the teacher shortage: Revisiting the lessons we've learned. *Phi Delta Kappan*, *98*(8), 8–18. Advance online publication. doi:10.1177/0031721717708289

Boyd, D., Grossman, P., Ing, M., Lankford, H., Loeb, S., & Wyckoff, J. (2011). The influence of school administrators on teacher retention decisions. *American Educational Research Journal*, *48*(2), 303–333. doi:10.3102/0002831210380788

García, E., & Weiss, E. (2019). *The teacher shortage is real, large and growing, and worse than we thought: The first report in "The Perfect Storm in the Teacher Labor Market" series.* Economic Policy Institute. https://www.epi.org/publication/the-teacher-shortage-is-real-large-and-growing-and-worse-than-we-thought-the-first-report-in-the-perfect-storm-in-the-teacher-labor-market-series/

García, E., & Weiss, E. (2019). *The role of early career supports, continuous professional development, and learning communities in the teacher shortage: The fifth report in 'The Perfect Storm in the Teacher Labor Market' series.* Economic Policy Institute. https://files.eric.ed.gov/fulltext/ED598210.pdf

Heins, E., Snyder, J., & Adams, T. (2016). *Teachers, school leaders, and public scholars developing an ecosystems approach to growing educator capacity.* Paper prepared for the 2016 meeting of the American Educational Research Association. https://edpolicy.stanford.edu/sites/default/files/docsonly/ilcaeraslides41016.pdf

Ingersoll, R. M., May, H., & Collins, G. (2019). Recruitment, employment, retention and the minority teacher shortage. *Education Policy Analysis Archives*, *27*(37), 1–42. doi:10.14507/epaa.27.3714

Ingersoll, R. M., & Smith, T. M. (2003). The wrong solution to the teacher shortage. *Educational Leadership*, *60*(8), 30–33.

Rinke, C. R. (2014). *Why half of teachers leave the classroom: Understanding recruitment and retention in today's schools.* Rowman & Littlefield.

Sass, D. A., Seal, A. K., & Martin, N. K. (2011). Predicting teacher retention using stress and support variables. *Journal of Educational Administration*, *49*(2), 200–215. doi:10.1108/09578231111116734

KEY TERMS AND DEFINITIONS

Administrator/Administrative: School principals and others in leadership positions who oversee teacher performance, establish building environments, and provide professional development.

Advocacy: The act of speaking up, asserting beliefs, and sharing experiences in an effort to change one's environment or circumstances in order to improve satisfaction and performance.

Beginning Teachers: Teachers who are new to the teaching profession (teaching years 1–5).

Burnout: Overall exhaustion and diminished enthusiasm and willingness to give full effort toward tasks. Burnout can occur at many different levels in education, including professional, instructional, and student levels.

Teacher Attrition: Teachers leaving the profession or moving between schools/districts.

Teacher Empowerment: Teachers are given safe spaces to collaborate, innovate, and develop and assume roles of leadership.

Teacher Retention: Teachers staying in classroom positions over time.

Well-Being: A sense of awareness and the implementation of practices in social, emotional, physical, and psychological health.

Chapter 2
Finding Wellness in Faraway Places:
An Educator's Journey

Paul Collins
Florida A&M University, USA

ABSTRACT

This chapter is designed to speak to those educators in the field who can relate to functioning on a mental, emotional, and physical low frequency based on the challenges of the workplace. The author unravels how he, as an educator, struggled to find balance in his own self-care practices while simultaneously devoting himself to helping students, and a school community, flourish. The requirements of becoming better as teachers and school leaders, supporting students and their families, and being agile in maneuvering organizational change can prove to be daunting at best. These are some of the challenges that are outlined. Nevertheless, this work will unpack some actionable strategies that have been helpful by being proactive, rather than reactive, in coping with the challenges that educators face.

INTRODUCTION

Mother to Son
By Langston Hughes

Well, son, I'll tell you:
Life for me ain't been no crystal stair.
It's had tacks in it,
And splinters,
And boards torn up,
And places with no carpet on the floor—
Bare.
But all the time

DOI: 10.4018/978-1-6684-2334-9.ch002

I'se been a-climbin' on,
And reachin' landin's,
And turnin' corners,
And sometimes goin' in the dark
Where there ain't been no light.
So boy, don't you turn back.
Don't you set down on the steps
'Cause you finds it's kinder hard.
Don't you fall now—
For I'se still goin', honey,
I'se still climbin',
And life for me ain't been no crystal stair.

The literature on the need for teacher self-care and wellness is lacking, but the conversation on this topic is more relevant than it has ever been during this inescapable historical moment accompanied by a Covid-19 pandemic. Such a historical moment illuminates the need for a well overdue conversation on teacher well-being. it is instinctively known that the notion of teacher wellness and notions of teacher self-care should be high on the educational field's totem pole of priorities. Nevertheless, such notions continue to await the attention and scholarly legwork necessary to shine light on and breathe new life into this timely educational topic. The enhancement of schools will be the result because this conversation is about prioritizing education's front line of defense against a myriad of negative outcomes.

Through the use of personal narrative, this work seeks to provide contemporary educators with powerful tools that, when implemented consistently, have proven to yield positively desirable results at the personal level. This manuscript will present educators with the author's personal journey through implementing Yale University's most popular course ever, which focuses on well-being (Santos, n.d.). The journey was fully online and allowed for an audited experience. Like so many in the field of education, the author too, found himself dealing with the implications of physical and emotional lows as he attempted to simultaneously motivate and inspire the nation's future citizens and leaders. The many trials undergirded by the general lack of societal respect of the field of education are exemplified by relatively low pay in comparison to other professions, long hours, ever-changing mandates, and increasingly challenging work environments, as the impacts of a global Covid-19 pandemic are being navigated by all. One can easily relate to the challenge of educator attrition, as so many brilliant educators tend to totally abandon the profession within the first five years.

The context mentioned above is a reality that the author, as an educator, had to address head-on during a time of an existential emotional and physical low point in his own career in the field of education. As a personal act of resistance in the interest of his own self-care, and an intentioned will to find balance and peace, he embarked upon a journey to discover the science behind the concepts of self-care and personal well-being. The author's exploration led him to what is now known as Yale University's most popular course ever—The Science of Well-Being. He had reached a point in his educational career where the ultimatum was crystal clear. He was either going to figure a way to function on a higher and healthier mental, emotional, and physical plane of existence as a professional educator, or he was going to exit the profession that he loved so dearly. Like so many in the field of education, the author's relationship with his profession was becoming toxic.

This Chapter is designed to speak to those educators in the field that can relate to functioning on a mental, emotional, and physical low frequency based on the challenges of the workplace. The author will unravel just how he, as a fellow colleague of the profession, struggled to find balance in his own self-care practices while simultaneously devoting himself to helping students and a school community to flourish. The requirements of becoming better at the craft, as teachers and school leaders, supporting students and their families, and being agile in maneuvering organizational change, can prove to be daunting at best. These are some of the challenges that are outlined. Nevertheless, this work will unpack some actionable strategies that have been helpful by being proactive, rather than reactive, in coping with the challenges that educators face.

It is essential that educators devote themselves to serving students well. It is a common refrain that they enter the profession because it is a calling. Educators are altruistic from the start. This also challenges those in the field to give themselves the permission to find balance in their own self-care while also caring so deeply for the lives that are positively impacted in schools. The Covid-19 pandemic has not made finding such a balance any easier. Nevertheless, this chapter is designed to be a strong voice in the discourse advocating and educating those needing such in understanding that the work around educator self-care and well-being must be central in working to recruit, maintain, and expand the profession. This Chapter will unpack an educator's personal journey and victorious fight to either figure out a way to function on a higher and healthier mental, emotional, and physical plane of existence as an educator—or exit the profession. The narrative is situated in a series of guiding and personal experiential outcomes stemming from a longitudinal personal journey in the study and practice of the research-based dimensions of the science for well-being (Santos, n.d.).

Who could have imagined that an American educator in search of his own sense of well-being would find the tools and a practice to support such while in another country during a global pandemic. The following guiding questions that serve as the framework for unpacking the author's longitudinal personal journey are:

1. Can understanding one's particular character strengths assist in educator wellness?
2. Is savoring the moment a useful construct to assist in teacher self-care?
3. How can expressions of gratitude and reflective/meditative time promote teacher well-being?
4. What part does acts of kindness and meaningful social connections play in teacher self-care?
5. How can exercise and a good sleep routine support teacher self-care?

Background

In completing a systematic review of teacher well-being relevant to this chapter, Hascher and Waber (2021) noted several key highlights such as social relationships being important to teacher well-being and that the outcomes of teacher well-being needed more research attention. Their systematic review spanned the course of nearly two decades, from 2000 to 2019. The work of these Switzerland-based researchers is helpful, but the needed research most relevant to this chapter must focus on the American educational systems. For example, Rebecca Richards (2020) highlighted the following based on a study conducted by the American Federation of Teachers:

In 2017, the American Federation of Teachers conducted an educator quality of work life survey that revealed the majority of teachers experience poor mental health, high levels of stress, and both mental and emotional exhaustion. This, in turn, hinders their ability to effectively support their students' social-emotional needs. Research has shown that ***teacher stress can negatively impact student conduct***—*leading to increased instances of disruptive student behavior and lower levels of pro-social behaviors in the classroom (Richards, 2020).*

Infographics produced by the Institute of Education Sciences (IES) titled, "How to HOW TO GROW Teacher Wellbeing in Your Schools,", which highlights the importance of teacher well-being and the notion of growing teacher well-being in schools. This heavily referenced infographic also provides guidance on where a teacher in need can start on their journey, with connections relevant resources. Of high importance is the Institute's attention given to school principals and other school administrators (IES, 2020).

Through research institutes, such as Brookings, Roberts and Kim (2019) note that broader approaches are needed at the research level in understanding well-being. They also highlight importantly that teachers should be included in the conversation in approaches to supporting their well-being. Another recommendation presented is that systems and organizations must work collaboratively in supporting teacher well-being. These represent excellent aspects of the research needs around notions of educator well-being. In this case, there remains the need for the work of teacher self-care as a part of assuring that attempts at reaching the goal of well-being, which not only stems from outside initiatives, but also from internal educator agency.

To better understand the implications of well-being as it relates to teachers' and administrators' perceptions of the evaluation process, Anderson et al. (2019) conducted a mixed-methods research study of more than 1,000 teachers and over 450 school administrators. Their quantitative results yielded that administrators perceived the process increased teacher well-being significantly more than the well-being of school administrators. In this study, teachers also noted the stressfulness of the evaluation process, which affected their well-being. This research also highlighted that both teachers and school administrators agreed that the main barrier to a better process was lack of time for all involved (Anderson et al. 2019). With the growing shortage of educators throughout the American school systems, this type of research, focusing on the key components of educator evaluations, becomes even more valuable to gain a better societal understanding of some of the factors that affect the well-being of not only teachers, but school administrators as well.

In her text, Allies (2020) outlines a practical approach to well-being for primary teachers and school leaders. This work provides a sound understanding of the concept of well-being to more thoroughly unpack its implications at the level of application. One will also find specific strategies in the support of educators in balancing the challenges of their professional work and non-work-related dimensions of life. Some of the strategies relate to thwarting the myriad of challenges stemming from educator workload issues, navigating self-esteem issues, an appropriate sleep regime, proper eating habits, and the implications of mindfulness. Additionally, ideas central to teachers and school leaders working to establish their own personal plan for well-being, is offered. Issues on the spectrum of a personal plan of action through implications for school policy possibilities on educator well-being, is presented (Allies, 2020).

In a study to explore the multimodal use of a diary as a positive tool to teacher well-being, Kelly (2021) reported that using such an approach yielded positive outcomes for teachers in their ability to flourish inside and outside of the classroom. Other research on educator wellbeing focused on the online blogging on English teaching challenges during the Covid-19 pandemic. This research revealed nine online challenges to the online pedagogical process. Seventeen coping strategies were identified in the results of this research that promoted teacher mental health and well-being (Abdel Latif, 2022).

Langford and Crawford's (2022) research on the topic of well-being highlights the general challenges of the educational field as teacher retention and turnover. Their case study investigates the views of 12 primary level teachers that have more than 5 years of teaching experience.

CONTEXT SETTING

There he was, a school administrator who had ascended to that rank after resisting the temptations of such, and departing a tenure-track faculty position to be impactful by remaining a classroom teacher for nearly a decade. He chose to navigate the profession in this manner even after having attained a doctoral degree in the field. There he was, mentally and physically exhausted, weary, and questioning the feasibility of remaining in the field of education. The question of exiting the profession after over 20 years of service was serious and weighed heavily. Perhaps a new setting could hold off the storm of discontent that had been building and had now reached a crescendo. The decision to continue on in light of personal un-wellness due to the toils of the profession or to exit the educational field was imminent and could not be put off any longer. Within this context, the author chose not to exit the profession. Instead, the decision was made to give educating without borders a try.

The idea of educating abroad was not a new one. The author had been considering such for a few years, as the discontent with the current state of his existence in the American educational system gradually increased. Getting to the point of actually acting on the idea did take a lot of time and much deep reflection. Where would he go? Which country was safe for expatriate educators? What about his wife and two children? How does one secure a job in the education profession in another country? These and so many other questions became central to his day-to-day thinking. This led to months of research on the Internet to identify the various countries of possibility. The author had to learn the nuances of foreign terminologies, such as "apostille," which is the process of authenticating official documents, such as university degrees and other pertinent documents needed by a country's officials in a country in which a person is seeking to work and reside.

This led him to a country on the other side of the globe, just months before the world would experience a global pandemic. The author's first approximately four months were heavily focused on acclimating to life abroad in the United Arab Emirates, while having no knowledge of the global Covid-19 pandemic just a few months away. Housing accommodations and some basic necessities were provided upon arrival in the new country. With the support of new colleagues, the author, his wife, and two children, ages 3 and 14, began to establish a new life.

A new life meant learning to visit currency exchange centers to convert American dollars into United Arab Emirates' dirhams, and understanding the value of the currency when exchanged for goods. Although English is widely spoken in the UAE, a new life meant navigating transactions with local businesspersons who may not understand, or minimally understand, English. One had to establish local phone services to communicate cost-effectively. Additionally, there was the need to figure out the logistics of transportation. The author and his family relied primarily on the Abu Dhabi taxi service as a means of initial transportation. This mode of getting from one location to the next was extremely safe and economical; less than $10 US afforded a person taxi transportation to most areas of destination within the island/city. The logistics of work for the adults and school for the children had to also be organized as a part of settling into another country.

While in the United Arab Emirates during the global Covid-19 pandemic, the author would find a better sense of well being through a focus on self-care and begin to thrive physically and emotionally. This is the context that led to this educator's newfound approach to personal well-being, even in his return to the United States of America to continue his work in the field of education.

While in the United Arab Emirates, the author was provided with an opportunity to participate in an International Baccalaureate Organization's Wellbeing and Student Leadership Professional Development training (International Baccalaureate PD, n.d.). This online professional development training consisted of four modules spanning the period of one month. The modules required participants to be truly engaged and involved in all of the activities/tasks and collaborate in the workshop discussions. It was not a "work at your own pace" online workshop. Because of the interactive nature of the course, it was imperative that participants logged on regularly, a minimum of three times per week. The beginning of the week for each module was full of posts, the middle of the week was for responding to the posts, and the end of the week was where closure occurred.

In wrestling with the implications of institutional well being, the author was forced to confront his own current state of well-being. He wanted to engage in the work of assisting students and their families from a place of strength. Hence, the work of self-care became self-evident and an essential pursuit. The author uses the reflective meaning-making framework of currere to assist in unpacking his journey.

CURRERE

The autobiographical approach of currere to curricularizing has been a useful tool of meaning-making in the field of curriculum studies for quite some time. As an introduction to and defining the method, Pinar states:

The Latin infinitive of curriculum—currere—I invoked in 1975 to emphasize the lived experience of curriculum, embodied potentially educational experience that is structured by the past while focused on the future. To study such experience—to expand the inner space of subjective non-coincidence with both past and future—I devised a method in four steps, or phases (Pinar, 2019, p. 50).

In further unpacking the method of currere, he shares:

In the first—the regressive phase—one returns to (not simply recalls) the past (or to aspects of it): for instance, one's school experience, the experience of an influential teacher or text, or one's ongoing relationship with an academic discipline. In the second—the progressive moment—one imagines the future (personal, social, political: intertwined as they may be). Why? Not only the past but also (fantasies of) the future structure the subjective and social present. In the third—the analytic moment—one studies these texts and the experiences they register to understand what before might have been obscured by one's submersion in the present. Incorporation of repressed or forgotten events into one's present understanding encourages an expanded subjectivity, now with room for what had been rejected or neglected before. In the fourth moment or synthetic phase, one pulls oneself together (for the moment at least) so as to act anew in the private and public worlds one inhabits. Such subjective synthesis or coherence can become the new site from which one can again regress to the past (should one work with the method again) (Pinar, 2019, p. 50)

It was the start of 2019, and he was finding much pleasure in reading former First Lady Michelle Obama's (2021) recently released book, *Becoming Michelle Obama*. The author had read both former President Obama's books years ago as he ran for president. Much of his inspiration to use the autobiographical method of currere was inspired by reading other people's autobiographical sketches. Autobiographical storytelling has always been of great interest to him. As a young boy, he could sit and listen to elders in his family and community recant aspects of their past for hours. The author thought it somewhat therapeutic to grapple with his own "becoming"

He is now on a path of writing a currere-oriented narrative focusing on what Poetter (2020) refers to as a focus on the curriculum fragments or small bits of memories that continue to influence the think/acting and personal/professional life binaries. This, in many ways, is very representational of the initial stages of the author writing his own story of a pursuit of well being couched in what is now is 20-plus years of experience as a professional educator that began to lose his way. The 'rewirements' established through research in the science of well being are key to understanding how to effectively turn self-care practices into life habits (Santos, n.d.). These rewirements will be used to assist in capturing the author's journey and provide practical recommendations for educator self-care.

In working to find his way back to a better mental, emotional, and physical state, notions of there being a science to well-being were intriguing (Santos, n.d.). The following is the author's use of currere to deeply examine some of the research-based practices that have proven beneficial on a personal level throughout the author's journey through the Science of Well-Being course (some regressive fragments), thinking about the future (the progressive), and the present quest for maintenance (the analytical and synthetical) (Pinar, 1975, 2012, 2019).

Regressive Fragment #1: Character Strengths to Assist in Educator Wellness

As counterintuitive as it may seem, the initial inroads to well-being and self-care started by being guided on a journey that led to the author's discovery of multiple key character strengths. Not certain of the connection between self-care and character strengths, the author followed The Science of Well-Being's online module for the week to the VIA Character Strengths Survey and Character Reports provided by the VIA Institute on Character (n.d). Once on the website, and after successfully completing the brief registration for access, he completed the self-assessment that took approximately 15 minutes. From the self-assessment, results are provided to assist in better understanding the assessment taker's best qualities. There was a personalized analysis provided that was accompanied by actionable recommendations on how to best apply the newfound character strengths to assist one in finding greater well being.

The VIA website provides helpful insight as to why understanding one's character strengths matter. In answering the question of, "Why Do Character Strengths Matter?" it states:

Character strengths are the positive parts of your personality that make you feel authentic and engaged. You possess all 24 character strengths in different degrees, giving you a unique character strengths profile. Research shows that understanding and applying your strengths can help: Boost Confidence, Increase Happiness, Strengthen Relationships, Manage Problems, Reduce Stress, Accomplish Goals, Build Meaning and Purpose, Improve Work Performance (VIA Institute on Character, n.d,).

In identifying the top four character strengths specific to him, the author began to use the tools provided through the course to self-monitor and engage with those character strengths on a daily basis. This may appear cumbersome and another addition to an educator's day, but the author found this to replace other non-essential daily activities by prioritizing this dimension of his self-care. In playing into and being mindful of his identified character strengths, more joyful moments became a part of his days. Like all good habits, rewiring ones daily actions, both cognitively and physically, will take effort and time.

In the spirit of working towards well being, educators are encouraged to take a small portion of their time to better understand this rewiring practice.

Regressive Fragment #2: Savoring for Educator Wellness

Savoring is the idea of being intentional about the notion of savoring meaningful moments in one's day is another aspect of the author's journey to well being by practicing self-care. If pressed, one could more than likely reflect back on times when they savored a/some moment(s) in life. But, this researched-based course journey unraveled scientific proof of the high correlation between savoring and well being. Most importantly is the notion of savoring intentionally and more systematically as a means of developing the practice to be recurring and a part of one's daily routine as a cognitive rewirement (Santos, n.d.). The author found noticing and more intensely appreciating the positives of the day, with intention, to be surprisingly enjoyable. Savoring as a practice was a key part of stress relief during the workday because it challenges one to live in the moment. All too many times, thoughts of worry about matters that ultimately prove to be inconsequential consume too many moments of an educator's day. Savoring the many good moments worthy of such, created more celebratory moments; which, in turn, proved to enhance the quality of a day.

Regressive Fragment #3: Expressions of Gratitude and Meditative Moments for Educator Wellness

Gratitude is being grateful and being thankful. It is all about perspective. The act of seeking out those moments to be grateful, regardless of how small, has proven to be a powerful personal rewirement learned through the Science of Well-Being course. What are you grateful for? This question is powerful and exponentially so when coupled with habituation. There are multiple ways presented as a part of rewiring one's mental habits presented in the course that can be implemented into the daily lives of educators. The author now engages in daily gratitude journaling. Although there have been days missed, and perfecting this psychological and emotional dimension of rewiring can cause challenge. New habits are difficult to establish. The author has found connecting this practice to a specific time in the day to be helpful, and consistency is increasing. That specific time is waking up from the previous night's sleep.

The combination of meditative time and gratitude journaling has become the first act of the author's day. Connecting these rewirements with the fact that one must wake up to start their day, can enhance the initial moments of the day dramatically. Especially considering the challenges that educators wake up to and must face on a daily basis to be effective and positive change agents in the lives of the children and families that they serve. The use of Google Docs or another writing application on a mobile phone to create a running gratitude log is logistically efficient, and can be completed in approximately 15 minutes when coupled with a personalized morning meditative exercise. This additional 15 minutes to an educator's opening moments of a day can thwart those deflated initial moments of a day that have so long been a part of an educator's week, leaving only the joys of "Thank God It's Friday" to look forward to.

Regressive Fragment #4: Educator Self-Care through Acts of Kindness and Social Connectivity

While residing in the United Arab Emirates, the author was once told by a wise gentleman that when he feel signs of deflation or depression, that becomes a signal for him to initiate the practice of doing nice things for others. He informed the author that this notion was common in those parts and not unique to him. It reminded the author of the Christian adage that, "It is better to give than to receive." This philosophical approach in conjunction with one being intentional in the maintenance of positive social connectivity with others has proven to be scientifically wonderful tools that can be used to enhance a person's well being (Santos, n.d.). Buettner's (2017) work on the world locations where the happiest, healthiest, and longest living humans on the planet, popularly known as Blue Zones, also aligns with the abovementioned benefits of positive social connectivity in support of well being.

To enhance intentionality in this regard, the author has begun to really pay closer attention to his emotional state. Where in the past, the oncoming signs of deflation or the onset of depression-like feelings, some vice such as emotional eating may have been unconsciously activated. Now, he strives to identify with the emotion and use it as a trigger to engage in acts of kindness toward others, while simultaneously engaging in social connectivity in a way that enhances the day of another human being. He has found those acts of kindness to be extremely beneficial to himself, and his connectivity with others enhanced. This is a rewirement that requires personal attentiveness to one's mental and emotional state in an intentionally frequent manner. Educators will find this beneficial because it challenges one to seek out ways to do and interact positively with those in their space so that negative and low frequency feelings, which can be brought on by a myriad of occurrences in a school day, can be challenged in a positive and intentional action of educator self-care.

Regressive Fragment #5: Exercise and Sleep as Educator Self-Care

As a youth, the author can readily recall experiencing the overflow of an educator's workday into personal and family time. His parent was a teacher and oftentimes brought work home that would extend into the evening hours and be completed in between carrying out the functions of post-workday personal and family life. The official hours of educators, inclusive of the intermittent breaks that are a part of an academic yearly calendar, has always been met with a general sentiment of being plush and justification for less pay relative to other professions. The author believes this to be an unfair sentiment and an ill-conceived conclusion.

In the field of education, there is much to be done in the area of research with a focus on educator workload. As an educator for more than two decades, the author notes that the line between official work obligations and personal time is too often blurred by the overflow of a day's official work obligations into what would otherwise be personal time. In finding wellness, this is a circumstance that must not be overlooked, as value of work and the guilt around pursuits of work/leisure balance can gradually lead to exploitative contexts in capitalist societal life (Weber, 2001).

Within the science of the well-being framework, a revisit to notions of adequate sleep and appropriate amounts of exercise are noted as critical to good self-care and overall personal wellness (Santos, n.d.). the common refrain of a person's health being an essential aspect of their wealth is worthy of attention, then this aspect of well-being cannot be underestimated, downplayed, or devalued by educators in pursuit of practical approaches to self-care and improved personal well-being. During this phase of work within the Science of Well-Being course, the author was challenged by his own work/personal life imbalance when juxtaposed to the research that explicitly reiterated what he already knew to be commonsensical. Establishing appropriate boundaries in one's life, where appropriate amounts of sleep and exercise becomes non-negotiable, has proven to be a valuable lesson on the journey to well being as a professional educator.

THE PROGRESSIVE: FORECASTING

In light of a global Covid-19 pandemic, the future of American K-12 education as it has existed will continue to be challenged. The continuous rethinking of the education profession will remain necessary (Apple, 2012). With the Covid-19 pandemic's forcing of human interaction into virtual spaces, newly discovered options to educational delivery models arose. This context will most certainly challenge pre-Covid traditional models of schooling. It will also challenge the ways in which educators envision technology's use in more efficiently engaging students while not compromising any of the rigor and integrity of their pedagogical practice.

Teacher attrition will continue to pose challenges to the profession (Madigan & Kim, 2021). This context has only been exacerbated by the Covid-19 pandemic (Loewus, 2021). Covid-19 challenged the profession to redefine itself and venture deeply into virtual spaces. New ways of approaching education were forced upon the profession and there is no un-experiencing the realities of the challenges, as well as, the future possibilities of having gone through a global Covid-19 pandemic. The author anticipates that future boundaries between official work responsibilities and personal life run the risk of blurring even more in the future. This should make the need for a keen focus on educator well being, and the successful maintenance of such, that much more of a priority. How well the educational leaders and school policy makers address this aspect of the profession will impact the future overall well being of the profession. The future implications are high for American K-12 education in general and those, more specifically, who want to positively impact children, families, and communities. The author stresses that they are worth high prioritization.

THE ANALYTIC: SELF-CARE AND WELL-BEING IN THE PRESENT MOMENT

As a general statement on the state of American public schooling, the current teacher workforce is facing many challenges. Districts across the country are struggling with hiring and retaining teachers (García & Weiss, 2019). Has the global Covid-19 pandemic forced educators going through similar challenges as the author to fully reconsider their options in securing a livelihood? This is a question not only germane to the education profession, as new ways of making a living in virtual spaces became an unintended consequence of approximately two years of social distancing, working from home, and distance learning for children. This phenomenon is causing many school districts throughout the nation to open their doors to begin a school year with employment vacancies; which is not in the interest of educator well being—at the outset of an academic year. The questions remain regarding the abovementioned. Will the number of professional educators nationwide increase? Will the number of professional educators nationwide simply remain the same? Or, will the number of professional educators nationwide decrease? There are no guarantees.

The author writes this manuscript after having found a stronger personal level of mental, emotional, and physical well being discovered after having travelled a long distance from his home country in an attempt to circumvent a full and complete departure from the education profession.

In this exploration, through the use of the method of currere, has allowed for educative pauses where the author reflected with the goal of gaining insight into well-being and self-care threaded through his past, present, and into the future (Dewey, 1986; Kuhnke & Jack-Malik, 2021). He is an educator who has experienced firsthand the multitude of joys and accompanying challenges that teachers have to navigate in the profession. He is also a survivor and an example of not exiting the profession after running into the reality of lowered mental, emotional, and physical levels, and choosing to remain in the classroom for about half of his more than 20-year career. He chose to remain a classroom teacher for almost a decade, even after having attained a terminal degree. He would like to believe that somehow, through the use of currere, others will be inspired. The author does realize that memories are not exact, experience reconfigurations can occur as time passes and become fictionalized, at least to a degree (Poetter, 2012). Even so, these are troubled times in the midst of a Covid-19 pandemic and social unrest is tearing at the fabric of attempts at a socially just democratic life. These troubled times demand voices from the numerical margins of our profession. Change can be initiated through storytelling, and currere is about the theorization of storytelling (Morris, 2019). This exercise is not simply theorized storytelling for academic romanticism. On the contrary, currere is a tool for the critically positive individual and the social change so desperately needed in the field of education.

SYNTHETIC: CONCLUDING, BUT NOT THE JOURNEY'S END

As alluded to at the outset of this chapter, the literature on the need for teacher self-care and is lacking, but the conversation on this topic is more relevant than it has ever been. The global Covid-19 pandemic has indeed proven to be an inescapable dimension of daily life. The enhancement of schools will be the result, because this conversation is about prioritizing education's front line of defense against a myriad of negative outcomes.

Through the use of personal narrative, this work provides contemporary educators with powerful tools that when implemented consistently, can yield positively desirable results at the personal level. Educators were presented with the author's personal journey through The Science of Well-Being course (Santos, n.d.). The author's journey was personal and not universal in the areas of the course where more attention might have been paid than to other areas. Hence, others will have similar, but not the exact, experiences depending on the closeness of their adherence to the myriad of aspects of the course experience.

The context mentioned above is a reality that the author, as an educator, had to address head-on during a time of an existential emotional and physical low point in his own career in the field of education. As a personal act of resistance in the interests of his own self-care, and an intentioned will to find balance and peace, he embarked upon a journey to discover the science behind the concepts of self-care and personal well being. Like so many in the field of education, the author's relationship with his profession was becoming toxic.

This chapter's purpose was to speak to those educators in the field that can relate to the author's articulated experiences. He unraveled just how he, as a fellow colleague of the education profession, struggled to find balance in his own self-care practices while simultaneously devoting himself to helping students and a school community to flourish. These were some of the challenges that were outlined.

The actionable strategies outlined have been helpful with being proactive, rather than reactive, in coping with the challenges that educators face.

It is essential that educators devote themselves to serving students well. And, if the refrain of education being a calling is to continue to have a strong resonance, then an educator's altruism must be from a balanced perspective and approach. Those in the field of education should give themselves the permission to find balance in their own self-care while also caring so deeply for the lives that are positively impacted in schools. Furthermore, this should be the case even more so during a global Covid-19 pandemic. Ultimately, this chapter was designed to be a strong voice advocating and educating those needing such an understanding that the work around educator self-care and well-being must be central in working to recruit, maintain, and expand the profession. This author's journey represents a victorious fight to figure out a way to function on a higher and healthier mental, emotional, and physical plane of existence as an educator, thereby thwarting the undesirable need to exit the profession.

Who could have imagined that an American educator in search of his own sense of well being would find a tools and a practice to support such while in another country during a global pandemic. The guiding questions that served as the framework for unpacking the author's longitudinal personal journey was: Can understanding one's particular character strengths assist in educator wellness? Does savoring a useful construct assist in teacher self-care? How can expressions of gratitude and reflective/meditative time promote teacher well-being? What part does acts of kindness and meaningful social connections play in teacher self-care? How can exercise and a good sleep routine support teacher self-care?

REFERENCES

Abdel Latif, M. M. (2022). Coping with COVID-19-related online English teaching challenges: Teacher educators' suggestions. *ELT Journal*, *76*(1), 20–33. doi:10.1093/elt/ccab074

Allies, S. (2020). *Supporting Teacher Wellbeing: A Practical Guide for Primary Teachers and School Leaders*. Routledge. doi:10.4324/9780429330698

Anderson, D., Cameron-Standerford, A., Bergh, B., & Bohjanen, S. (2019). Teacher evaluation and its impact on wellbeing: Perceptions of Michigan teachers and administrators. *Education*, *139*(3), 139–150.

Apple, M. W. (2012). Rethinking Education, Rethinking Culture, Rethinking Media: Rethinking Popular Culture and Media, edited by Elizabeth Marshall & Ozlem Sensoy (Milwaukee: Rethinking Schools, 2011). Educational Policy, 26(2), 339–346. doi:10.1177/0895904811417593

Buettner, D. (2017). *The blue zones solution: Eating and living like the world's healthiest people*. National Geographic Books.

Dewey, J. (1986, September). Experience and education. *The Educational Forum*, *50*(3), 241–252. doi:10.1080/00131728609335764

García, E., & Weiss, E. (2019, April 16). *U.S. schools struggle to hire and retain teachers: The second report in "The perfect storm in the teacher labor market" series*. Economic Policy Institute. https://www.epi.org/publication/u-s-schools-struggle-to-hire-and-retain-teachers-the-second-report-in-the-perfect-storm-in-the-teacher-labor-market-series/

Hascher, T., & Waber, J. (2021). Teacher well-being: A systematic review of the research literature from the year 2000–2019. *Educational Research Review, 34,* 100411. . 2021.100411 doi:10.1016/j.edurev

IES. (2020, February). *Infographic: HOW TO GROW Teacher Wellbeing in Your Schools.* IES—REL Regional Educational Laboratory Program. https://ies.ed.gov/ncee/edlabs/infographics/pdf/REL_PA_How_To_Grow_Teacher_Wellbeing_in_Your_Schools.pdf

International Baccalaureate PD. (n.d.). *Professional development.* International Baccalaureate®. https://www.ibo.org/professional-development/

Kelly, L. (2021). Playing with the diary: how crafting a multimodal and sensory diary can have a positive impact on teacher wellbeing. *Reflective Practice, 23*(1), 1–16. . 2021.1973986 doi:10.1080/14623943

Kuhnke, J. L., & Jack-Malik, S. (2021). Roofs, Nesting Instincts, and Student Evaluations of Teaching During a Pandemic. *Currere Exchange Journal, 5*(2), 44–52.

Langford, S., & Crawford, M. (2022). Walking with teachers: A study to explore the importance of teacher wellbeing and their careers. *Management in Education.* Advance online publication. doi:10.1177/08920206221075750

Loewus, L. (2021, May 4). Why teachers leave—or don't: A look at the numbers. *Education Week, 5.* https://www.edweek.org/teaching-learning/why-teachers-leave-or-dont-a-look-at-the-numbers/2021/05#:~:text=And%20yet%20about%208%20percent%20of%20teachers%20leave

Madigan, D. J., & Kim, L. E. (2021). Towards an understanding of teacher attrition: A meta-analysis of burnout, job satisfaction, and teachers' intentions to quit. *Teaching and Teacher Education, 105,* 103425. doi:10.1016/j.tate.2021.103425

Morris, M. (2019). Currere or the Erasure of the Author. *The Currere Exchange Journal, 3*(1), 5–17. https://cej.lib.miamioh.edu/index.php/ CEJ/article/view/10

Obama, M. (2021). *Becoming.* Crown.

Pinar, W. (1975). Currere: toward reconceptualization. In W. F. Pinar (Ed.), Curriculum theorizing: The reconceptualists (pp. 396–414). Academic Press.

Pinar, W. F. (2012). *What is curriculum theory?* Routledge.

Pinar, W. F. (2019). Currere. In Key Concepts in Curriculum Studies (pp. 50–52). Routledge.

Poetter, T. S. (2012). *Teaching again: A professor's tale of returning to a ninth grade classroom.* Information Age Publishing.

Poetter, T. S. (2020). The thicket. *Currere Exchange Journal, 4*(2), 1–15. https://cej.lib.miamioh.edu/index.php/CEJ/article/view/128

Richards, R. (2020, May 21). *Improve teacher wellbeing with self-care strategies and formalized peer connections.* EAB. https://eab.com/insights/blogs/district-leadership/improve-teacher-wellbeing/

Roberts, A., & Kim, H. (2019, May 6). *To promote success in schools, focus on teacher well-being.* Education Plus Development. https://www.brookings.edu/blog/education-plus-development/2019/05/06/to-promote-success-in-schools-focus-on-teacher-well-being/

Santos, L. (n.d.). *The Science of Well-Being.* Dr. Laurie Santos. https://www.drlauriesantos.com/science-well-being

VIA Institute on Character. (n.d.). *Bring Your Strengths to Life & Live More Fully.* https://www.viacharacter.org/

Wearing, J., Ingersoll, M., DeLuca, C., Bolden, B., Ogden, H., & Christou, T. M. (Eds.). (2019). *Key Concepts in Curriculum Studies: Perspectives on the Fundamentals.* Routledge. doi:10.4324/9781351167086

Weber, M. (2001). *The Protestant Ethic Debate Max Weber's Replies to His Critics, 1907–1910.* Liverpool University Press.

KEY TERMS AND DEFINITIONS

Character Strengths: The positive parts of your personality that make you feel authentic and engaged.

Gratitude: The mental and emotional posture of being grateful. Gratitude can also be expressed physically by the acting out of the mental and emotional posture of gratefulness.

Rewirements: Practices of self-care and well-being that, when done consistently and with intentionality, over time tend to make lasting changes at the emotional, mental, and physical/acting levels of functioning.

Savoring: Engaging in a way of thinking about a particular moment or context of joy, pleasure, and/or fulfillment with the intention of increasing that moment's intensity and duration.

Self-Care: The act(s) of taking care of oneself through behaviors that support mental, emotional, and physical wellness.

Social Connectedness: The experience of feeling connected to others. Positive social connectedness involves interacting with others and the byproduct of such yielding feelings of being valued and cared for at the interpersonal level.

Well-Being: The state of being healthy, happy, and comfortable in a myriad of given contexts. Well-being is germane to issues of mental, emotional, and physical states of functioning.

APPENDIX

Figure 1. This visual representation of the cyclical currere phases recommended to assist educators engage in documenting their own journey of professional self-care and well-being
Adapted from: Pinar (2019)

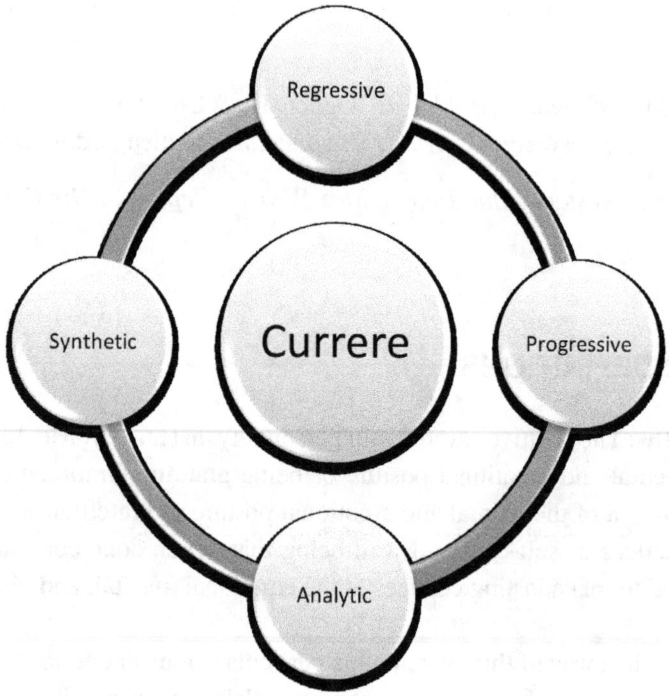

Chapter 3
Critical Dialogue at the Intersections of Race, Education, and COVID-19

Cristofer G. Slotoroff
https://orcid.org/0000-0003-4078-6637
Morris Hills Regional School District, USA

Ashley Gibson
Baylor University, USA

ABSTRACT

In this chapter, two public school teachers and recent doctoral graduates recount and reflect upon the ways in which their critical dialogues inform their rendering of the stressors weighing on educators since the onset of the COVID-19 pandemic in early 2020. The teachers—one, a Black woman in Texas, the other a White man in New Jersey—explore how their shared, liberatory, educational goals are compromised by institutional pressures, economic uncertainties, uneven enforcement of localized curricular policies, and ongoing resistance to healthcare initiatives instituted to combat the spread of COVID-19. To accomplish this, the authors highlight how race, identity, and pedagogy are disparately addressed in their respective workplaces. The authors conclude by suggesting that increased space for continued critical dialogue may help other educators to make sense of what are often tumultuous, hasty changes made since COVID-19 first affected American schools.

INTRODUCTION

"I HAVE COME to believe over and over again that what is most important to me must be spoken, made verbal and shared, even at the risk of having it bruised or misunderstood. That the speaking profits me, beyond any other effect." - Audre Lorde

DOI: 10.4018/978-1-6684-2334-9.ch003

For those unfamiliar with educators' struggles during the COVID-19 pandemic, consider a quick scroll through posts within the Facebook group called "Teachers Against Dying." If the group's moniker is not, in itself, adequately evocative, the group's (5000+) members' posts might be. These reveal the fear, disarray, and discontent we felt as we tried to make sense of our profession, our craft, and our dwindling humanity. At least one of us wrote a will, just in case. Such is the extent to which the COVID-19 pandemic rendered us—and by "us," I mean educators—more powerless than we already were. In "Teachers Against Dying" and in the countless ad-hoc online groups like it, in group texts with our colleagues, in Zoom sessions, via FaceTime, on the phone, and socially distanced at the park, we needed to talk: to each other, to the nameless void that is the Internet, to anyone and everyone who might be listening. The COVID-19 pandemic continues to dehumanize educators, but dialogue is therapeutic. Dialogue is liberating. Dialogue is necessary. This article explicates such dialogue between colleagues.

Audre Lorde writes about the importance of transforming silence into language. Under already challenging professional circumstances, educators are often silenced by their superiors. In a field that necessitates humanity, such silence is dehumanizing. It remains important to speak the truth in moments that raise concerns, and in the face of surmounting challenges to the profession of teaching. Our collective silences can do little to protect us, so we may as well speak (Lorde, 2007). When we, educators, humanize our ways of being in the world through our language, we engage opportunities to transform.

As the COVID-19 pandemic alters our lives, it also gives us ample reason to revisit our normative patterns. Educators must reimagine paths to dismantle unjust status quos and challenge oppressive systems while navigating individual and collective traumas. Educators are navigating these circumstances at the myriad intersections of life; they engage in critical dialogue that has the power to heal and transform the landscape of US K-12 education.

This chapter is one example of that critical dialogue. The dialogue here comprises two voices: one is a Black woman, a 13-year veteran classroom teacher, and a former school administrator in Texas. The other is a White man and a practicing classroom teacher of 11 years in New Jersey. Each voice shares personal experiences navigating the intersections of their shared participation in a doctoral program, their professional responsibilities, race, culture, and region, and other challenges present in the day to day of classroom responsibilities and local legislation that impacts teaching.

Right now, it is difficult to discern "normality" in any facet of our lives. As emerging scholars and as educators, our perspectives are essential to this moment. In this chapter, we share our personal experiences before and during the pandemic to elucidate how crisis education looks, feels, and transpires. We describe our relationship as colleagues and educators, and we offer a shared discourse between two scholar teachers, in two different places, with two different ethnic backgrounds, in two different roles, who appreciate each other's positions as recent graduates from a doctoral program. We offer commentary on the social and cultural implications of the pandemic for educators. We speak at the intersections of our personal identities, and our relationship as classmates and friends. We hope our shared experiences shed light on how we are all showing up during this pandemic, and perhaps what we can do to empathize with teachers everywhere who are coping with the day-to-day realities of how our vocation and, thus, our lives remain ever-changing.

AS EXPERIENCED IN TEXAS

There continues to be a startling absence of humanization in the Texas public education system. Historically and currently, teachers have not and are not spared in this dehumanizing paradigm. As a Black woman educator in K-12, I continually perceive how issues of power manifest in public education. Even under normal circumstances, I am—along with a troubling amount of Texas Teachers—too often rendered powerless. During the COVID-19 pandemic, these realities are only exacerbated. This is more tragic considering the pandemic's potential as a catalyst for improving education, at large. There was perhaps some encouraging empathy shown to educators in the Pandemic's early days. Then, teachers were placed high atop a pedestal of civic glory. Now, nearly one year later, Texas teachers (too often, silently) catalogue countless public backlashes and probing conversations concerning professionalism or effectiveness. This is education's dehumanization in practice (Freire, 2018). When so many have lost so much, teachers are nonetheless expected to sacrifice all: their time, their mental health, and their livelihood, for the sake of educating the nation's youth. Still more troubling is realization that this is not a malfunctioning system; this is a system functioning exactly as honed and designed.

Present Challenges

Above all, the pandemic is a missed opportunity to humanize the profession. Educators' dehumanization—already disproportionately amplified within marginalized populations—is part and parcel of a derelict notion of American class oppression (Brown, 2017; Freire, 2018; Hooks, 1994; Love, 2019). Teachers are regarded first as public employees, subsidized in large part by local taxes. To that end, the American connotations of receiving public dollars are historically unflattering. Just as the "worth" of librarians or postal workers is questioned, so too is that of teachers: those trusted, respected, lauded, and—yes—essential professionals to whom we entrust our collective futures.

My colleagues across my district and across my state work to tow the lines for decision makers who mask their negligence by scapegoating educators. There is a pressure to comply that In response to such marginalization, teachers have few avenues for meaningful recourse. This is my main concern with US public education, but particularly Texan public education. Teachers lack the necessary agency to combat their dehumanization at the hands of institutional forces. While teachers' accountability is never far from public discourse, there are rarely means by which the powerful may be put in check.

This mutual accountability ideal necessitates openness to change, but before exploring the nature of required changes in pursuit of said ideal, it is worth explaining institutional openness to change as a construct. As a veteran classroom educator, I immediately assumed a teacher-centered approach to my administrative service. My district hired me to serve as a culture and climate specialist, to primarily focus on improving culture through the use of restorative practices. Such culture comprises not only teachers' and students' morale, but also administrative buy-in and willingness to challenge dominant views. My position is designed to affect meaningful change, but I eventually discerned my district's preference for maintaining an established order, for reinforcing antiquated occupational norms. When I challenged such norms with what (I know to be) best practices, I met resistance. So ingrained was cultural complacence that whenever I challenged district practices, I was preemptively told not to bother. The culture was a hierarchy of calcified compliance and unquestioned, top-down authority. I realized that organizations lacking a power-sharing ethic may never truly adopt restorative practices with fidelity. Restorative practices require a sense of community predicated on interdependence. In a culture based on individuals' power, I noticed that no one was willing to give up or even share their power.

Who Will be First to Tell the Truth?

The pandemic has only made the "powerful" versus "powerless" dichotomy clearer. I am part of a Facebook group called "Texas Teachers for Safe Reopening," and it is often a nearly constant din of educators' screams into a proverbial echo chamber of other powerless educators. Since Texas teachers may not meaningfully unionize, we are at our legislators' mercy. Those seeking explicit, progressive political involvement in such a "red state" too often experience harrowing consequences. The irony is disturbing: to be explicitly partisan in a democratic society is, allegedly, antithetical to public education. While the pandemic rages, a glaring testament to teachers' powerlessness is Texas's continued insistence on standardized testing. Though so many have gone without so much; standardized testing remains a priority: decision makers must continue to appraise teachers' worth. Again, since we re-imagine the notion of schooling on a nearly daily basis, this could be a watershed moment to realign, repurpose, and effectively allot empathy and humanity in imaginative and innovative ways. Alas, our leaders maintain the status quo: why seek the humane, the practical, that which centers human lives when it might knock one from his perch? It is sad and it is frustrating, but I remain hopeful with the onus to become a scholar, a force for transformative justice in my field. To enact such justice, we cannot afford to check our politics at the door: to maintain this norm as the status quo preserves only those who wield power.

AS EXPERIENCED IN NEW JERSEY

Collegial Interactions

One of our critical dialogues' most stark revelations has been the extent to which my co-author and I have to calibrate our moral compasses before making countless daily decisions. On a collegial, peer-to-peer level, I work closely with a teacher who is at the beginning of her career, and I find that my most useful advice is, somewhat paradoxically, to keep as low a profile as possible. I find myself advising her to interact with as few other employees as possible. "It's safer that way," I say. Before the onset of the COVID-19 pandemic, this simply would not be the case. Before the onset of the COVID-19 pandemic, I did not have to be a teacher *and* a surrogate administrator, school officer, custodian, and disciplinarian. Now, however, just as the pandemic eroded many professional relationships across industries and nations, I mourn the death of collegiality in the public high school where I work.

Though I enjoy the protection of a labor union, like all unions, my own is only as good as its members' collective binding. As of this writing, we remain without a contract. In addition to the incrementally increasing, simmering animosity toward the parties who will sit across the table from our union's negotiations team, it is worth noting the degree to which our own members—my colleagues—are distrustful of one another. One of the wedges that divides our membership (and, I can only imagine, countless others,) is the role that the pandemic's safety measures play in our day-to-day, occupational lives. Our state requires non-vaccinated teachers to undergo weekly COVID-19 testing. As word inevitably travels within the school as to who is and is not vaccinated, who has or has not had a booster shot, these flames of tension are fanned. In addition, while New Jersey still requires all of those in the school buildings—faculty, staff, and students—to wear masks, some teachers still—in spite (or, perversely, perhaps *because*) of their positions as role models and trusted adult professionals—flagrantly spurn this rule. These teachers, of course, draw the ire of the masked teachers. Finally, each time a masked teacher is thrust—most usually because of a colleague's persistent and egregious disregard for this now-longstanding, state-mandated policy—into the uncomfortable position of enforcing the mask mandate, our collegial fabric is more completely torn.

It is difficult to quantify the extent to which this diminished collegial trust is systemic, permanent, or simply the timely byproduct of my school's circumstances, but it is validating to be able to share my experiences with my co-author: another educator, a peer, and one to whom I do not have to explain the context of these troubling changes. When I am at work, however, I have noticed how—perhaps as a pre-emptive, self-defense mechanism—my colleagues seldom speak to one another for more than a few minutes at a time. Some have young children still ineligible for vaccinations. Others (like this author) may live with immunocompromised family members or an immunocompromised partner. A once thoughtless opportunity to have a collegial interaction has effectively become a serious, calculated decision to spend a prep period masked, distanced, and—if one is speaking to an unvaccinated colleague—perhaps increasing the risk of a COVID-19 infection. Accordingly, when we *do* find time to communicate with one another, our interactions are overwhelmingly transactional in nature. We no longer share stories, commiserate, validate, empathize, swap materials, recall successes, lament failures, laugh and cry at this strange passion to which we have dedicated ourselves. Instead, we orient ourselves to one another in detached, cursory ways based primarily on what we can grant or withhold to one another at a moment's notice: a few spare copies of a novel, a ream of printer paper, a working dry-erase marker, a stack of multiple choice quiz forms, or some help with a finnicky video projector.

Teacher-to-Administrator Interactions

It is difficult, at times, to compartmentalize the increasingly permeative occupational tensions between administrators and the district's unionized faculty and staff. Institutional messages—over school announcements, in emails to the faculty, on the verbal and person-to-person level—of positivity, appreciation, the importance of mental health, or the critical function that teachers serve within our society must also be reconciled with our less competitive wages, our lack of a contract, and the day-to-day strain of enforcing health mandates without ample support. Stagnated contract negotiations mean teachers are asked by our union not to volunteer for the many unpaid roles that teachers usually and enthusiastically fill throughout the year. In return, at the end of the school day, I now see an administrator positioned near the exit of our building to ensure that teachers are not leaving a minute early. Such tension, eventually, becomes toxicity.

On a personal level, once routine duties have become deeply taxing, despondent chores. This year, I am assigned—despite my protestations that I live with an immunocompromised person—to perform 80 minutes of work duties every other day (as I have been for the past eight school years) that is now almost exclusively disciplinary and conducted in the immediate vicinity of many unmasked students. First and, again, despite my protestations, I supervise a ninth and tenth grade lunch period in which there are at least a hundred unmasked students eating and socializing. For these forty minutes, I am (along with a custodian,) often the only adult in the room. This is a departure from years past, and (I assume) the product of a staffing shortage or an unwillingness to hire more support staff. During these lunch periods, my responsibilities are as follows: I am to write students passes to the library, I am to circulate throughout the room to ensure that students are throwing their trash away, I am to make sure that students are not walking around the cafeteria once they have finished eating, and I am—on paper, at least—to make sure that students are wearing their masks when they are not eating. I have noted to my higher-ups the absolute futility of this last directive, but it has fallen on deaf ears: I simply cannot perform these tasks, with any fidelity, at the same time. My repeated requests for administrative support during lunch periods have gone unaddressed. For these first 40 minutes, to maintain any semblance of sanity or tranquility, to maintain a shred of my vocal chords' viability after shouting untold directives to students through my own mask (or two), is a fool's errand. This 40-minute lunch period is followed by a 40-minute hall duty, during which I spend most of my time asking or, oftener, begging that my students comply with the masking regulations in place since the beginning of the year.

In an educational sense, such is the disconnect between administrators and teachers that pre-COVID-19 measuring sticks are still used to measure students' (thus, their teachers') performance. In the beginning of this 2021–2022 school year, I (along with the other AP English teachers from both schools within my district) was asked by my supervisor—a genuinely brilliant, deeply caring woman I admire, and one who I wholeheartedly believe was asking in good faith—why students' AP exam scores were lower this past year. After many of my colleagues noted, as a possible cause, the presence of a deadly global pandemic that moved parts of the school year online and killed or uprooted the lives of more than a few within our own community, I asked whether other subject area scores were similarly lagging compared to those of years past. When my supervisor responded in the affirmative, I could not help but wonder the reason for this information's omission. I do not believe such an omission was intentional, let alone malevolent, but I do believe that it was indicative of how normal it has become to silo analyses of teachers' "performances" to departmental test scores at the expense of the "bigger picture." In this case, the "picture" being the presence of "an ongoing global pandemic that continues to kill millions of people."

These at-best detached, or at-worst adversarial teacher-to-administrator interactions amount to stressors that COVID-19 has exacerbated. In spite of this, I optimistically and faithfully regard my superiors as human beings and decent professionals who want the best for the school's students and the community at large. Nonetheless, it is, day by day, harder to square this assessment with teachers' ever-heavier burdens, ever-stagnating wages, and ever-absent support. Critically, I respect and admire my superiors' intellect and powers of observation. In light of this, it is problematic, therefore, to consider how often I—along with my colleagues—am asked to "be strong," "to work through this difficult time," to "maintain a sense of camaraderie by working together," and "keep occupational concerns out of the classroom" when those asking me to do this are those who have the power to improve my circumstances.

Teacher-to-Student Interactions

Most oppressive and most harmful are the ways in which my interactions with students are compromised as a result of COVID-19's increased pressure on teachers. These interactions are magnified because my students—all students—deserve so much better than what I can give them right now. As the COVID-19 pandemic enters its third year, my students remain, fortunately, the reason that I continue to teach. Whenever I teach them, I feel optimistic about the future, I am visibly and vocally supported in my efforts, and I feel deeply appreciated. In these regards, teaching is a welcome respite from an otherwise difficult working environment. Still, it is with my students that I most acutely feel the limitations of my available time, the futility of my professional efforts, and the degradation of my emotional well-being. For well over a decade, I have been flattered and eager if asked by a student to write a recommendation letter. I have approached students' requests for college essay help with as much zeal, passion, and circumstantial awareness as that which I apply to the cover letters that I submit to prospective employers. I have just about always been happy to spend a lunch period helping a student to understand coursework from another humanities class. This year, regrettably, I have discontinued all of these efforts.

To be clear, it feels *awful* to tell a student who has enough faith in me to ask for my help that "I simply cannot find the time to do this," but my school's and indeed my profession's reaction to COVID-19 has marginalized teachers as human beings. Since all of us wear masks, since only some of us socially distance to the extent that it is possible, since only some of us are vaccinated, and since there is simply no location inside of the school building safe enough to eat lunch without exposing oneself to other unmasked, possibly unvaccinated students and teachers, I eat each day in my car. I used to be able to check emails, grade papers, or offer extra help during a prep period or a hall duty, but now my students—who are equally stretched by an education system that too often pretends the COVID-19 pandemic's emotional and social effects have subsided—are just as exasperated and devoid of time as I am. Many simply want to know "how to get a good grade." Who could blame them? I cannot. Perhaps even more regrettably, my students have responded to my policy with a respectful, knowing glance over a masked face. They say what administrators do not: "I totally get it." I continue—as I always have and always will—to believe them. On my better days, I convince myself that they value their teacher's—an adult's—vulnerability in admitting that times are tough to the extent that I cannot help them. It may be a delusion, but it is one with which I have taught myself to live.

Existential, Occupational, Bureaucratic Forces

Extrinsic, uncritical, educational scrutiny from pundits and parents has become as commonplace as it is consistently misinformed, decontextualized, and delivered in soundbites borne of earlier televised soundbites. Such discourse has become a perennial fixture of the educator's professional life. To be clear, no educator I know is afraid of genuine, meaningful, and frank critique. Teachers like to talk about teaching. When mounting rent payments, mortgage payments, utility bills, car payments, and a two-bedroom house's worth of student loan debt are at stake, the school board meeting zeitgeists and resultant kneejerk administrative curricular reviews must, inevitably, take shape through the lens of one's job security.

My time at work is spent working to the extent that eating my lunch is, in the interest of my health and the health of those I love, a solitary endeavor in my car that comes at the expense of productivity. Since our departmental faculty room was eliminated a few years ago to create an additional office for support staff, and since our remaining faculty rooms are small, poorly ventilated, and crowded, there is no location except for one's own classroom to enjoy a "mask break" to lesson plan, grade papers, or eat. It is nearly a trope at this point to note that hardly any teachers take the full length of their lunch periods to eat. I was not any different. Now, since I am not in the building unless I am teaching, there is no additional time for my students because there is no additional time for myself.

Existentially, the pandemic's adverse educational effects on my vocation have even managed to transcend my place of employment. Since I cannot reasonably expect my wages to keep pace with inflation, let alone surpass it, and as our union has warned us of unfavorable changes that may yet come to our healthcare, I have had to—despite being a tenured teacher—look for employment elsewhere. I picked up a second job, through an online education company, grading students' papers within a prestigious university's non-degree certificate program. I was lured into this by the university's prestige, but I quickly came to find out that I would not be interacting—in any capacity—with anyone affiliated with the school. In this regard, I could not help but feel like I was perpetuating a disingenuous endeavor:

scores of students, around the world, had signed up for this class at a prestigious university only to be clandestinely scored and evaluated by a high school teacher in New Jersey. Worse still, though the publicly traded company who hired me has several thousand employees and substantial institutional connections within the pantheon of higher education, I was not paid (for my months of work) until several weeks past the company's self-imposed, contracted pay date. When I was paid, it was only after I reached out no fewer than ten times to various parties within the company, and it was only after I asked to whom I should address a certified letter demanding that the company honor the contract they wrote that their funds were deposited in my bank account.

At the state level, in a testament to a paradoxical irony of hyperbolic magnitude, The State of New Jersey's bureaucratic labyrinth of a certification system has precluded my career (in public education) from further advancement. From my current vantage point, this is because I have decided to become more educated. This year, my credentials for supervisor, school administrator, and principal were all denied by the State. I won my appeal for the supervisory credential this past spring, but—after noting (ostensibly because of the pandemic) my applications as "in process" from mid-August to late November—the fact that I (along with my co-author) earned my doctoral degree from Baylor University in Texas—in the field of education, focused in "Leadership and Organizational Change"—is not recognized by the State of New Jersey as equivalent to earned credits (in a non-matriculated, non-degree program, for instance,) that are explicitly geared toward educational leadership in this state. Despite the $380 application fee for the latter two certifications, despite my passing scores on each certificate's respective exams (that totaled an additional sum upwards of $700 for the privilege of taking them), despite my Master of Arts in Teaching degree (with an accompanying thesis analyzing the merits of various textual readability formulae), despite my 11+ years teaching in two New Jersey public high schools, despite the (deeply timely) 240-or-so page research dissertation that I wrote on the social and emotional implications of a 1:1 student-to-device implementation in a public school, despite the fact that I have written or revised no fewer than five district-level curricula over the course of my career, despite the fact that I have led professional development focused on optimizing teachers' use of digital resources, despite the fact that I have advised a gold medal-winning literary magazine and coached State Sectional Champion girls soccer teams, and despite the fact that I hold both a supervisory certificate and two instructional certificates that certify me to teach grades K–12 in any New Jersey public school, I am—as of this writing—not qualified to be a school principal or district-level administrator. I remain in the process of formally appealing this decision, which comes—as all bureaucratic endeavors of this nature must—at the expense of time I could be spending on my students, my family, or myself.

IMPLICATIONS

Our critical dialogue revealed two implications. First, we acknowledge that even if the pandemic (hopefully) wanes, and (if) public education returns to its pre-pandemic guise, educators' felt dehumanization will not disappear. Thus, liberatory educational practice entails counteracting such dehumanization. To help teachers to keep their humanity intact during the pandemic, Helmke (2020) emphasized how school administrators can help teachers by making an effort to "go beyond normal efforts," "manage expectations," provide "mental health support," and "model caring communities" (pp. 37–39). We hear echoes of our own professional dialogue in these words: Helmke's suggestions are pragmatic and realistic, but they are—perhaps most critically—tailored to individuals in their practice. To humanize is to acknowledge our individual circumstances' value and validity. Administrative efforts of this nature are validating.

Second, to counteract educators' dehumanization during the pandemic, ongoing dialogues are helpful when they are proactive, responsive, and liberatory in recognizing participants' humanity. Ongoing dialogues of this nature are critical to liberatory education. When a Michigan school staff member suggested that proactive entreaties were important for faculty members just as they are for students (Gill, 2020, p. 27), this employee's principal started sending emotional wellness check-ins each Monday. This is an important action: When schools closed for in-person classes, previously open lines of communication were closed along with schools' classroom doors. Re-opening these lines of communication liberates educators as this article intends: during a crisis (and during crises), authentic and collaborative discourse is more than commiseration or camaraderie, it the construction of understanding in practice.

CONCLUSION

When the pandemic struck, teachers' challenges only multiplied. Institutional mandates from our schools amounted to added occupational stresses. Both of us, in effect, try to educate toward a more inclusive, more equitable future while we try to be whole people. We remain subtly and overtly impeded. Still, we continue our critical dialogue in pursuit of transformative justice. To navigate this pandemic together in shared dialogue is to teach ourselves how to both find the words to survive these times and to balance our professional priorities with our drive to educate (Pliner et al., 2011). What is beautiful is that we have each other as friends and thought partners. We hope that what we have shared here helps to bind other educators together toward hope and liberatory practices across the varied intersections of our lived experiences.

When my co-author and I talk, we often do what many educators are doing right now: we cry on one another's shoulders. At the same time, we are both aware of our agency as future scholars, as leaders right where we are. In Texas and in New Jersey, I am always refreshed after our conversations as classmates and as friends. These dialogues are the spaces in which the real work takes place; these are conversations between lifelong educators who care about what it means to be fully human. We aspire to allow others to join us, to progress, and to do more than merely survive.

In painting what at times may be a harrowing portrait of what it is like to be a public educator right now in the United States, in writing this chapter with the knowledge that many—for reasons too innumerable to list in a space like this one—are working with far more diminished resources, with far less experience than we possess, we dare to ask: what should we do? What *can* we do?

We can speak to our experiences and our ambitions, but where opportunities for advancement ought to be most likely, we find roadblocks: positions filled by those who are closest to the appointing administrator, supervisory position postings that ask for a decade of experience (or worse: those that "prefer retired administrators"), hierarchical powers diametrically opposed to any potential hires who could—rightly or wrongly, but dependably and superficially—be regarded as "controversial" or "unorthodox." Predictably, one's propensity to ask pointed questions only marks a viable avenue for career advancement in the most exceptional of scholastic circumstances. In a way, this dynamic aligns neatly parallel to teachers' ageless, canonical dictum: *Just close the door and teach.* Administrators do the administrative equivalent: tune out the noise, the trends, the initiatives, the cutting edge, and go with "what works." Effectively (and admittedly): like teachers, school administrators do not have an easy job right now. When scrutiny is high, it is not surprising that so many prefer the known quantity that years of experience represents.

So, then, to further our liberatory goals without hindrance and—candidly—to find a way to supplement our stagnated incomes, we have looked outside of our teaching careers to start our own education consulting companies. In addition, we have worked, pursued, or continue to pursue administrative positions while we prospectively, hypothetically, and vigorously lament any eventual absence of *classroom teaching* in our lives. Through these dialogues, we have taught each other and learned from each other: how to start and maintain an LLC, how to network in a career so often sequestered from other professional realities, how to make our classroom practices restorative, just, equitable, and—again—*liberatory*. Nonetheless, we remain upwardly mobile, carving out the path that is hopefully more self-sustaining and enriching. We are accustomed to carving it without pay and with considerable effort, we are accustomed to carving it both for and at the expense of our students. We feel forced to apply for administrative roles, postdoctoral positions, grants, consulting opportunities, professional development seminars, and conferences because we are compelled to do better for our students and for our world, but—for once—also for ourselves.

Still, we wonder in our dialogues with one another, and within our classrooms every time that we too *just close the door and teach*: is it fate that we too may become the ones "at the top" who just "do our jobs?" Might we be the ones who, in turn, *tune out the noise, the trends, the initiatives, the cutting edge, and go with "what works"*? How do we meaningfully disrupt, challenge, and tangibly shift what is broken about ourselves and what we do?

In all likelihood, the greatest educational enigma is the strictly retrospective clarity of these questions' answers. Put simply: we will only know these when we, inevitably and accomplished, look backward for clues as to what led us to our destinations. What we can say now, with certitude, is that while COVID-19 mutates, spreads, and cruelly deprives its victims of oxygen to the lungs, it does the same to public education. Educators are the esoteric oxygen that breathes life into teaching and learning, and without ample time or opportunity—for dialogue, for sense-making, for compensation, for rest, for space to exhale, for healing capacity, for restoration—the body deteriorates until it becomes a shell of itself.

REFERENCES

Brown, A. M. (2017). *Emergent strategy: Shaping change, changing worlds*. AK Press.

Freire, P. (2018). *Pedagogy of the oppressed (50th anniversary edition)*. Bloomsbury Academic.

Gill, J. (2020). Long-distance leadership: Principals support teachers as they dive into remote learning. *Learning Professional*, *41*(3), 26–29.

Helmke, S. (2020). Address the stress: How leaders can support teachers in an extraordinary year. *Learning Professional*, *41*(5), 36–37.

Hooks, B. (1994). *Teaching to transgress: Education as the practice of freedom*. Routledge.

Kaden, U. (2020). Covid-19 school closure-related changes to the professional life of a k–12 teacher. *Education Sciences*, *10*(6), 165. doi:10.3390/educsci10060165

Lorde, A. (2007). *Sister outsider*. Crossing Press.

Love, B. (2019). *We want to do more than survive*. Beacon Press.

Pliner, S. M., Iuzzini, J., & Banks, C. A. (2011). Using an intersectional approach to deepen collaborative teaching. *New Directions for Teaching and Learning*, *2011*(125), 43–51. doi:10.1002/tl.432

Chapter 4
Social Self-Care:
The Necessity of Turning Outward

Nalanda Ray
Amity University, Kolkata, India

Anindita Majumdar
https://orcid.org/0000-0002-5836-0047
Woxsen University, Hyderabad, India

ABSTRACT

In a world dominated by augmented reality (AR) and hyper-digitization, the education system is on the verge of revolution. However, this rapid change has come at the expense of the pillars of knowledge-providers (i.e., educators). Based on past literature reviews, this chapter identifies the predominant sources of stress and declined well-being of teachers. These include the wave of AR, the COVID-19-triggered online transformation of classroom teaching, and the increasing diversity within classrooms. Their impact has been studied under two classifications—declined personal (reduced self-efficacy and accelerated stress) and social well-being (isolation and alienation). This chapter proposes the 'Me Within We' model of social self-care to enable teachers to experience a high level of well-being by fostering belongingness through empathic relationships and the establishment of group identity. Future researchers are urged to empirically investigate the holistic efficacy of various dimensions of educator self-care—including social, physical, emotional, and spiritual.

INTRODUCTION

As you grow older, you will discover that you have two hands, one for helping yourself, the other for helping others. -Maya Angelou

The significance of self-care transcends the benefits which are yielded by just one individual. Instead, it has a ripple effect on a macro-level. Broadly speaking, self-care refers to the act of looking after one's own well-being — which is an optimal amalgamation of their psychological, emotional, physical,

DOI: 10.4018/978-1-6684-2334-9.ch004

spiritual, and social domains. In a world now dominated by hyper-digitization, there is an increase in the number of potential stimuli that could affect one's health and well-being. Added to this, some of today's biggest companies are now aggressively investing in augmented reality (AR), such as Facebook's recent $10 billion backing into its AR venture (Wilton, 2021). To adapt to these changes in society, the education system is rapidly modifying itself to shape into these technologies. Although they may prove to have multiple advantages for a classroom environment, it is inevitable that they cumulatively add on to the number of modalities that teachers and educators will have to adapt to fast. This could potentially increase their stress and detrimentally affect their well-being due to the constant need to cope with the constant transitions in their environment (Tzima et al., 2019). While the world may not be slowing down any time soon, it is, therefore, crucial to focus on resilience-building and self-care among teachers.

Self-care among educators and teachers has always been essential — especially because it stretches far beyond the outlined 9 to 3:30 job (Steele, 2018). The irony lies in the fact that the job description of teachers is not restricted to teaching. If it were to be simply teaching, the profession of teachers could be unequivocally replaced by education companies such as Khan Academy and BYJU's. However, the role of educators covers the vast sea of teaching, mentoring, care-taking, and honing a child's emotional, physical, social, and cognitive well-being (UNESCO). Furthermore, with awareness surrounding teenage suicide increasing, educators have the additional role of monitoring their student's emotional welfare and their vulnerabilities, and risk of suicidal tendencies and ideation. With educators' burnout increasing for these reasons, it not only proves to have a detrimental effect on their well-being but also on that of their students and dependents.

As the term focuses on the 'self', people often overlook the necessity of turning outward for internal fulfillment. To address this area of concern, the primary focus of this chapter is on social self-care. The reason for this may be attributed to the undying and everlasting salience that one's social world holds over them. Canadian-American psychologist Paul Bloom once said that "humans are social beings, and we are happier, and better when connected to others". Therefore, considering that our social world lays the brick and mortar of personal development, self-care and reassurance, educators require consistent societal reinforcement to sustain their well-being. While psychological and physical self-care may revolve around building personal resilience, social self-care ensures that this resilience is psychologically sustainable via an educator's environmental stimulus. Especially in a profession that deals with the sustenance of an entire generation's current and future mental health, professional, and personal success, it is of utmost salience for society to bring its attention to the well-being of educators.

BACKGROUND

Contemporary Social Stressors for Educators

With augmented reality (AR) being one of the most recent pillar-in-the-making for the education sector, it is salient to investigate its impact on educators and teachers, as they play a key role in proliferating the integration and acceptance of such technology in classrooms. Studies have found that a majority of them find the constant need for training to adapt to the rapid changes in classrooms as a result of technology very stressful (Tzima et al., 2019; Varanasi, 2021). Closely associated with this is the recent resurgence of the term 'technostress', which refers to the consequent decreased mental well-being of an individual who is unable to adapt to technology (Ragu-Nathan et al., 2008). Although there has been limited research into the role of technostress in education (Fuglseth and Sørebø, 2014), it has been found that it has a negative impact on not just their well-being, but also on the job performance of teachers (Wang and Li, 2019; Estrada-Muñoz, 2021).

The coronavirus pandemic has further magnified the negative health impact of the technological world on educators' well-being. This is especially because it has accelerated the transition of traditional teaching methods into online modes of teaching practically overnight (Rapanta et al., 2020). This transition, in addition to the existing stressors of the pandemic, has increased the burden that teachers now face (Pate, 2020). First, one of the most significant issues that have arisen as a result of this, is how educators have to juggle both online classes and their life at home, which has demolished the boundaries between professional and personal life. Specifically, the changing roles that they have to play between being a teacher, parent, partner, and caretaker of elderly parents, has made it difficult to demarcate the different domains of their life (Houlden and Veletsianos 2020; Loziak et al., 2020; Ilić-Kosanović, 2021; Syrek, 2021). Second, the coronavirus pandemic has caused educators to reach their burnout threshold quicker than they would have otherwise. Much of this has been attributed to the increasing number of stressors that they now face (Pressley, 2021). These include inadequate directions from superiors, the extra hours required to prepare for and adapt to online teaching, lack of social connections, the uncertainty of work, and increased working hours (Loziak, 2020; Hong et al., 2021).

The third cause of stress for educators, which has grown steadily over the past few years, lies in the environment of their work. In terms of its environment, even before the pandemic emerged, the complexity of classrooms has been increasing (Ramachandran, 2005). One of the most significant aspects in this area is the inclusivity of diversity in the education sector — which includes socio-economic, cultural, linguistic, and/ or ethnic diversity. Especially in light of digitization, the world has become increasingly diverse (Jha and Shenoy, 2016), which has been reflected in classrooms as well. While such multidimensionality marks a progressive milestone, it also contributes to a more complicated environment, as teachers are expected to cater to a host of subjective needs. Resultantly, the excess workload, personalized attention, and lack of training have heightened teachers' feelings of burnout, depersonalization, and stress, and reduced their self-efficacy (Glock et al., 2019; Amitai et al., 2020). Therefore, while diversity in these areas is necessary for the holistic growth and success of an integrative classroom environment (Glock et al., 2019), educators are often forced to face the brunt of societal growth without adequate training and social support.

Therefore, three of the most significant social stressors that have led to the depreciated well-being of educators include the integration of AR in the education sector, the impact of the pandemic and amplified workload, and the increasing complexity and diversity of classrooms.

MAIN FOCUS OF THE PAPER

Based on the literature review and current trends in behavior, the following have been identified as fallout areas of the cumulative impact of the rapid integration of AR, the impact of the COVID-19 pandemic, and the increasing complexity of classrooms:

Decline in Personal Well-Being

Personal well-being refers to the self-satisfactory state of one's own existence (Musek and Polic, 2014). The negative effects of the changing environment of the education sector can be seen to have extensive implications on two broad areas of declined personal well-being — i.e., self-efficacy and burnout.

Reduced Self-Efficacy

A teacher's belief regarding their ability to carry out classroom tasks successfully and appropriately plays a significant role in the academic performances and well-being of students (Klassen and Tze, 2014; Barni et al., 2019). Additionally, other contributory factors to personal well-being such as job satisfaction and job stress are also impacted (Caprara et al., 2003). However, the recently forced dependence on the digital world and changing dynamics of classrooms have had unforeseen ramifications in the level of self-efficacy of educators.

First, with the mode of teaching changing rapidly, teachers now have a lot to learn and adapt to in order to effectively be able to conduct classes with the same success rate as they could during traditional modes of imparting knowledge (Mannila et al., 2018). However, with the perpetual upgradation of technology on a round-the-clock basis, it may be extremely difficult and overwhelming to cope with it. Especially with the pandemic expediting this rate of change, it has become burdensome for teachers to gain digital competency (Hatlevik, 2016). Therefore, a large percentage of educators have faced the short end of the stick, whereby not only are they trying to consistently adapt to the demands of society, but to also perform optimally in other areas of their lives. This has led to reduced levels of self-efficacy and, consequently, self-esteem and confidence among teachers who find it strenuous to keep up with such the demands of AR and online teaching — especially in the absence of adequate training and attention from their institutions.

Accelerated Stress and Burnout

In the States, 27% of teachers have reportedly considered quitting their profession due to the stress and hiked burden of their jobs during the coronavirus pandemic (Dickler, 2021). However, the pandemic has simply unmasked a trend that was already brewing. Polls from PDK International in 2019 suggest that 50% of teachers considered leaving their job, while 48% felt as though they were not valued by their community. Most reasons for quitting revolved around undergoing high amounts of stress and low pay. Additionally, Smiley (2020) states that the life quality of teachers may be significantly hampered due to the stress and anxiety that they face — including the onset of enduring mental health problems. Hence, with there being a significant rise in the mental strain of educators and teachers, the focus of society needs to transition into *preventative foresight.*

Added to this, the diversity in classrooms, while a milestone of inclusive classrooms, has generated cumulative pressure on teachers to pay personalized attention to each student from different backgrounds. For instance, a country like India is primarily characterized by linguistic, and consequently, cultural diversity. According to the Eighth Schedule of the Constitution, the country hosts 22 official languages (Singh, 2020), and therefore, multilingualism is a woven part of India's culture (Bhaskaran, 2017). This pluralism has now translated into a predominant feature of classroom environments. Educators are therefore required to cater to the needs of each and every linguistically diverse group while ensuring that classroom material is universally comprehensible to all students. This workload has created immense pressure on educators (Cardozo-Gaibisso and Harman, 2019).

Closely associated with the concept of stress is *burnout,* which is a feeling of saturation and exhaustion as a result of prolonged exposure to stress. As iterated previously, the immense hike in workload especially during the pandemic, low pay, imbalance in work-life dynamic, and lack of digital-competence training, have all contributed to the collective burnout of the educators (Alderton, 2021).

Decline in Social Well-Being

Social well-being, which is the meaningful interactions and positive relationships that we form with those around us, lays the foundation for an educator's sense of belongingness and helps build their social identity. With humans being instinctively social by nature, the extent to which we connect with others determines our adaptivity and motivation to function cohesively. This is the fundamental area which the current effects of hyper-digitization threaten. As a result of the physical isolation that teachers face, their consequent feeling of belongingness is now declining — which could have extensive ramifications on the formation and sustenance of their social identity.

Singular Existence: Isolation and Alienation

Lortie (1975) proposed three types of isolation for educators — egg-crate isolation, psychological isolation, and adaptive isolation (Ostovar-Nameghi and Sheikhahmadi, 2016). For the purpose of this study, the first, and third types of isolation have been focused upon. Egg-crate isolation refers to the alienation that an educator may feel as a result of their physical separation from their peers and co-workers because of the concrete structure of schools and the separated classrooms. This phenomenon may now be generalized to the context of online teaching during the pandemic. Zoom and Microsoft Team classrooms have completely obliterated a teacher's physical association to their classroom and with their peers, and instead, replaced it with a 14-inch screen. With there being limited communication with people from their own profession and no connectivity, apart from that of their broadband network, social identity crises and feelings of alienation and detachment are inevitable.

The other major type of isolation, which is arguably the most relevant one at present, is adaptive isolation. It refers to the seclusion that teachers feel due to their inability to meet the demands of contemporary teaching methods. One of the most detrimental aspects of today's e-learning and online classrooms is the stress that educators face due to their lack of training in building digital competence. Resultantly, many teachers may implement their available knowledge of face-to-face classes in online modes of teaching, without understanding the personalized approach that must be taken across different modes (Delgado, 2020). Therefore, while many educators do find e-learning tools extremely effective (Zalat et al., 2021), their optimal utilization of those tools is often hindered due to their lack of training. This disparity between wanting to teach effectively but being unable to do so due to adaptation constraints stands as a major source of isolation among educators across the world.

Therefore, the collective experience of personal burnout and stress, and isolation tamper with the essence of human nature — which is to socialize with others and establish a sense of belongingness with like-minded individuals.

SOLUTIONS AND RECOMMENDATIONS

The implications of a demotivated and stressed teacher travel far beyond their own personal lives, especially because they hold the key to the growth and success of future generations across the globe. Whether it is the values they proliferate, the way they impart knowledge, how they carry themselves, to the empathy they show in class, students tend to internalize and shape themselves in accordance with the exposure they receive. In light of these, the self-care and well-being of educators must be prioritized. While extensive self-care has been a concept closely associated with and popularized by the palliative care industry (Mills et al., 2018), it has not gained equitable attention in the education sector. This has to change, for the sustenance and positive health of every population that is dependent upon knowledge accumulation.

Social self-care is one of the most important aspects of the self-care domain because it accounts for the environmental cues and modifications that can help sustain one's personal self-care. In a way, it provides positive reinforcement for educators to remain engaged in their work without compromising their well-being. Social self-care strategies focus on the angle of establishing interpersonal relationships, catering to environmental stimuli, and utilizing social reinforcements to build upon one's resilience. Therefore, turning outward is key.

Figure 1. Proposed 'me within we' model of social self-care

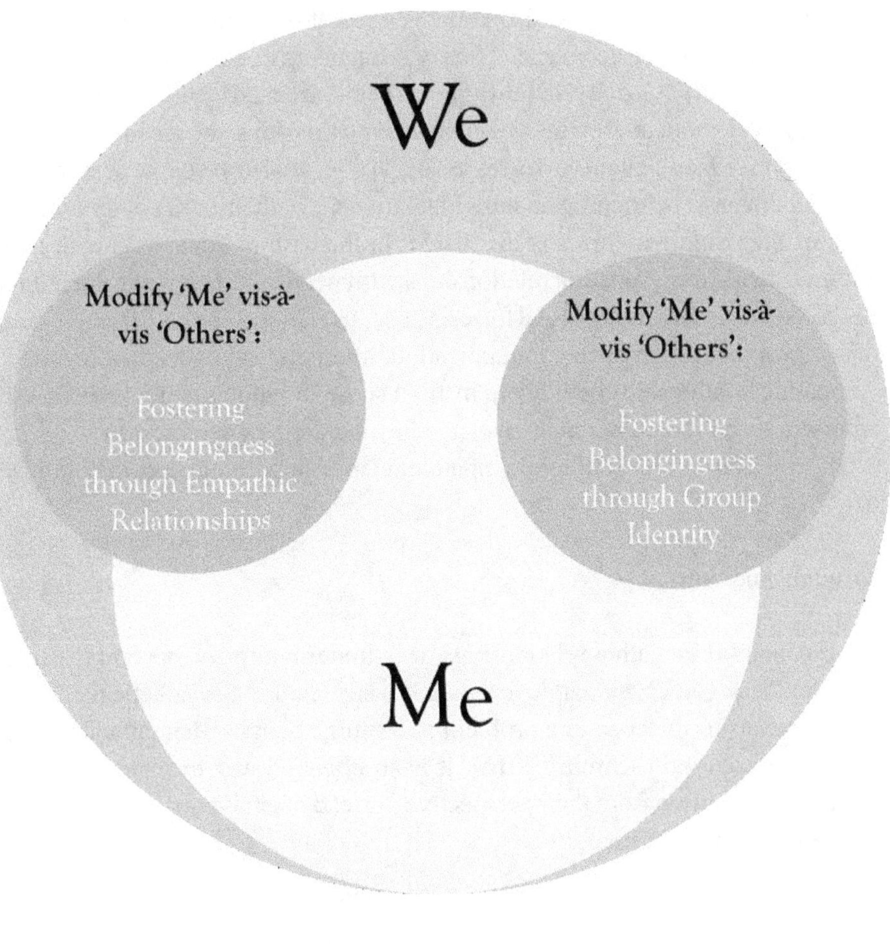

Turning Outward to Modify 'Me' Vis-à-Vis 'Others'

The present chapter proposes this theoretical foundation of social self-care to emphasize the necessity of environmental variables to enhance our sense of self and well-being in relation to other people or groups. Therefore, it assumes that optimal self-care may be achievable, but is contingent upon our relationship with others. It has two dimensions — first, to foster belongingness through empathic relationships, and second, to foster belongingness through group identity.

Fostering Belongingness through Empathic Relationships

The pioneer psychological theory of motivation, i.e., Maslow's 'Need Hierarchy' theory (1943), outlines the necessity of the belongingness paradigm in fostering teacher self-care (Leahy and Wolfe, 2021). Specifically, social self-care may be the most appropriate way to achieve this sense of belongingness because they both believe in the 'self' existing within their social surrounding. To elaborate on this, social self-care emphasizes the importance of leaning into our social relationships to establish our own well-being. Similarly, belongingness prioritizes leaning into our social relationships and groups to establish a sense of social self. Therefore, if both concepts are synthesized, one could indulge in social self-care by building positive social relationships to increase their belongingness and reduce feelings of isolation, alienation, and loneliness.

Creating meaningful connections with people can have a therapeutic effect (Soler-Gonzalez et al., 2017) for educators, who deal with hyper-isolation as a result of online classrooms, in that they have been found to increase one's self-esteem and efficacy (Greenberg et al., 2001). In particular, the role of empathy in establishing positive social relationships has been validated by numerous studies, all of which believe that it is the key element to growing positive interrelationships and an outlet for the accumulated stress that educators may face (Yuguero-Torres et al., 2017). It also helps in preventing burnout and excessive emotional drainage by training an individual to manage their levels of emotional involvement in various facets of life (Yuguero-Torres et al., 2015). In the case of educators, with their heightened stressful emotions, establishing empathic relationships with people in their environment may be greatly beneficial. This could involve investing in and fostering social relationships with friends, family members, neighbors, and/ or peers. Through open communication, interpersonal understanding, and perspective-taking, these empathic relationships could help instill a sense of belongingness among educators, who would have otherwise been forced to remain isolated beyond their 14-inch screen.

To increase the prevalence of meaningful empathic relationships, educators may follow these strategies (Carpenter, 2020):

1. Vision through Audition

To establish meaningful empathic relationships, it is important to see beyond the information that one's eyes may offer them. Hence, empathic listening is a key feature. Empathetic listening may provide educators with the means to understand a problem to its full extent — thereby increasing the odds of finding an appropriate solution (Schmitz, 2016). It is an effective way to mute one's own biases and observe someone else's situation from their perspective, instead of analyzing it through the smokescreen of one's own experiences and schemas.

2. Interpersonal Sharing of Feelings

The entire basis of empathy rests upon the shared understanding of another person's feelings and emotions. Therefore, the interpersonal sharing of feelings is one of the most indispensable components of building empathic relationships. It refers to the openness with which one expresses themselves to another person, and in turn, how this is reciprocated in order to establish an empathic relationship. There is an element of vulnerability, which can act as a cathartic point for educators, who may then share their inner feelings and honest state of mind to encourage a flow of relatability.

3. Observation of Nonverbal Cues

Nonverbal cues and communication often express much more personal emotions, judgments, and feelings, as compared to their verbal counterparts. Since it is a direct tool into the understanding of one's raw, and often unconscious, feelings, the careful observation of one's nonverbal gestures could be an impactful way to establish an empathic relationship with them.

Fostering Belongingness through Group Identity

Another way by which a sense of belongingness may be instilled within teachers is by establishing and widening their group identity. Social support and being a part of a group have been shown to reduce one's levels of stress (Haslam and Reicher, 2006; McKimmie et al., 2019), as well as increase one's ability to cope and adapt to social change — which is a skill required in today's age of rapidly transitioning technology. This has been predominantly attributed to the reciprocal support that in-group members provide each other and the sense of belongingness that invites feelings of purpose and motivation.

While this chapter has focused on much of the environmental stressors that AR and digitization have brought about, there is no doubt that such modes of communication can be used to contribute toward the sustained social well-being of educators. A recent trend among educators is to use social media platforms to connect, relate to, share ideas with, and observe the life and teaching styles of other educators in their profession (Carpenter and Green, 2017). These social media platforms, ranging from Facebook, Instagram, Twitter, and WhatsApp, have had a significant impact in creating a global community of educators and thus, have widened their group identity across geographical borders. Alongside enabling educators to support and interact with each other, social media provides them with a platform for finding like-minded individuals (Leahy, 2021). This promotes stress-release by acknowledging the similarities in struggles and challenges that many others in their profession face. Therefore, encouraging the widespread of social networking sites among educators can prove to be an effective way by which they can cater to their well-being. By the same logic that relatable memes can reduce stress and anxiety, other relatable audio, visual, or written content may have a similar effect on educators (Joshi, 2018).

Teachers could also engage in collective "study groups", which may enhance both their career growth and reduce their feelings of alienation (Ostovar-Nameghi and Sheikhahmadi, 2016). The idea behind *Teacher Study Groups* is that they would serve as a hub for the exchange of honest, relatable, and novel information, which may both amplify group identity with like-minded and similar people, and discuss current practices, theories, and ideas for classroom engagement. Their therapeutic nature could have long-lasting effects on the acclimatization of teachers to digitized classrooms. Simply knowing that someone is not alone while going through something may help instill a sense of togetherness and social bonding among educators.

FUTURE RESEARCH DIRECTIONS

The importance of social self-care among educators and teachers cannot be understated. No longer is it an option — social self-care has become a necessity. It provides professionals with the ability to scan their environment for reinforcements that can help them sustain their internal resilience built via other self-care strategies. By providing such strategies and bringing this much-needed dialogue to the forefront, this chapter may aid educators to prioritize their own mental, physical, emotional, and social well-being. In turn, this will help foster a more positive classroom environment for students and teachers alike. In today's world, with EdTech on the rise, society must acknowledge the boundless advantages that educators provide for the future generation — which stretches far beyond textbook teaching.

Social self-care as a terminology has not gained much recognition yet. Hence, future researchers should focus on extending further techniques of social self-care to help vitalize the term and spread awareness among the education sector and society alike. Additionally, researchers could investigate the holistic efficacy of social, emotional, psychological, spiritual, and physical self-care by synthesizing their collective impact on increasing the well-being of educators. This could help widen the scope of the present chapter's proposed 'Me Within We' model of social self-care.

Alongside this, it is of utmost salience to explore ways by which educators' adaptation to AR-integrated and online classroom environments can be made smoother. This includes research into effective training procedures in partnership with various institutions so that they can be implemented efficiently. Without institutional support, the well-being of educators will not be able to surpass the threshold of 'self'. In order to support its growth on a larger scale, collaborative effort is necessary.

CONCLUSION

Teacher self-care is crucial for the sustained growth of the education sector. Specifically, social self-care is arguably one of its most salient dimensions, because it ensures the long-term preservation of personal well-being and other types of internal self-care by providing environmental stimuli and external sources of reinforcement. While social stressors, especially those related to technology, will only increase rapidly with time, educators should implement social self-care strategies to preserve their own well-being. Not only should this be limited to self-implementation, but schools and other educational institutions should actively direct their resources to ameliorate the condition of teachers.

The implications of educator social self-care stretch far beyond their own well-being. On a micro-level, it aids in the welfare of teachers to help them perform optimally in classroom environments — regardless of the modality. However, on a macro-level, due to the significant exposure that students gain from their educational institutions, the values and outlooks that teachers hold are often transferred into them without any conscious effort. To prevent the unintentional negative values and added stress from being inculcated by learners, educator self-care must be prioritized. Through the implementation of social self-care strategies highlighted in the present chapter's proposed 'Me Within We' model, it may be possible to encourage teachers to turn outward to help their inner self and, in the long run, aid the sustenance of the entire education sector.

REFERENCES

Alderton, M. (2021, July 31). *Teachers are feeling burned out. artificial intelligence can help*. Retrieved from https://www.usatoday.com/story/life/2021/07/31/education-can-enhanced-through-technology-like-ai/7939422002/

Amitai, A., Vervaet, R., & Houtte, M. V. (2020). When teachers experience burnout: Does a multi-ethnic student population put out or spark teachers' fire? *Pedagogische Studiën*, (97), 125–145.

Barni, D., Danioni, F., & Benevene, P. (2019). Teachers' self-efficacy: The role of personal values and motivations for teaching. *Frontiers in Psychology*, *10*, 1645. Advance online publication. doi:10.3389/fpsyg.2019.01645 PMID:31354604

Bhaskaran, R. P. (2017). Language complexity and Multilingual education in India – a Policy Perspective1. *Issues and Ideas in Education*, *5*(2), 199–214. doi:10.15415/iie.2017.52013

Brackett, M., & Cipriano, C. (2020, April 7). *Teachers Are Anxious and Overwhelmed. They Need SEL Now More Than Ever.* EdSurge. https://www.edsurge.com/news/2020-04-07-teachers-are-anxious-and-overwhelmed-they-need-sel-now-more-than-ever

Caprara, G. V., Barbaranelli, C., Borgogni, L., & Steca, P. (2003). Efficacy beliefs as determinants of teachers' job satisfaction. *Journal of Educational Psychology*, *95*(4), 821–832. doi:10.1037/0022-0663.95.4.821

Cardozo-Gaibisso, L., & Harman, R. (2019). Preparing in-service teachers to work with linguistically and culturally diverse youth. Handbook of Research on Engaging Immigrant Families and Promoting Academic Success for English Language Learners, 361-377. doi:10.4018/978-1-5225-8283-0.ch018

Carpenter, D. (2020, February 14). *3 ways to build real empathy for others in your life*. Verywell Mind. Retrieved from https://www.verywellmind.com/how-to-develop-empathy-in-relationships-1717547

Carpenter, J. P., & Green, T. D. (2017). Mobile instant messaging for professional learning: Educators' perspectives on and uses of Voxer. *Teaching and Teacher Education*, *68*, 53–67. doi:10.1016/j.tate.2017.08.008

Delgado, P. (2020, November 2). *Teacher training, the Great Challenge of Online Education - Observatory: Institute for the Future of Education*. Retrieved from https://observatory.tec.mx/edu-news/teacher-training-challenge

Dickler, J. (2021, March 1). *More teachers plan to quit as Covid stress overwhelms educators*. CNBC. https://www.cnbc.com/2021/03/01/more-teachers-plan-to-quit-as-covid-stress-overwhelms-educators.html

Estrada-Muñoz, C., Vega-Muñoz, A., Castillo, D., Müller-Pérez, S., & Boada-Grau, J. (2021). Technostress of Chilean teachers in the context of the COVID-19 pandemic and Teleworking. *International Journal of Environmental Research and Public Health, 18*(10), 5458. doi:10.3390/ijerph18105458 PMID:34065219

Fuglseth, A. M., & Sørebø, Ø. (2014). The effects of technostress within the context of employee use of ICT. *Computers in Human Behavior, 40*, 161–170. doi:10.1016/j.chb.2014.07.040

Ghavifekr, S., & Pillai, N. S. (2016). The relationship between school's organizational climate and teacher's job satisfaction: Malaysian experience. *Asia Pacific Education Review, 17*(1), 87–106. doi:10.100712564-015-9411-8

Glock, S., Kleen, H., & Morgenroth, S. (2019). Stress Among Teachers: Exploring the Role of Cultural Diversity in Schools. *Journal of Experimental Education, 87*(4), 696–713. doi:10.1080/00220973.2019.1574700

Glock, S., Kleen, H., & Morgenroth, S. (2019). Stress among teachers: Exploring the role of cultural diversity in schools. *Journal of Experimental Education, 87*(4), 696–713. doi:10.1080/00220973.2019.1574700

Greenberg, L. S., Watson, J. C., Elliot, R., & Bohart, A. C. (2001). Empathy. *Psychotherapy (Chicago, Ill.), 38*(4), 380–384. doi:10.1037/0033-3204.38.4.380

Haslam, S. A., & Reicher, S. (2006). Stressing the group: Social Identity and the unfolding dynamics of responses to stress. *The Journal of Applied Psychology, 91*(5), 1037–1052. doi:10.1037/0021-9010.91.5.1037 PMID:16953766

Hatlevik, O. E. (2016). Examining the relationship between teachers' self-efficacy, their digital competence, strategies to evaluate information, and use of ICT at school. *Scandinavian Journal of Educational Research, 61*(5), 555–567. doi:10.1080/00313831.2016.1172501

Hong, X., Liu, Q., & Zhang, M. (2021). Dual stressors and female pre-school teachers' job satisfaction during the covid-19: The mediation of work-family conflict. *Frontiers in Psychology, 12*, 691498. Advance online publication. doi:10.3389/fpsyg.2021.691498 PMID:34168602

Houlden, S., & Veletsianos, G. (2021, October 14). *Coronavirus pushes universities to switch to online classes - but are they ready?* Retrieved from https://theconversation.com/coronavirus-pushes-universities-to-switch-to-online-classes-but-are-they-ready-132728

Ilić-Kosanović, T. (2021). Work-life balance of teaching staff at higher education during COVID 19 pandemic. *Serbian Journal of Engineering Management, 6*(1), 63–71. doi:10.5937/SJEM2101064I

Jha, P. N., & Shenoy, P. V. (2016). Digitization of Indian Education process: A hope or hype. *IOSR Journal of Business and Management, 18*(10), 131–139. doi:10.9790/487X-181003131139

Joshi, A. (2018, October 17). *Memes can help people cope*. The Daily Evergreen. https://dailyevergreen.com/38952/opinion/memes-can-help-people-cope/

Klassen, R. M., & Tze, V. M. (2014). Teachers' self-efficacy, personality, and teaching effectiveness: A meta-analysis. *Educational Research Review, 12*, 59–76. doi:10.1016/j.edurev.2014.06.001

Leahy, J., & Wolfe, J. (2021). *Teacher Self-Care: A Guide for Educators* (Dissertation). Spiral.

Loziak, A., Fedáková, D., & Čopková, R. (2020). Work-related Stressors of Female Teachers During Covid-19 School Closure. *Journal of Women's Entrepreneurship and Education, 3-4*. Advance online publication. doi:10.28934/jwee20.34.pp59-78

Mannila, L., Nordén, L., & Pears, A. (2018). Digital Competence, teacher self-efficacy and training needs. *Proceedings of the 2018 ACM Conference on International Computing Education Research*. 10.1145/3230977.3230993

McKimmie, B. M., Butler, T., Chan, E., Rogers, A., & Jimmieson, N. L. (2019). Reducing stress: Social support and group identification. *Group Processes & Intergroup Relations*, *23*(2), 241–261. doi:10.1177/1368430218818733

Mills, J., Wand, T., & Fraser, J. A. (2018). Exploring the meaning and practice of self-care among palliative care nurses and doctors: A qualitative study. *BMC Palliative Care*, *17*(1), 63. Advance online publication. doi:10.118612904-018-0318-0 PMID:29669559

Musek, J., & Polic, M. (2014). Personal Well-Being. Encyclopedia of Quality of Life and Well-Being Research. doi:10.1007/978-94-007-0753-5_2148

Okeke, C. I., & Mtyuda, P. N. (2017). Teacher Job Dissatisfaction: Implications for Teacher Sustainability and Social Transformation. *Journal of Teacher Education for Sustainability*, *19*(1), 54–68. doi:10.1515/jtes-2017-0004

Ostovar-Nameghi, S. A., & Sheikhahmadi, M. (2016). From teacher isolation to teacher collaboration: Theoretical Perspectives and empirical findings. *English Language Teaching*, *9*(5), 197. doi:10.5539/elt.v9n5p197

Pate, C. (2020, May). *Self-Care Strategies for Educators During the Coronavirus Crisis*. https://selcenter.wested.org/wp-content/uploads/sites/3/2020/05/Self_Care_Strategies_for_Educators_During_the_Coronavirus_Crisis.pdf

Pressley, T. (2021). Factors contributing to teacher burnout during COVID-19. *Educational Researcher*, *50*(5), 325–327. Advance online publication. doi:10.3102/0013189X211004138

Ragu-Nathan, T. S., Tarafdar, M., Ragu-Nathan, B. S., & Tu, Q. (2008). The consequences of technostress for end users in organizations: Conceptual Development and empirical validation. *Information Systems Research*, *19*(4), 417–433. doi:10.1287/isre.1070.0165

Rai, S. (2021, April). *Teaching and the New Education Policy*. The Tribute. https://www.tribuneindia.com/news/schools/teaching-and-the-new-education-policy-240818

Ramachandran, V. (2005). Why School Teachers Are Demotivated and Disheartened. *Economic and Political Weekly*.

Rapanta, C., Botturi, L., Goodyear, P., Guàrdia, L., & Koole, M. (2020). Online university teaching during and after the COVID-19 crisis: Refocusing teacher presence and learning activity. *Postdigital Science and Education*, *2*(3), 923–945. doi:10.100742438-020-00155-y

Schmitz, T. (2016, October 28). *Empathy - empathetic listening*. The Conover Company. Retrieved from https://www.conovercompany.com/empathy-empathetic-listening/

Scott, E. (2020, August 3). *5 Self-Care Practices for Every Area of Your Life*. Verywell Mind. https://www.verywellmind.com/self-care-strategies-overall-stress-reduction-3144729

Singh, H. (2020, July 14). *Official languages in Indian Constitution*. https://www.jagranjosh.com/general-knowledge/official-language-in-indian-constitution-1438068790-1

Smiley, A. (2020, February 7). *Why School Wellness Isn't Just for Kids: Many Teachers are Stressed and Depressed*. Occupational Health & Safety. https://ohsonline.com/articles/2020/02/07/why-school-wellness-isnt-just-for-kids-many-teachers-are-stressed-and-depressed.aspx

Steele, D. (2018, May 24). *Teaching's far from a 9-to-3:30 job: Here's what our day really entails*. ABC News. https://www.abc.net.au/news/2018-05-24/teachers-pay-teaching-profession-hours-duties-education/9786176

Syrek, C., Kühnel, J., Vahle-Hinz, T., & Bloom, J. (2021). Being an accountant, cook, entertainer and teacher—all at the same time: Changes in employees' work and work-related well-being during the coronavirus (COVID -19) pandemic. *International Journal of Psychology*. Advance online publication. doi:10.1002/ijop.12761 PMID:33826148

Tzima, S., Styliaras, G., & Bassounas, A. (2019). Augmented reality applications in education: Teachers point of view. *Education Sciences*, *9*(2), 99. doi:10.3390/educsci9020099

Varanasi, R. A., Vashistha, A., Kizilcec, R. F., & Dell, N. (2021). Investigating technostress among teachers in low-income Indian Schools. *Proceedings of the ACM on Human-Computer Interaction*, *5*(CSCW2), 1-29. 10.1145/3476081

Wang, X., & Li, B. (2019). Technostress among university teachers in Higher Education: A study using Multidimensional person-environment misfit theory. *Frontiers in Psychology*, *10*, 1791. Advance online publication. doi:10.3389/fpsyg.2019.01791 PMID:31447734

Wilton, T. (2021, October 26). *Facebook to Invest $10B this Year in VR and AR to Help Fuel the Metaverse*. Academic Press.

Zalat, M. M., Hamed, M. S., & Bolbol, S. A. (2021). The experiences, challenges, and acceptance of e-learning as a tool for teaching during the COVID-19 pandemic among University Medical Staff. *PLoS One*, *16*(3), e0248758. Advance online publication. doi:10.1371/journal.pone.0248758 PMID:33770079

KEY TERMS AND DEFINITIONS

Augmented Reality: A technology using which reality can be modified by including additional digital sensory stimuli like sounds and visuals.

Burnout: A body's feeling of exhaustion and fatigue due to prolonged exposure to different kinds of stressors. These could be emotional, physical, social, or psychological stressors.

Diversity: In the context of this chapter, it refers to the cultural, ethnic, socioeconomic, and linguistic variations of students within classroom environments.

Isolation: The state of being alone and cut off from others.

Personal Well-Being: One's sense of self-satisfaction with their own existence.

Self-Care: The act of taking care of one's own wellbeing by promoting their mental, physical, social, psychological, and spiritual health.

Social Self-Care: The act of taking care of one's own wellbeing through maintaining positive social relationships and by establishing meaningful connections and developing one's social identity.

Social Well-Being: One's feelings of belongingness and content by being a part of social groups and/ or by establishing positive and meaningful social relationships.

Chapter 5
COVID-19 Recovery in Schools and Self-Care for Teachers

Jia Borror
Nova Southeastern University, USA

Sarah Ransdell
Nova Southeastern University, USA

ABSTRACT

This chapter is about the nature of COVID-19 recovery and what teachers can do to support themselves and their students through these challenging times. The nourishment and well-being of teachers is necessary so they can support students as they focus on meeting their learning goals. The pandemic has created many new obstacles that must be overcome in order to come out triumphantly on the other side. This chapter provides a wide variety of research-based approaches for teachers to implement that take into account the mind, body, and spirit. Recommendations, considerations, and tips for going back to the classroom, whether virtual or online, are also addressed.

INTRODUCTION

Teacher self-care is needed to recover from the pandemic and is more important than ever before. Because teachers dedicate so much of their time and energy to students, it may be difficult to carve out time for themselves, but incorporating intentional acts of self-care can reduce anxiety, stress, high blood pressure, and a multitude of other health-related issues. Teachers must care for themselves before they can support their students, even in the best of times. Covid-19 has brought about the worst of times, at least in anyone's recent memory. This chapter is about optimizing the incredible strengths of teachers during some of the darkest days. Teachers determine student progress more than any other single factor (Engin, 2020). Positive teachers help to create positive students. Borror (2020) wrote about teacher self-care at the beginning of the pandemic and indicated that teachers need to identify their stressors, build a strong system of support amongst family, friends, and colleagues, and incorporate time for spiritual practices like reflection, prayer, or meditation. Overall health and well-being must be considered for the optimal

DOI: 10.4018/978-1-6684-2334-9.ch005

nourishment of teachers. The following practices should also be incorporated to optimize self-care: establish a positive mindset (an attitude of gratitude), find a balance in one's personal and professional life, nurture relationships that are satisfying and provide a sense of belonging, and create consistent routines for sleep, exercise, and nutrition to ensure good physical health. This chapter will provide suggested recommendations for teachers to care for their mind, body, and spirit, as well as tips for going back to the physical classroom, online classroom, or some combination of both in the aftermath of the pandemic.

Teachers, students, and parents will recover from the Covid-19 pandemic, but it won't be an easy task, especially with the number of infections still fluctuating due to multiple variants in circulation. The nature of Covid-19 recovery has been unpredictable, so teachers must forge ahead and do what they can to improve the process for themselves and their students. During and after the pandemic, teachers should focus on their own internal healing and self-care strategies before turning the focus to their students. Engin (2020) has shown that teachers who have self-efficacy are self-motivated. Administrators may not always be available to direct or motivate them, so teachers must do it for themselves. Teacher self-care improves self-motivation and student learning. Teachers need to prioritize their individual needs first and foremost, in the same way that airplane passengers put their own masks on before assisting children or others that need extra help. With Covid-19 face masks now sharing the space with those oxygen masks that drop from the ceiling of a plane, teachers must be prepared to follow the correct sequence. Let's start with a discussion of the profound effect the pandemic has had on educators and their students around the world and the challenges they are currently facing.

THE SHIFT TO COVID-19

In March of 2020, teachers had to quickly shift from in-person to online teaching while adjusting to virtual instruction amidst rampant school closures. Teachers worked relentlessly during this time, understanding that the shift to virtual education provided a silver lining, as online learning resulted in less infections for themselves and their students. However, connecting with students and keeping them engaged took on a whole new meaning. Online teaching and learning have been difficult transitions for both teachers and students alike. Learning loss among students during the 2020-2021 school year, sometimes referred to as the Covid-19 slide, has been documented even though teachers continued to work extremely hard. Many students fell behind during the pandemic due to a variety of reasons such as a pause in their academic instruction, the transition to strictly online learning, and limited resources to name a few (Farzan & Taylor, 2020). Students faced a multitude of other challenges with online learning as well, including limited social interactions with peers, short attention spans, connectivity issues, equipment failure, and deficient devices such as old cellphones. Additionally, some students needed more attention, time, or encouragement than online instruction was able to provide. Students who fell behind and lost their confidence were supported and guided by their teachers who reminded them that they could succeed if they did the work and didn't give up.

Solving problems in an online environment and dealing with challenges remotely has been quite stressful for teachers. It is hard, but not impossible, to offer one-on-one assistance to students online; however, it is an additional task in an already challenging situation in which many teachers were not properly trained or prepared. Teaching online requires both knowledge and skills about the hardware and software being used, multiple strategies to engage students, and innovative techniques that may be completely different than anything teachers have ever learned or implemented before. Borror et al. (2020)

found that virtual instruction requires more emphasis on visual enhancements and creativity for student engagement and comprehension. Considering all of these factors, teachers must work even harder to prepare and succeed.

Although Covid-19 vaccinations are available for all teachers and students ages five and older, they have divided Americans in unexpected ways. There is a lot of controversy surrounding the vaccine, side effects, and who should be required to get them. Vaccines are now mandated by the government for many federal workers and contractors, as well as for private companies and organizations with 100 or more employees. Lawsuits and pushback from those who disagree with these mandates are ongoing. A few states have mandated vaccines for teachers, while others encourage them by offering financial incentives. The Centers for Disease Control and Prevention (CDC) and the World Health Organization (WHO) both recommend getting vaccinated to limit the transmission of Covid-19 and to reduce the risk of getting the virus in the first place. Media reports of Covid-19 related deaths for both vaccinated and unvaccinated individuals have many people feeling unsettled and dealing with anxiety and trepidation. The FDA approval of the Pfizer Biotech vaccine makes it easier to require it to promote the health and well-being of others, but hesitancy should be respected until the moment it jeopardizes the health of others in any way. In a study by Kerekes et al. (2021), participants in six countries including the United States were more likely to accept the idea of vaccination when the vaccine had a high rate of effectiveness and low risk of fever. Other studies investigating vaccine acceptancy rates among various demographics have mixed results based on age, socioeconomic status, gender, political affiliation, and education level.

The research is clear about ways to reduce transmission. Vaccination, ventilation, handwashing, and masks are better than not, and each mitigation strategy adds to the model independently (Giardina et al., 2021). In other words, they all matter. Simulation of elementary school students with Covid-19 transmission shows that each of these behaviors reduce infection, so all strategies should be instituted. For certain schools, districts, and public spaces that require face masks, a popular sentiment is that it shows respect for those around you by reducing the risk of transmission. Teachers wear their face masks to honor the health and safety of their students and students wear face masks to honor their teachers' health and safety. This sentiment can be found in New York City's subway on the inside walls of the trains as a type of public health announcement. If it can be done on public transport, then it can be done with teachers and students.

Teachers can't teach if they are sick, and student learning will be impacted in a negative way. Once there is no ambiguity about what the teacher expects to reduce infections, they can focus on teaching and learning. With mask mandates starting to loosen within school districts around the world, one perspective is to err on the side of caution. If teachers have underlying health conditions, elderly or sick family members who live in their households or are just uncomfortable about the increased risk of exposure, then they should continue to wear face masks. Although they may not be able to require their students to wear them, other measures such as the use of hand sanitizer in the classroom, frequent reminders to wash hands, encouraging students to stay at home when they are not feeling well, and physical distancing whenever possible can be taken. The reality is that indoor masking cannot continue forever.

Now that the 2021-2022 school year is underway, teachers, parents, and students are dealing with the challenges of returning to school in the aftermath of a pandemic. These uncertain times continue to present countless challenges related to the coronavirus in what is now considered the new normal. When the teacher or one of the students fall ill, they must quarantine for up to 14 days. An entire class under quarantine can cause quite a disruption to the teaching and learning process. So, what can teachers do to remain calm amidst the chaos and encourage the same demeanor among students? First things first.

Review the prevention strategies to reduce Covid-19 when in the classroom. If students are fearful about Covid-19, then desensitize it and get that topic out of the way. Mask mandates, physical distancing, and quarantine rules continue to change, and neutral space is hard to come by in a Covid-19 ravaged world. Many students have had to deal with emotional trauma or the physical loss of a parent or loved one. For parents who may have lost a job, family members must deal with the repercussions of that such as food insecurity and lack of funds to pay the bills. Students come to class with the burdens of everyday life compounded exponentially with coronavirus ills, and teachers have their own share as well. It may be hard for students to think about or talk about but providing them with an opportunity to share their experiences and connect with classmates going through similar circumstances can make a huge impact. Social connections can help to reduce depression and anxiety, regulate emotions, and increase self-esteem in both children and adults.

CREATE A WARM CLASSROOM ENVIRONMENT

In the everchanging social climate of Covid-19, teachers must offer a neutral and safe place in the physical or virtual classroom where there is no judgement, just a positive outlook and a warm learning environment in which they imagine the best of each student in their care. Judgement must be reserved for learning objectives only. Sowani and Lavalekar (2020) recommend that teachers should establish and maintain a positive and supportive classroom climate to enhance student motivation and engagement. Part of this entails allowing students to have a say in what they are learning and the activities they engage in. Students greatly benefit from a consistent daily routine and encouraging messages that teachers provide by showing their love of the students and subject matter. Teachers can maintain their own sanity by keeping students focused on academics and not dramatics. Teachers must exude a calm demeanor and an authoritative presence to gain respect. By removing fear with facts and sustaining a sense of inner peace, teachers can model how to control their emotions by demonstrating tranquil and peaceful interactions with students and coworkers throughout the day. The two-year-old, the 13-year-old, and the college student will respond well to a sense of calmness emanating from the teacher.

Calming music played softly right before the official start of class might be one way to create a peaceful classroom environment. Playing soothing music can provide students with a few minutes to relax, minimize stress about anything that may have happened before they arrived to class, and help them to feel more optimistic. White (2007) found that playing classical background music in an elementary school classroom helped increase positive behavior among students and kept them motivated and on task. Further, Hicks-Moore (2005) found that calming music helped to reduce agitated behaviors in older adults during mealtime. Providing students with an opportunity to listen to soothing music or to participate in an opening activity to start their morning in a positive way can set the stage for a productive and happy day.

Even while wearing face masks, teachers and students can express joy. The smallest student might project peace and calm while wearing a mask, in part, because they've known nothing else. Partnering with students in their educational journey provides an opportunity for both teachers and students to bring their knowledge and experience to the table and learn from one another. Sharing one's passions and interests can help teachers establish closer relationships with students and connect with them in a more meaningful way. For example, if a teacher communicates their passion for travel by telling stories and sharing pictures of an enjoyable vacation, it may inspire students to share their interests and goals as well. When students feel as if they have a voice and a choice in their education, agency is created. Agency, play, and other types of seeking behavior improve resilience in children and young adults (Masten & Motti, 2020). The student with agency can make choices as an active stakeholder in their own learning environment, and the teacher with agency can make the classroom environment serve their own needs for teaching.

The two-year-old depicted below is wearing a mask with ease and even a bit of excitement for the new school experience as he attends his first day of preschool amid the Covid-19 pandemic. Even at two, he learns to wear a mask. When masks are no longer needed, the idea of a mask will never leave those who have had to endure wearing them for months on end. There will be more pandemics and disasters because that is our history. But teacher self-care and student self-care can be mutually beneficial, symbiotic, and healing. Wellness helps all people; teachers need it to keep up with little bodies of energy in the classroom and students need it for self-control.

Figure 1.

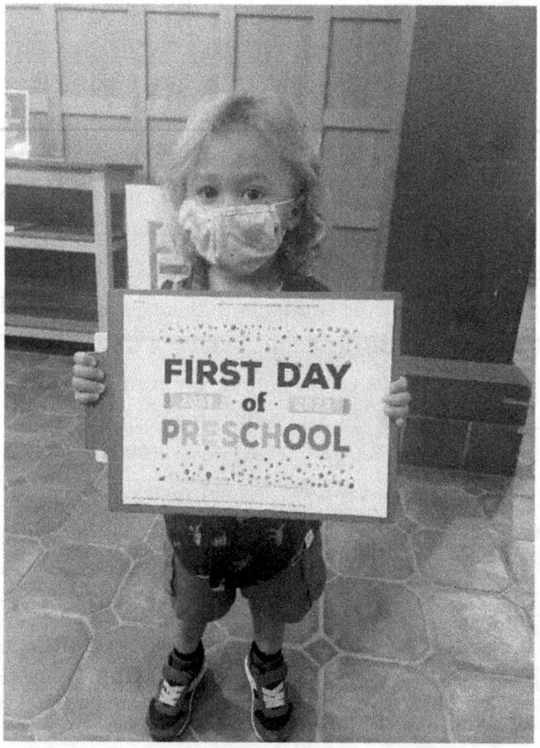

WELLNESS ASPECTS FOR TEACHERS

A mind-body-spirit approach encompasses all aspects of wellness for teachers. However, the focus of overall health and well-being may be quite different from one individual to the next. For some it means eating healthy, nourishing foods, and getting plenty of sleep. For others, it means incorporating a spiritual practice such as mediation, prayer, yoga, or spending time in solitude. A consistent exercise or skin care routine may be the most important aspect of wellness for some. It is important to understand that incorporating small self-care strategies such as these can help teachers feel more balanced overall. Teachers must strive to take care of the inside and the outside of their bodies to receive optimum benefits. An occasional massage, facial, or manicure can also provide a sense of relaxation and rejuvenation during periods of stress. Furthermore, taking care of the outside can positively impact the way one feels on the inside.

An Attitude of Gratitude

Gratitude is an essential component for teachers' overall well-being during the current social climate created by the pandemic, and this starts with having an optimistic mindset and being grateful for all the things they already have. Starting each day by writing down three things one is grateful for, or even sharing them with a close friend or confidant, can make a world of difference in the way one experiences life. Making it a conscious habit to set aside a few minutes each day to focus on the positive things in one's life will help teachers feel happier and more fulfilled. When operating from a place of abundance, feelings of fear, frustration, and anger will dissipate, and more opportunities will arise. Rather than focusing on the things that are not going in the right direction and complaining, take control of the situation and look for a solution. When a negative thought comes up, think of two positive thoughts to overcome it. Celebrate whenever possible, especially to acknowledge the small steps taken toward accomplishing one's goals and aspirations. Most people celebrate when they achieve something big, but it's also important to acknowledge the little accomplishments along the way. Another way to express gratitude is to show appreciation to others by sharing a compliment or letting someone know how much they mean to you.

Meditation

Meditation can be beneficial for both teachers and students because it centers the body and the mind on the act of breathing deeply and physical awareness in the moment. Teachers experience job-related stress from heavy workloads, student discipline issues, frequent evaluations by administrators, and continual changes to the curriculum. Olivo (2015) found that mindful meditation exercises for a few minutes each day can help boost confidence in teachers while reducing stress and enhancing the ability to focus and concentrate. This can be accomplished by sitting quietly in a comfortable position, closing the eyes, and observing the flow of the breath. Students may also experience stress due to any number of reasons including test anxiety, bullying, pressure from teachers and parents, or issues at home. Research shows that benefits of mindfulness interventions for students include increased focus, reduced anxiety, and an opportunity to relax (Strapp & Lambert, 2020). Setting aside a few minutes during the day to incorporate a mindful meditation in the classroom can lead to positive changes for both teachers and students.

Physical Fitness

Physical exercise is an important part of overall wellness with numerous benefits associated with it: stress relief; improved mood and concentration; increased strength and confidence; and lower body mass index (BMI). Yoga has therapeutic effects which can reduce physical and emotional stress, as well as promote flexibility and a sense of calmness and self-awareness (Woodyard, 2011). Incorporating a consistent yoga practice can also strengthen muscles and bones and reduce the risk of osteoporosis (Cronkleton, 2021). There are so many other options to incorporate exercise and movement as well. Walking, running, swimming, dancing, group fitness classes, weightlifting, boxing, spinning, CrossFit, and Pilates are popular ways to burn calories and reap the benefits of physical exercise. Sometimes the hardest part is starting, but once you do, the enhanced mental and physical aspects will be noticeable. Include exercise as part of your daily or weekly routine by scheduling it on your calendar to avoid any excuses as to why you can't do it. If you set aside time to make the investment in yourself, you will be less likely to fail. After repeatedly engaging in your exercise of choice, you will make it a regular habit, so stick to your plan and soon it will be an essential part of your life that you can't live without. Once you get those endorphins flowing, you will feel so much better about accomplishing your goal of incorporating exercise into your life and doing something positive for yourself.

A student with good physical health will need consistent routines for exercise and movement as well. Providing an opportunity for students to incorporate exercise during the school day can impact their learning, behavior, and mental health. Barile (n.d.) reported that exercise optimizes attention and motivation in students and gets the brain ready for learning. Chair yoga is an easy option to use in the physical or virtual classroom since students are usually seated in a chair and need breaks when they get wiggly or uncomfortable after long periods of instruction. A short yoga routine can be incorporated during the school day by the teacher leading the students through a series of poses such as the seated twist, cat-cow stretch, and slow neck rolls, or by following along to a video. By the logic of yoga, the inner peace the teacher gains from practicing yoga can be directly experienced by the students, and vice versa. Reciprocal effects are compounded effects. One of the authors, a lifelong teacher and learner, expresses pre-pandemic joy in the photo below while doing goat yoga (Ransdell, 2020).

Set Intentions and Use Affirmations

It is often customary to set an intention at the beginning of a yoga class, which helps the practitioner to create a shift in their mindset to focus on behaviors they want to incorporate in their practice. For example, one might set an intention at the beginning of a yoga class to focus on the breath. Setting intentions can be used in a variety of other situations as well, directing the way one would like to act or feel. A teacher may set an intention related to their personal or professional goals such as, "Today I will go for a walk after dinner to work on my physical health," or "I will contact the local university to inquire about classes for my graduate degree this week." Setting an intention guides the teacher to envision how they will act and feel when working towards a new goal. Once the intention has been set, affirmations can help to remind teachers of their intentions. While walking, the teacher can affirm their intention by repeating, "I am strong" or "I am healthy." After contacting the local university to inquire about graduate programs, an affirmation might be, "I am smart and capable." Creating a ritual to set an intention each day can easily be incorporated as part of one's morning routine, just like making coffee. By setting aside a few minutes in the morning to state one's intentions, it will help to keep the focus on the actions and mindset needed to achieve them. When affirmations are added to this process, goals are kept in the forefront, mood is boosted, and changes can be manifested.

Figure 2.

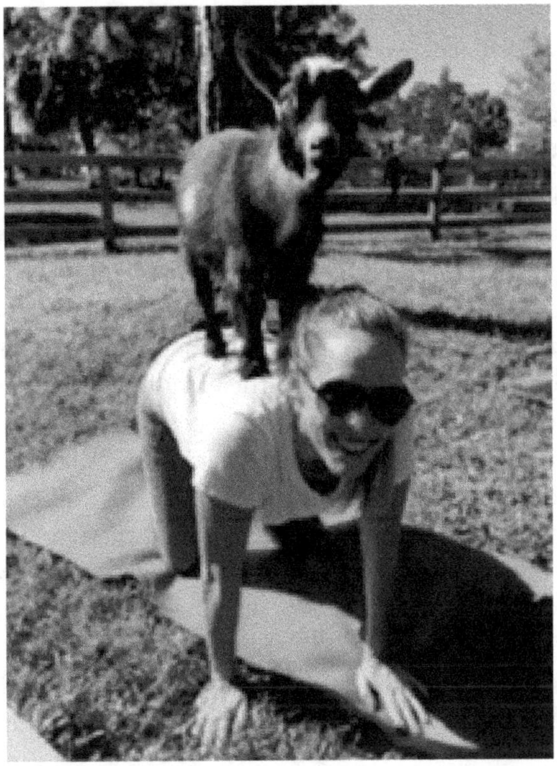

Develop a Reflective Practice

A daily or weekly reflective practice can provide an opportunity for teachers to think about different aspects of their lives that can be improved. Think about what's been working and what has not. Ask questions such as, "What was my most engaging lesson this week? Which teaching strategies were most effective? What was the most challenging situation I had to deal with? What could I have done better in that situation? How can I improve next time?" Reflection can be targeted to personal or professional goals and be accomplished through journaling, or sharing with a close friend, family member, or counselor. It can also take place while walking, exercising, being in nature, listening to music, or even spending time in solitude. Small changes to one's regular routine or practices can make a big impact. If one change doesn't work, try something else instead. For example, going to bed an hour earlier each night may provide teachers with more energy and stamina the next day. This is a simple step that can make a huge difference in one's outlook. Incorporating a reflective practice along with setting intentions and stating affirmations has the potential to effect change in the practitioner as knowledge, skills, talents, and new possibilities are reviewed, considered, and implemented. For those who prefer to put their thoughts on paper, reflective journal templates and notebooks can be found online to guide and inspire teachers. Having a dedicated journal or notebook also helps to hold one accountable and keep track of their goals.

Make Connections and Build Relationships

Collaboration with colleagues can make a significant impact on teacher perspective, efficacy, and confidence. When teachers work together, they establish significant personal and professional relationships which contribute to improved teacher performance, better learning experiences for students, higher student achievement, and overall school improvement. It is important to note that connecting and collaborating with others in person may be more difficult to achieve during the pandemic as social interactions have been limited and can cause stress and anxiety, but virtual options can be considered. A study about teacher collaboration and professional development indicated that benefits such as increased confidence, ongoing support, development of new knowledge and skills, establishment of new relationships, wider social networks, and improved student achievement can result from teacher collaboration (Boice et al., 2021). Although finding the time for collaboration may be difficult, the rewards far outweigh the disadvantages.

Relationships that are satisfying and provide a sense of belonging or community should be nurtured. These are the types of relationships where one person isn't making all the effort. Healthy relationships include honest and kind communication, as well as a sense of appreciation and acceptance. Relationships can provide emotional support during times of need and a distraction from daily life. Harter and Arora (2008) reported that Americans are the happiest when they spend six to seven hours a day socializing with others. Conversely, those who spend their time alone without any social interactions are the least happy and report feeling stressed and worried. The best way to gain a new friend is to be a friend, so take the initiative to reach out and share something about yourself and get to know more about the other person. Remember to stay open-minded, look for similarities, and be authentic.

Adopt a Pet

Approximately 68% of households in the United States have a pet, and studies indicate that pets can help reduce feelings of loneliness and increase feelings of emotional support (NIH, 2018). Research has also shown that having a companion pet such as a cat or dog helps to increase positive feelings when experiencing stress, which can lead to high blood pressure and raised cortisol levels, as well as an increased heart rate (Janssens et al., 2021). There's a sense of comfort in knowing that you have a loyal companion at home waiting to greet you with unconditional love. A benefit of having a dog is the increase in physical activity one will experience by walking it several times a day. However, if a dog is too much responsibility or a trigger for allergies, fish are another option. Simply watching fish swim around in a tank can promote a sense of calmness (Janssens et al., 2021).

Animals can help students improve their social skills, reduce stress and anxiety, and promote sharing and cooperation. Prior to the pandemic, the authors volunteered to read with preschool students on a regular basis accompanied by reading dogs who offered unconditional acceptance of all children in attendance at a small private preschool in South Florida. The preschoolers always looked forward to the reading dogs' visit and followed directions by sitting cross-legged on the carpet to take turns having the dogs sit on their laps during story time. For those students who were hesitant about getting too close the dogs, they were instructed to sit further away until they were more comfortable moving closer. The picture below is of Norton and Nugget, the reading dogs, who wore their school shirts proudly during a visit with the children. Research shows that when children read to dogs, it helps them develop a love of reading, increases confidence, and improves reading skills (Siejka, 2016).

Figure 3.

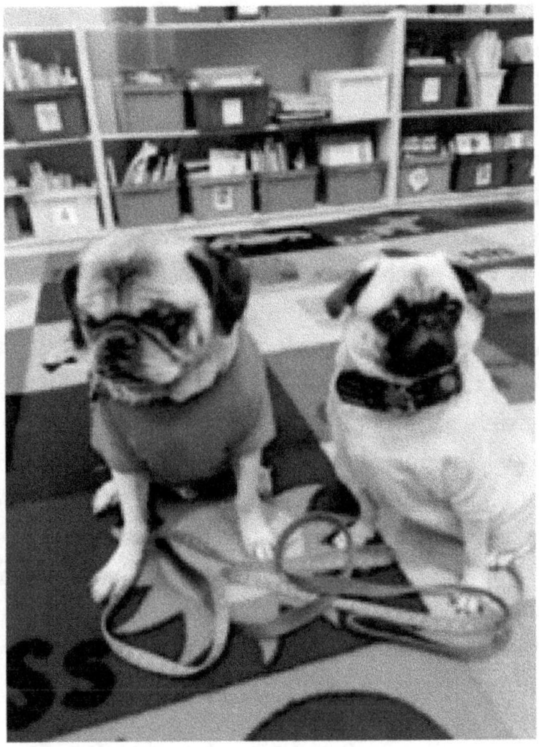

Find a Balance in Personal and Professional Pursuits

In order to maintain healthy relationships with others, it is critical to take time for yourself. Giving too much of your time and energy away can be detrimental to your emotional well-being. Whatever it is that brings you joy, set aside time to do just that. Teaching requires continual professional development to advance and stay informed of the newest developments, theories, and best practices. But perhaps there is another aspect of your career you would like to develop or explore. Endless opportunities exist that will provide a sense of purpose and satisfaction in your professional endeavors and ultimately benefit your students as well. Whether this is accomplished through self-exploration, reading, workshops, joining a new group, or higher education, follow your passion and continue to develop your professional strengths and interests.

Hobbies and personal interests cannot be pushed aside either. Pursue your dreams and try something you've always wanted to do by stepping outside of your comfort zone. You'll never know if you like something new unless you give it a try. Whether it's dancing, cooking, crafting, reading, volunteering, gardening, scuba diving, painting, or photography, there are so many options. Finding a new hobby that you enjoy will help you to relax and take your mind off the daily stresses of life while staying mentally engaged. Research has shown that taking up a hobby provides cognitive stimulation and is associated with lower levels of depression in both men and women (Fancourt et al., 2020).

Resilience

Teaching is a calling, and resilience is a type of calling too in that it can be learned and developed. Resilient teachers are those that can handle adversity and challenges such as a pandemic or a hurricane or a school shooting by practicing self-care. Being ready for anything is an asset to any profession, but it is a higher calling for those entrusted with the mental and cognitive well-being of students. Keeping a positive outlook, coming up with a plan of action, refusing to give up, continuing to work hard, staying flexible, and collaborating with others are excellent strategies for building resilience. Masten and Mosti (2020) found that resilience is very much dependent on an entire system working together to be ready for crisis and change. The resilience of children in disasters depends on many systems and adaptive capacities within the child and within the student-teacher relationship. Disasters can overwhelm many of the systems that children and families depend on, either simultaneously or in a devastating cascade of challenges. However, disasters also mobilize responses across many systems and motivate better responses in the future. Covid-19 is uncovering many gaps in how well communities are prepared to meet the needs of children and families during the pandemic as well as the cost to collective resilience of health and socioeconomic disparities. It is imperative to respond now to the pandemic disaster with the best knowledge available on what matters for children and what works to protect them. However, it also is crucial to learn as much as possible from this disaster to prepare for future shocks, both expected and unknown. Teachers play a big part in anticipating and defending against change that affects their students in negative ways.

Sleep and Nutrition

The time we spend sleeping accounts for one third to one quarter of our lifetime (Johns Hopkins Medicine, n.d.). Sleep is necessary to maintain proper brain function, process information, regulate metabolism, and for memory processing. There are many health-related problems associated with lack of sleep such as depression, migraines, high blood pressure, and increased risk of illness (Johns Hopkins Medicine, n.d.). Establishing a consistent routine for sleep will help to reinforce your body's sleep-wake cycle. The recommended number of hours varies by age, but adults need approximately seven to nine hours per night. Avoiding large meals, alcohol, caffeine, technology, and exercise too close to bedtime will help to ensure a good night's rest.

A balanced diet is essential to maintain a healthy weight and lifestyle. Nutrition is often neglected because teachers are on their feet most of the day with little time to eat a nutritious meal. Fast food and processed foods may be quick and easy, but in the long run they will be detrimental to one's overall health and wellness. The CDC (n.d.) recommends adding a rainbow of colors to your plate with fruits and vegetables such as leafy greens, oranges, blueberries, bananas, and tomatoes. Additionally, it is important to eat whole grains, protein, calcium-rich foods, and limit sugars, saturated fat, sodium, and alcohol. The benefits of healthy eating include strong bones and muscles, lower risk of heart disease and diabetes, stronger immune system, better mood, more energy, and longer life span (CDC, n.d.).

Mental Health

Between the isolation and physical distancing requirements many people experienced during the pandemic, mental health must be prioritized. Research has shown that those who struggled with mental health issues such as anxiety and depression prior to the pandemic are struggling even more now (Czeisler, 2020). According to Mental Health America (n.d.), an organization established to promote mental health and prevent mental illness, one out of every five adults (approximately 50 million Americans) have a mental health condition and 50% of them go untreated. Counseling sessions with a trained professional, whether virtual or in-person, can help individuals by providing a safe and supportive environment where positive changes can be experienced. Developing a rapport with the counselor or therapist is essential so that individuals feel comfortable sharing their struggles, thoughts, and personal information.

Laughter

The saying "Laughter is the best medicine" is true. Whether it's a comedy show, a YouTube video, a funny movie, or talking with a friend who makes you laugh, laughter can be an excellent form of self-care to take your mind off the stressful aspects of daily life. Laughter is beneficial for overall health and well-being. It relieves tension, releases endorphins, helps to protect against heart attacks, promotes a positive outlook, strengthens relationships, and boosts immunity (Robinson et al., 2021). Integrate humor and laughter into your life whenever possible. It will put you into a more relaxed and positive space to deal with any challenges that come your way. Sometimes it may be hard to laugh during life's difficult times, but thinking of a funny memory, sharing a good joke, or framing some photographs of happy times with friends and family members is a great place to start.

Vision Boards

The use of vision boards for teachers can be helpful as they direct one's focus to goals and aspirations through positive words and images. A vision board is an excellent way to remember what to do to stay on the Covid-19 teaching and learning recovery track. A vision board can help with self-regulation by promoting confidence and motivation. TTT4U (n.d.) is a site that describes some of the key elements in creating one and recommends that teachers create both a personal and professional vision board. The necessary materials for a traditional vision board include magazines, scissors, a poster board, and glue. Professional vision boards can be created at the beginning of each school year to define goals that you want to accomplish during the year related to leadership, student achievement, parent partnerships, or anything else associated with teaching and professional development. Start out by making a list of professional goals you'd like to include on your vision board and then find pictures, words, phrases, and quotes from magazines that align with them. Next, cut out the images, glue them to your vision board, and display it in a location where you will see it every day as a constant reminder to continue making progress toward your goals, dreams, and aspirations.

There really are no parameters as to the correct way to create a vision board. LaBorde (2020) explains that a vision board can be any type of display with images that represent the things you want to have in your life or the person you want to be. It is a creative process that can be utilized with students, parents, colleagues, or administrators that allows them to visualize what they want to accomplish and where they see themselves in the future. A vision board can be created on a cork board, a magnetic board, a dry erase board, or digitally on a computer (LaBorde, 2020). For example, an online vision board assignment in the form of a book cover could be a creative way to have middle school students share how they envision themselves starting over in a new situation. A book cover such as *New Kid* by Jerry Craft can be projected as an example to a large group of students on a screen. *New Kid* is a middle school book about staying true to yourself while trying to fit in somewhere new. Students can envision their best self. Will that best self be calm and relaxed? Will that best self be the best student or best person they can possibly be? Envisioning it will make it easier for them to achieve.

TEACHER INITIATIVES DURING THE PANDEMIC

Online read aloud over Zoom was implemented by one of the authors as a volunteer in a Covid-19 ravaged kindergarten class, with some students online and others in the classroom space. In a public elementary school classroom in South Florida, the teacher wore a mask at that point late in 2020 and early 2021, but the young students did not. The students could attend to the book, but it was challenging for the author because she often could not see the students. The classroom camera was difficult for the teacher to adjust properly, as she did not have sufficient training to use it. The author displayed a stuffed animal reading along with her via Zoom and the students spontaneously brought out their own stuffed animals from their desks. It was so calming that many put their heads on their desks, sighed, and some even sucked on their thumbs. For small amounts of time with a really good book like *Caps for Sale*, calm and authority could be maintained over the miles and Internet hardware. *Caps for Sale* provides a wonderful story about frustration, success, and lessons learned. While searching for the book details, the author found a YouTube video of a narrator reading the book. YouTube provides hundreds of such read along books to use in the elementary classroom, whether that's virtual or in-person. Reading aloud to students is beneficial because it helps to increase their vocabulary and comprehension, exposes them to various genres and topics, models fluency and diction, and promotes a love of reading. It also provides an opportunity for students to sit back, relax, and be transported to another place and time, if only for a short while.

One of the authors also volunteered to virtually assist a young adult during the pandemic who was aging out of the foster care system in South Florida while trying to obtain her GED, the equivalent to a high school diploma. The General Educational Development (GED) tests are a group of four subject tests which, when passed, provide certification that the test taker has high school-level academic skills. The student was struggling with the math subtest of the GED but was determined to succeed, even with her spotty internet service. Although the student's life was filled with chaos and uncertainty, she exhibited resilience by continuing to practice even when things got tough. The author taught the student how to be a smart test taker by treating the learning like a video game, making it competitive and fun. Rather than focusing on the trauma that was happening in her life, she shifted her focus to studying math and passed with flying colors.

Test takers who understand the test do better. The enemy was the fear of math in this case. Fear was reduced by understanding the culture of the test: don't leave any blank questions; the score is simply the number correct; guess if you must. With her newfound confidence and knowledge, the student became calm and skilled even when her internet failed due to the insufficient bandwidth. She succeeded because she was resilient and found another solution. Instead of using Zoom, she stayed on the phone to talk about the math problems and look at photos that the author sent. The student was able to learn math that she had long associated with chaos and fear. Now it is associated with success and she will be better equipped for 2021 and beyond. She can calculate the 20% tip in a restaurant in her head. She can use per capita measurements, like cost per yard, to determine which of two deals is a better bargain. She may even like the new power it affords her in the world. In the future this young adult may instruct her own children on how to solve a math problem, or she may be encouraged to pursue higher education goals, or even become a teacher herself.

The initiatives described above are only two of the volunteer opportunities that one of the authors participated in during the pandemic, so it was no surprise that she was recognized by the Florida Distance Learning Association (FDLA) with the Distinguished Service Award for 2021. By following her interests and passion to help students reach their full potential, she was rewarded for her excellence. This relates to teacher self-care because it is the best feeling in the world to see a student succeed and make their teacher proud. In this case, the teacher was restored with faith in the power of her teaching and inspired to continue teaching students about math and statistics.

CONCLUSION

Teachers face many occupational stressors in their daily lives, so it is essential that they become masters of self-care. Prioritize what you need to manage stress and avoid burnout because taking care of yourself is one of the best things you can do for your students. It is the hope of the authors that this chapter has provided you with some validation for the strategies you are currently implementing to take care of your physical, emotional, and mental health. The authors also encourage you to consider some new self-care strategies presented in this chapter as you continue your journey to enrich the lives of all the students you are blessed to teach and inspire now and in the future.

REFERENCES

Barile, N. (n.d.). Beyond the classroom. *Exercise and the brain: How fitness impacts learning.* https://www.wgu.edu/heyteach/article/exercise-and-brain-how-fitness-impacts-learning1801.html

Boice, K. L., Jackson, J. R., Alemdar, M., Rao, A. E., Grossman, S., & Usselman, M. (2021). Supporting teachers on their STEAM journey: A collaborative STEAM teacher training program. *Education Sciences, 11*(3), 105. doi:10.3390/educsci11030105

Borror, J. (2020). Developing as a teacher. In Teacher Self-Care. Cambridge Scholars Publishing.

Borror, J. Ransdell, S., Binaco, J., & Feeser, A. (2020). The impact of transitioning to online learning and virtual conferences on students and educators during the coronavirus pandemic. *Distance Learning Journal, 18*(1).

CDC. (n.d.). *Healthy eating for a healthy weight.* https://www.cdc.gov/healthyweight/healthy_eating/index.html

Cronkleton, E. (2021). Yoga for osteoporosis: 5 beneficial poses. *Healthline.* https://www.healthline.com/health/osteoporosis/yoga-for-osteoporosis#12

Czeisler, M. E., Lane, R. I., Petrosky, E., Wiley, J. F., Christensen, A., Njai, R., Weaver, M. D., Robbins, R., Facer-Childs, E. R., Barger, L. K., Czeisler, C. A., Howard, M. E., & Rajaratnam, S. M. W. (2020). Mental health, substance use, and suicidal ideation during the Covid-19 pandemic – United States, June 24-30, 2020. *MMWR. Morbidity and Mortality Weekly Report*, *69*, 1049–1057. doi:10.15585/mmwr.mm6932a1 PMID:32790653

Engin, G. (2020). An examination of primary school students' academic achievements and motivation in terms of parents' attitudes, teacher motivation, teacher self-efficacy and leadership approach. *International Journal of Progressive Education*, *16*(1), 257–276. doi:10.29329/ijpe.2020.228.18

Fancourt, D., Opher, S., & de Oliveira, C. (2020). Fixed-effects analyses of time-varying associations between hobbies and depression in a longitudinal cohort study: Support for social prescribing? *Psychotherapy and Psychosomatics*, *89*(2), 111–113. doi:10.1159/000503571 PMID:31658464

Farzan, A. N., & Taylor, A. (2020). Students in England fell behind by average of three months during shutdown, study finds. *Washington Post.* https://www.washingtonpost.com/world/2020/09/01/studentsengland-fell-behind-three-months-coronavirus-study/

Giardina., . . . (2021). When do elementary students need masks in school? Model-estimated risk of in-school SARS-CoV-2 transmission and related infections among household members before and after student vaccination. MedRxiv. doi:10.1101/2021.08.04.21261576

Harter, J., & Arora, R. (2008). Social time crucial to daily emotional well-being in U.S. *Gallup.* https://news.gallup.com/poll/107692/social-time-crucial-daily-emotional-wellbeing.aspx

Hicks-Moore, S. (2005). Relaxing music at mealtime in nursing homes. *Journal of Gerontological Nursing*, *31*(12), 26–32. doi:10.3928/0098-9134-20051201-07 PMID:16375095

Janssens, M., Janssens, E., Eshuis, J., Lataster, J., Simons, M., Reijnders, J., & Jacobs, N. (2021). Companion animals as buffer against the impact of stress on affect: An experience sampling study. *Animals (Basel)*, *11*(8), 2171. doi:10.3390/ani11082171 PMID:34438629

Johns Hopkins Medicine. (n.d.). *The science of sleep: Understanding what happens when you sleep.* https://www.hopkinsmedicine.org/health/wellness-and-prevention/the-science-of-sleep-understanding-what-happens-when-you-sleep

Kerekes, S., Ji, M., Shu-Fang, S., Hao-Yuan, C., Harapan, H., Rajamoorthy, Y., & Wagner, A. L. (2021). Differential effect of vaccine effectiveness and safety on COVID-19 vaccine acceptance across socioeconomic groups in an international sample. *Vaccines*, *9*(9), 1010. doi:10.3390/vaccines9091010 PMID:34579247

LaBorde, S. (2020). *What is a vision board?* https://makeavisionboard.com/what-is-a-

Masten, A. S., & Motti-Stefanidi, F. (2020). Multisystem resilience for children and youth in disaster: Reflections in the context of Covid-19. *Adv Res Sci, 1*, 95–106. doi:10.1007/s42844-020-00010-w

Mental Health America. (n.d.). *The state of mental health in America.* https://mhanational.org/issues/state-mental-health-america

NIH. (2018). *The power of pets: Health benefits of human-animal interactions*. https://newsinhealth.nih.gov/sites/nihNIH/files/2018/February/NIHNiHFeb2018.pdf

Olivo, E. (2015). Two simple mindful meditation exercises for teachers. *The Guardian*. https://www.theguardian.com/teacher-network/2015/dec/06/two-simple-mindful-meditation-exercises-for-teachers

Ransdell, S. (2020). *Teacher Self-Care*. Cambridge Scholars Publishing. http://www.cambridgescholars.com/teacher-self-care

Robinson, L., Smith, M., & Segal, J. (2021). *Laughter is the best medicine*. https://www.helpguide.org/articles/mental-health/laughter-is-the-best-medicine.htm?pdf=13511

Siejka, A. (2016). Tail waggin' tutors. *Children & Libraries, 14*(2), 32–33.

Sowani, D. A., & Lavalekar, A. (2020). Exploring psychological well-being of college students in relation to college classroom environment. *International Journal of Education and Management Studies, 10*(4), 428–433.

Stapp, A. C., & Lambert, A. B. (2020). The impact of mindfulness-based yoga interventions on fifth-grade students' perceived anxiety and stress. *International Electronic Journal of Elementary Education, 12*(5), 471–480. doi:10.26822/iejee.2020562137

TTT4U. (n.d.). *How to create a teacher vision board to visualize your goals*. https://www.teachandtaketime4u.com/2018/03/08/create-teacher-vision-board/

White, K. N. (2007). *The effects of background music in the classroom on the productivity, motivation, and behavior of fourth grade students*. https://files.eric.ed.gov/fulltext/ED522618.pdf

Woodyard, C. (2011). Exploring the therapeutic effects of yoga and its ability to increase quality of life. *International Journal of Yoga, 4*(2), 49–54. doi:10.4103/0973-6131.85485

KEY TERMS AND DEFINITIONS

Affirmation: A positive statement that helps motivate one to achieve a desired change.

Agency: The capacity of teachers or students to take ownership in the teaching and learning process by making choices that contribute to their growth.

Goal: A specific and measurable outcome one strives to achieve.

Intention: A statement about one's commitment to actions related to an intended accomplishment.

Pandemic: Worldwide outbreak of a disease.

Reflection: The process of looking back at prior events, actions, or thoughts in an effort to make future improvements.

Resilience: The capacity to remain strong and bounce back after dealing with a challenge or difficulty.

Chapter 6
Human Capital Development in Youth Inspires Us With a Valuable Lesson:
Self-Care and Wellbeing

Ansar Abbas
https://orcid.org/0000-0003-4521-1920
Airlangga Universtias, Indonesia

Fendy Suhariadi
https://orcid.org/0000-0001-9679-2185
Airlangga Universtias, Indonesia

Dian Ekowati
https://orcid.org/0000-0001-9726-4720
Airlangga Universtias, Indonesia

Rakotoarisoa Maminirina Fenitra
Airlangga Universtias, Indonesia

Mochammad Fahlevi
https://orcid.org/0000-0002-1419-8308
Bina Nusantara University, Indonesia

ABSTRACT

Human capital is the bundle of information, skills, and talents individuals build for personal well-being and economic productivity. Human capital provides long-term benefits for future generations. It is vital for economic growth, social capital, and the development of networks. Human growth is a challenging and never-ending process. However, the importance of early childhood and youth development is ever crucial. Because youth are susceptible to biological growth, academic and career advancement, and long-term planning, stress can come to them in various forms and sources. Stress represents an undeniable reality of life, particularly in youth concerning the academic sphere. Taking care of oneself represents a regularly practiced concept to relieve stress. Learning about self-care helps carefully maintain and improve short and long-term health and well-being. Its cohorts to improve overall health and well-being thus required scholarly attention to find the new way to benefit children and youth development.

DOI: 10.4018/978-1-6684-2334-9.ch006

INTRODUCTION

Developing nations have made significant gains in human capital in recent decades. Enormous problems have threatened human economic development and competition in the global system. Consequently, the western world is making enormous efforts to develop models geared toward balanced youth growth. Recent Southern European migration has been characterized by significant flows of higher-skilled young people (Staniscia et al., 2021). Stress is a condition that affects everyone at some time in their life. However, it manifests differently in various people and is interpreted by the one experiencing it. One of the most obvious facts is that psychologists feel that stress is detrimental to an individual's health. For example, stress is hazardous for children and adolescents. Academic obligations, peer pressure, and other factors contribute to a wide range of continuing stresses for students in secondary and higher education settings (Pascoe et al., 2020). Another phenomenon that has significantly impacted students' life course shift is a societal change caused by the covid-19 pandemic (Husky et al., 2020; Wang et al., 2020). Therefore, adolescents and young people are subjected to increased healthcare services, counseling, and advisory services (Dalky & Gharaibeh, 2018). However, in particular, young people require special attention regarding stress development and education to become masters of stress awareness and prepared to manage stress.

Many countries have encountered the need for human capital development during the past decade, which has become increasingly prevalent due to global change. The Fourth Industrial Revolution includes the emergence of digital technology, which marks the shift from an industrial economy to a digital economy. Society is one of the change reasons. Technology has aided human development by influencing how governments respond to constituent needs in social services and public service delivery. The rapid spread of technological innovation necessitated a more adaptable next generation to keep pace with the rapidly shifting global system. Because of this, academics must use mastery and machinimas theories to formulate ways to produce a more resilient generation that can oversee hardship on its own in the future. Much literature has been produced on young people's propensity to stress.

This chapter discusses the notion of youth development and argues that it is critical to have a thorough grasp of it. The following section has described its relationship to human capital development. As crucial as describing stress theories is making connections between stress notions and childhood, adolescent development, and educational stressors. Further Academic life, stress, and wellness are linked to achieving a consensus and understanding to build their connection. Future directions that may be learned to develop mindful methods for various situations are explained as the chapter proceeds to its end.

Purpose of the Study

According to the development of a transactional stress model, coping strategies are essential in delaying a stress reaction. Specifically, academic stress and the possible relevance of psychological well-being as an individual determinant of coping methods in the academic context are under investigation. The study has several specific objectives, including identifying students based on their level of psychological well-being during academic life and identifying its precautions in real life. Human capital development aspects must be kept in mind during academic life. Well-being educational strategies and how to equip with self-care are combined as objectives of this chapter.

Justification of the Study

Manifestations and the idea of well-being are complicated and widely used in health and personal development. It is important to remember that one's well-being is dependent on both the individual and the environment and that the environment might be essential during childhood and youth. It is widely acknowledged that the settings of family, school, and peers are vital for successful growth. It is also undoubtedly critical that human capital development occurs in a conducive setting. Knowledge about self-care education is critical. Research should shed light on how self-care mastery can be gained or provided.

Significance of the Study

Stress is the element that can harm human life and Individuals. It has been considered a critical source of psychopathology, dysfunction, and failure in both academic and real-world research when it comes to psychology. Adolescence has not exempt from this but is more vulnerable due to several critical and underdeveloped aspects of the human body and mind. It could injure psychological well-being, but its repercussions are far more devastating from individual to social, psychological, and economic factors. This chapter covers unique aspects of academic life stress that may permanently lead to natural life stress in individual life.

Research Questions

Applying how to manage stress has varying implications on academic, personal, and professional success, psychological well-being, and quality of life. This study postulates how academic stress, life stress, and human development differed in self-care perspectives. Student learning, adjustments, and personal mastery may be hindered if they do not employ various self-care methods. There are several ways in which adolescent development may be improved against change and stress subjects. It includes affirmations that reflect their innate needs or cultural shifts that they should be ready to embrace. Dietary mindfulness and learning commitments from the source of stress in their lives are included as matters of awareness youth should be prepared to know from the self-point of view.

LITERATURE REVIEW

1. Human Capital and Youth Development

Human capital development has piqued the curiosity of academics for decades. Understanding how human capital development occurs is frequently linked to educational and value-added abilities in persons with potential benefits for them and society. When Schultz (1961) said that human capital is one of the most critical parts of today's economy, it was because of the development of classical economics in 1776. The scientific theory of human capital was established in the concept of human capital (Fitzsimons, 1999). It marked the first time that notion had been formalized as a theoretical framework. Human capital was recognized as one of the essential components for national economic success in the modern economy (Schultz, 1971). Several academics have attempted to explain how human capital can contribute to sociopolitical progress and freedom in a variety of circumstances since its establishment and expansion (Becker, 1993; Coleman, 1988; de Oliveira et al., 2000; Klepinger et al., 1999; Neuman, 1986; Temple, 1999; Woodhall, 1987). Many governments and organizations have sought innovative and inventive strategies to preserve a competitive advantage due to recent concerns such as globalization, a knowledge-based economy, and technological advancement. The competitive advantage is often achieved by having a flexible, knowledgeable, skilled workforce and a pleasant work attitude. As a result, a company's success is dependent on employees with greater individual skill levels. Therefore, individuals are highly valued assets that may be recognized within human capital, becoming increasingly significant. Suppose the young people of today are the future. In that case, their human capital is worth a lot if they are talented and quick people who care about their own and other people's well-being. Alternatively, if they are fragile, they will burden the nation due to their mental incapacity.

As youths graduate, many hope to find a successful profession; they are the world's future. Three out of four people feel they would get the job they desire, and four out of five want to work in a high-skilled field. Because employment is not solely based on a person's education or degree, young people are dissatisfied with their jobs, with only one in every five working in a high-skilled area. The issue of young people's skills and employability has piqued UNICEF's interest. Educators are examining critical components of the school-to-work transition to understand the issue better. They include it in UNICEF initiatives, including educating youth about employment and facilitating their entry into productive job opportunities. The aspect is related to gaining personal mastery, being socially informed, and having well-being; research is essential. Several programs, such as the Global Transferable Skills Framework and Generation Unlimited, are in the works. What is the definition of a child's well-being? The historical conceptions of well-being in children are two issues that must be addressed to understand better what defines well-being in educational environments. It is necessary to investigate the effects of educator and leadership well-being on educational results. They established a community-wide strategy to ensure everyone's health and well-being, Analyzing the positive influence of a well-being approach on educational training to improve them. It is vital to understand children's lives before and after entering and graduating from high school and college.

At this moment, both youth development and human capital development are taking place simultaneously. Stress is the origin of all problems. It is vital to understand what is creating the stress in the first place if one wants to avoid harmful behavior (Abbas, Ekowati, et al., 2021a). The literature suggests an increasing demand for positive effective leadership management of well-being (Abbas, Saud, Ekowati, Usman, et al., 2021; Abbas, Saud, et al., 2020). In addition, iterative research reveals that environmental, biological, social, and psychological elements have a role in forming social fabric and diversity management (Abbas, Ekowati, et al., 2021b; Abbas, Saud, Ekowati, & Suhariadi, 2021). Between these two lines, the social fabric of the mind is vital (cf. Chance, 2015). Knowing their minds and bodies will allow youths to be more conscious of their problems and barriers to well-being. A human capital development perspective should consider youth development, stress causes, theories to explain them, and other developments. This is one approach to understanding how to master youngsters during their growth from a self-care and well-being standpoint in order for them to become productive individuals and future generations.

2. Youth, Development

A combination of biological and psychological changes or development is known as youth development. Youth development is aided by activities and experiences that develop social, ethical, emotional, physical, and cognitive skills. It helps youth prepare for the trials of puberty and adulthood while also allowing them to reach their best potential. Furlong (2013) noted that youth is a formative experience that can influence an individual's level of dependency, manifesting itself in various ways depending on one's cultural background. Cultural standards or traditions influence an individual's personal experience. At the same time, the level of dependency a youth has on their family affects how they still rely on them emotionally and financially. Others define youth as the period of one's life in adolescence or early adulthood. It is frequently referred to as the period between childhood and adulthood (maturity). It is also defined as "the appearance, freshness, strength, enthusiasm, so on that is distinctive of a young person." In addition, it does not describe youth as a stage that can be associated with specific age ranges. Nor does it define youth as a stage that can be tied to specific behaviors, such as holding part-time jobs or having sexual encounters (Cohen, 1997; Volberg et al., 2011; White & Wyn, 2004; Woodman, 2003)—beginning with the recognition that the social conditions that shape the human experience of growing age. Transition and development are terms used to describe the stages of youth based on social and psychosocial assumptions in many instances. The concepts of transition and development are strongly associated with one another. Both presume a linear movement from one recognized status to another. For both, youth is just a stage of life that is still growing and developing. Youth development can be taken into the following two accounts:

a. Developmental approaches significantly impact young people because they help construct a universal, normative set of behaviors and attitudes that correspond to their effective integration into adult society.
b. Transitioning to adulthood is determined by social and psychosocial processes, which can be put "at risk" by adverse social conditions. People who know what they are doing can also change social and psychological conditions. They can try to get the process back on track to follow predetermined, "normal" rules in the case of deprivation.

To conceptualize the issues that influence youth development, one must first recognize that the experiences of age are influenced by social and psychological conditions, such as the function of the state, among other factors, and that youth and the state help shape these meanings. All these characterizations are predicated on the assumptions that (a) there is a normative transitional process from which young people experience, (b) youth is a linear process or position on a life course, and (c) culture, economy, and social psychology or politics are the essence to the development process, respectively. Most literature about youth development is based on implicit references to popular conceptions of generations. The generations have come to be seen as the implicit norm. It has become customary to compare the changes of this generation (from school to employment, leaving home, and creating nuclear families) to the transitions of previous generations. This timeline questions young people's life patterns and choices throughout history by challenging accepted preconceptions about what ought to be. According to the United Nations, youth are defined as those between 15 and 24. All United Nations statistics are based on this age range, with education cited as a basis for these numbers. United Nations also acknowledges that this varies without regard to other age categories indicated by member nations, such as those between 18 and 30. Young adults aged 13 to 19 can be distinguished within the United Nations system, an essential distinction between 20 and 29. While seeking to enforce some uniformity on statistical procedures, the UN is well aware of the inconsistencies between approaches within its standards. The 15–24 definition, i.e., measure adopted in 1981, defines children under 14, under 18, i.e., defined in the 1979 Convention on the Child's Rights.

High schoolers develop at a wide range of rates, just as they do in middle and high school. However, the 1979 Convention on the Child's Rights defines children as those (Furlong, 2013). This age range belongs to adolescents who are primarily in high school or pre-university stage education, and the development of children takes off throughout their high school years. Youth develops into high school students who begin to appear more mature while also developing the ability to think about plans. During this stage of development, the difference in growth between boys and girls is pronounced.

Furthermore, there is a significant variance in physical milestones between different children. Boys are reaching the age when they develop rapidly, while girls are only beginning to slow their growth. Many females are likely to have reached their full height by the time they graduate from high school, if not earlier. On the other hand, boys are frequently still growing and acquiring muscle power. During these development years, students are required to combat several physical forefronts. Many high school students experience 1) Possess a voracious appetite, 2) a Need to get more sleep, and one may be drowsy in class, and 3) thrill, e.g., learning to drive, they have visual-spatial coordination to gauge distance and speed accurately and respond swiftly, while they have increased social needs as well.

From this perspective, adolescents' experiences turn into the need and chances to demonstrate responsibility, earn independence to meet social needs, and obtain real-life experience. Depending on the situation, the adolescent may get some work experience that immediately applies to their future profession or adds to their experience. Real-life or working experience evident advantage is earned money. However, much of that money is discretionary spending rather than savings (Bachman & Schulenberg, 1993). Combating several fronts, this is the mid-to-late-adolescent years, where independent thinking begins. Adolescents are not preparing for more than just their own lives; they begin to consider how the rest of the world functions. That transformation is a long-term process. It does not occur in a single sitting. Teens are likely to do the following during their high school years: they demonstrate a growing ability to think, make intelligent judgments, and independently distinguish between reality and fiction. Readings and real-life experiences expand their thinking to include more abstract concepts, such as comparing what could be. In this development, they may consider and devise strategies for dealing with hypothetical circumstances that may arise by themselves. They also begin to develop their own goals for the future and consider other people's opinions while making their decisions. They have started aiming for the life where they could be reached in recent years (Costa, 2001). At this very point, students' well-being and self-care emerge with utmost importance due to increasing complexity and emerging stress due to the following reasons.

a. Youth must understand the ramifications of choices, not only today but also in the future. They may face difficulties choosing what is right and what Is wrong for them related to the future. i.e., related to their academic disciplines, career, personal aims, friends, and society. Suppose they are uninformed of the psychological and physiological changes that occur as people age. In that case, they may face complications or paradoxes in their decisions, which will cause stress.
b. They also develop a strong sense of right and wrong and shape their judgments based on their experience and moral principles. Prioritizing moral principles, i.e., what a moral should be and what they experience in real-life happenings, push harder to occupy one stance.
c. They must choose, express, or write about a wide range of topics with a high level of sophistication in science, social studies, literature, and learning about the history of the world.

d. They learn to find, use, and compare information from various sources.
e. They are experiencing emotional and psychological meanings related to themselves and their surroundings. Thus, they are more vulnerable to stress at this age.

This view aligns with Piaget's stage theory that illustrates how children's cognitive abilities grow throughout time. Cognitive development entails changes in the way the brain works and its abilities. Psychologist Piaget believes that early cognitive growth consists of processes based on actions, which later change mental operations. According to Jean Piaget's theory of cognitive development, children progress through four distinct phases of mental development. While his theory is concerned with understanding how children acquire knowledge, it is equally concerned with understanding the nature of intelligence (Badakar et al., 2017). As a result, Piaget argued that children have an active role in the learning process, behaving much like tiny scientists conducting experiments, recording observations, and learning about the environment. A child's ongoing interaction with the world adds new knowledge, builds on existing knowledge, and alters long-held views to suit newly learned information. Therefore, researchers consistently investigate the links between health-promoting self-care practices, self-care self-efficacy, and self-care agency. A study aimed to determine the links between these concepts and the specific influence of spiritual growth, a component of health-promoting self-care practices (Callaghan, 2005). He noted that school nurses are especially concerned about the impact of gender and religion on adolescents' health and ability to care for themselves. Adolescents need to know about and access community social support networks, such as faith-based groups, to identify and meet gender-specific health and self-care needs, especially spiritual health needs. Their medical problems or disabilities may influence adolescents' health and self-care. Because of this, this demographic has more significant levels of self-care self-efficacy due to social support from family, school nurses, and other health professionals (Callaghan, 2006). Helliwell and Putnam (2004) explained the context of social well-being and said. Education continues to be what might be referred to as an instrumental variable, with higher levels of subjective well-being being associated with higher levels of education by simple correlations. However, the effects of higher levels of education tend to disappear. Early education is part of social development. The literature demonstrates that ability to talk about, argue, and think critically to solve significant problems of a young child is high when interacting with others to achieve common goals (Ardalan, 2017; Haywoode, 2018).

This section's critical thinking review reminds us that enormous variables have a role in youth development in the early stages of adolescence. Making new acquaintances and learning how to connect with others in these situations also educates children about their responsibilities as citizens in a democratic society. Educating youngsters about their obligations as citizens in a democratic society is vital for their development. In order to help children become responsible people who can express themselves, identify and solve problems, negotiate roles and comprehend the influence of their actions on others. However, the literature does not emphasize teaching young people about natural health and kinesthetic awareness. For this reason, social studies is an integral part of the early childhood curriculum (Krechevsky et al., 2016; Krechevsky et al., 2014; Mardell & Carpenter, 2012). However, there is a minor focus in the literature on teaching young people about natural health and education that inculcates them an understanding of their bodies.

3. Stress and its Theories

Theories that are concerned with the specific relationship between external demands (stressors) and bodily processes (stress) can be divided into two categories: approaches to 'systemic stress' that are based on physiology and psychobiology (Selye, 1976b; Viner, 1999) and approaches to 'psychological stress' that are developed within the field of cognitive psychology (Folkman & Lazarus, 1988; Lazarus, 2006; Lazarus & Folkman, 1984).

Several scientists and journalists attribute endocrinologist Hans Selye's work to popularizing the stress theory. After a series of animal studies, he showed that a wide range of stimuli (such as heat, cold, and hazardous substances) might elicit expected consequences when forced and prolonged. Based on the work of Selye, these nonspecifically induced alterations are what comprise the stereotyped (i.e., particular) response pattern associated with systemic stress. On page 64 of his book, Selye describes stress as a state manifested by a syndrome that consists of all the alterations in a biological system caused by nonspecific stimuli (Selye, 1976a). The General Adaptation Syndrome (GAS) is a stereotyped reaction pattern that progresses through the following stages.

- An initial shock phase and a subsequent countershock phase are both parts of the alarm reaction. During the shock phase, autonomic excitability increased adrenaline output, and gastro-intestinal ulceration was observed. During the countershock phase, defense processes begin to operate for the first time and are characterized by increased activity. This stage has characterized the disappearance of alarm reaction symptoms, which implies the organism has adapted to the stressor.
- On the other hand, resistance to noxious stimulation increases while resistance to other stressors decreases simultaneously. If the adverse stimulation continues, resistance eventually gives way to the state of fatigue in the organism. Because of the exhaustion of the organism's ability to adapt to the stressor, stage symptoms resurface, but resistance is no longer viable. If the stimulation continues, irreversible tissue damage occurs, and the organism eventually succumbs.

Both subjects are fundamental to psychological stress theories, such as those developed by the Lazarus group, which is one example (cf. Arnold, 1960; Janis, 1989; Lazarus, 1966). On the other hand, Selye does not detail the mechanisms involved in the cognitive transformation of noxious events into the subjective experience of being upset. Furthermore, Selye does not consider coping mechanisms as critical mediators of the stress–outcome relationship, which is a flaw in his thinking.

According to the transactional model of stress and coping developed by Folkman et al. (1987). Individuals employ adaptation to manage internal and external pressures that exceed their resource capability. According to the transactional model of stress, coping strategies are essential in delaying the onset of a stress reaction. Specifically, the possible relevance of psychological well-being as an individual determinant of coping methods in the academic context was investigated in this research. The study has two specific objectives: (a) to identify distinct profiles of students based on their level of psychological well-being; and (b) to investigate the differences between these profiles in terms of the application of three coping methods (positive reappraisal, support-seeking, and planning). Several later models, most notably the transactional model (Sameroff & Fiese, 2000), place a far greater focus on contextual influences in developing a child's physical and mental health. The transactional model views neurological, psychological, and social development as dynamic processes resulting from intricate interactions between the child and the caring environment rather than static processes. The ability of child and parent needs to be adjusted according to developmental change proceeds which are critical to developmental health. The quality of the caregiver-child relationship is regarded as critical to the child's well-being. Hence, assistance for parents responsible for the care of their children is essential for the child's growth in health. Despite being widely acknowledged in child development, the transactional model has not yet been thoroughly combined with the fundamental principles of the medical model to generate an integrated model that would govern the administration of child healthcare services in the United States. The transactional model has not yet been thoroughly combined with the fundamental principles of the medical model. It meant to generate an integrated model that would govern the administration of child healthcare services in the U.S. Instead of focusing entirely on the kid in isolation. The current pediatric healthcare delivery system is built on an antiquated logic model that emphasizes the child's interaction with the environment rather than the child in isolation. The result is that while parenting guidance and support are gradually being incorporated into child health monitoring guidelines, these activities continue to be under-or unreimbursed to a significant extent. With an emphasis on stress theories, biological and psychological components are explained and investigated. However, it is essential to realize that biological elements induce psychological issues and adversity. As a result, psychological variables have received more attention in the research. Conversely, the argument to support the idea of including biological changes that may lead to psychological peculiarities in youth development studies is valid from an educational point of view. Individuals who are persuaded to understand the causes of stress buildup will be more equipped to articulate it to someone.

4. Childhood, Youth Development, and Academic Stress

While prior research has had a significant role in understanding maturity, called youth or emerging adulthood, its paradigm conceptualizes developments among adults 18 to 25 (Arnett, 2000). Children who have earlier age than eighteen years are often considered a child. Depending on the perspective, childhood is widely regarded as either a normal biological stage of development or a contemporary concept or fabrication. Aspects of childhood theories include how the concept of the child or childhood is employed in society. They include questions such as what a child's nature is, what childhood's purpose or function is, and how the concept of the child is employed in society. A strong interaction between ideas and technology, like with any invention, was developed inside a framework of social, political, and economic necessities to create the concept of childhood in the first place. Child development theorists deal with solid contrasts exposing the development through time of a child's psychological or emotional significance as viewed from maturity. Several theorists posit that child development concept are frequently highly colored or emotive. It has prompted some scholars to investigate the possibility of allowing children themselves to reflect on their own childhood experiences (Birren & Cunningham, 1985; Cunningham, 1998; DeMause, 1995; Elder, 1998; Freud, 1953; Panter-Brick & Smith, 2000). Children or young people frequently choose to continue their college or college-level education. Developmental psychologists are now looking at young adults' developmental and educational transitions as a well-defined, separate stage. Emerging adults had previously been seen as covering other phases of development. Students' stress is regarded as a process of a transaction between the new and challenging environment they experience and their personal and societal resources. Students' stress students are regarded as the last transition period before adulthood (Towbes & Cohen, 1996).

Psychological and physical distress could express itself differently, including mood, sleep, and food disorders. Although the little study has shown that there is pathology, numerous students have separate sub-symptomatic discomforts, which are rarely discussed. 15% of students had suicidal thoughts, the second largest cause of death (after traffic accidents) among persons between 18 and 24 (Boujut et al., 2012). Despite the various reports, including sonority, exhaustion, headaches, and backaches among students of the first year, psychological illnesses, such as depression and suicide, and behavioral abnormalities (e.g., eating habits, addictive behavior). It also includes various other risk factors, including psychoactive intake, which tends to grow over time; students might plan to avoid stress through several coping mechanisms (Deb et al., 2015; Huan et al., 2008; Yan et al., 2018).

Students under 18 are under significant stress and frequently suffer development challenges, which is entirely reasonable. Given that this growth occurs in two stages, first physical development and then intellectual development, knowledge should be available to identify stress areas.

5. Academic Life, Stress, and Well-Being

Several opportunities and obstacles are presented by years in which pupils learn in schools, schools, and universities. According to the Institute of Public Policy Research analysis, almost five times as many students told their colleagues of a mental health condition ten years ago. As a result, the demand for counseling services in the past five years has risen; 94 percent of UK higher education providers questioned by IPPR, e.g., Institute of Public Policy Research. According to the Higher Education Statistics Agency statistics, the number of students who have dropped out of university due to mental health issues has quadrupled, which is worse. It is a mental and psychological health issue for pupils.

Also, students need to learn how to live their lives. It includes settling in a new place, making new friends and relationships, and managing new financial and budgetary tasks. In addition to academic success, social media were also highlighted as a potential source of stress and worry. Another research indicated that popular social media like Instagram and Facebook could boost feelings of insufficiency among 14-24-year-olds. It is also recognized as a worry within universities. Many students indicate that their sensation of popular and social success is under strain. Such peer pressure could have deadly repercussions if it has been set free. Peer pressure occasionally can lead to hazardous drug-related activity, and a growing percentage of students seek suicide support or self-harm. Fortunately, mental health and well-being have been understood and approached changes as much as today's children's difficulties. Well-being and mental health are more recognized as problems that touch all of us and exist at a level of seriousness and complexity than problems that could harm a few individuals. The readiness of well-known people to communicate openly about their well-being and mental health difficulties helps stigmatize and open things up. Promoting students' well-being helps produce a better overall experience that benefits all.

A state of emotional exhaustion, a tendency toward depersonalization, and a sense of low personal accomplishment typically occur among people in the helping professions is referred to as burnout. In short, it is a syndrome characterized by emotional exhaustion and a sense of diminished personal accomplishment. Burnout can be defined as follows: (Maslach, 1982; Maslach & Jackson, 1981). However, this paradigm has been broadened to include occupations less focused on people, such as accounting and finance, in recent years. It has also been found that burnout symptoms can manifest themselves in situations other than education or work, such as in sports or relationships (Bakker et al., 2008; Demerouti et al., 2001; Maslach et al., 2001). Students have been demonstrated to suffer from academic stress, according to various researches (Abbas, Ekowati, et al., 2020; Abbas, Eliyana, et al., 2020; Dada et al., 2019; Qi, 2019; Tagurum et al., 2017; Yan et al., 2018). When it came to academic burnout and life challenges, the first of the questions posed about the present situation among students was about how many students were experiencing these issues. Second, it was asked whether disparities in academic burnout and life pressures among different genders and different years of education. There were some disparities in stress levels between males and females and between years. Overall, students stated that the stress associated with future growth was the most distressing concern (Lin & Huang, 2014).

We can state categorically that juvenile stress development is entwined with socioeconomic inequalities, notwithstanding academic stress. It is realistic to establish appropriate activities by which children may confront these challenges. However, for young people to coordinate and react to changes, they must first be aware of what is happening around them.

CONCLUSION

Lerner and Overton (2010) noted that the theory of mind is an innate potential talent in humans that requires years of social and other experience to develop fully. Individuals may build successful theories of mind. According to Neo-Piagetian theories of cognitive development, the theory of mind results from the human mind's more extraordinary hypercognitive ability to register, monitor, and depict its functioning. Empathy is a related notion that refers to the recognition and comprehension of the mental states of others, including their beliefs, desires, and, most importantly, emotions. This is frequently referred to as the ability to "place oneself in the shoes." Recent neuro-ethological animal behavior research implies that even rodents may have ethical or sympathetic capacities. While empathy is characterized as adopting an emotional perspective, the theory of mind is defined as a cognitive perspective (Hynes et al., 2006). According to recent developmental psychology studies, the infant's ability to imitate others is at the root of both theory of mind and other social-cognitive abilities such as perspective-taking and empathy. According to Meltzoff (2011), the infant's natural sense that others are "like me" enables it to perceive the equivalence between physical and mental experiences visible in others and those felt by the self. In imitation, the child uses his experiences to comprehend the motions of others who turn toward an object of interest. Others have questioned the role of imitation in advanced human social-cognitive skills like cognition and sympathizing. Horowitz (2010) discovered that adult respondents copied an experimenter demonstrating a novel task less closely than children. According to Horowitz, the actual psychological state behind imitation is unknown and cannot infer generalizations about human mental processes. While most studies have been done on infants, the theory of mind constantly develops throughout childhood and into late adolescence as the prefrontal cortex synapses (neuronal connections) develop. The prefrontal cortex is assumed to be involved in decision-making and planning (Laghi et al., 2016).

Children sequentially develop a theory of mind skills. The ability to realize that others have different desires is the first skill to learn. Soon after, children can recognize that others hold different opinions. Recognizing that others have access to various knowledge bases is the next skill to learn. This sequence depicts the general trend in skill acquisition. More attention is placed on specific skills in some cultures, causing more valued skills to grow before others deemed less significant. In this sequence, children learn that people may hold incorrect beliefs and that others can conceal their emotions. Individualistic societies, such as the United States, emphasize realizing that others have different perspectives and values. This talent may not be as crucial in a collectivistic culture such as China. Unless a greater understanding of global challenges, cultural transitions, and current influences is fostered, no culture can advance. (Etel

& Yagmurlu, 2015). From birth, properly developing newborns exhibit social communication through their efforts to interact with others and compel others to interact with them.

Behaviors such as cooperative visual attention, social referencing, and pretend play constitute developmental stages in the Theory of Mind development. Mindreading research is an essential resource for describing the cognitive mechanisms that develop the human capacity for self-awareness. However, some argue that contrary to Theory Theorists' claims, evidence suggests that the potential for self-awareness is not dependent on the Theory of Mind. We can argue that it is much more plausible to believe that self-awareness can be derived from a Monitoring Mechanism dependent on the Theory of Mind. Thus, it should be included in the pedagogy of self-care behavior for understanding the self in a better way. Consolidating relevant social skills is an essential aspect of typical development. It allows people to form and sustain cordial social relationships and supports community adaptability throughout their lives.

The formation of social skills is a complex developmental process that involves the maturity of a wide range of underlying cognitive abilities known as social cognition (Abbas et al., 2022). Term TOM (theory of mind) refers to the ability to impute mental states to self and others, including desires, knowledge, beliefs, and intentions, to predict behavior. This concept was induced in academic debate in 1970; since then, the theory of mind has remained a central focus of developmental and social psychology and speech therapy (Premack & Woodruff, 1978). It was recognized to demonstrate flexible and explicit TOM. Infants must construct distinct abstract representations of reality and traverse between them to identify their states from those of others using various clues, thereby behaving as theorists. Since then, this subject has become one of the most researched developmental cognitive sciences. TOM and other social cognitive conceptions have recently garnered attention in social neuroscience, resulting in a considerable body of consensus literature regarding the brain networks supporting TOM. It could be utilized in an academic setting to develop a self-care behavior to cope with stress. The act of anticipating the behavior of others or oneself by assuming what others want, think, or believe. These inferences, which amount to a theory of mind, are universal in human adults to the best of our understanding. Although it is plausible to presume that some experience influences their existence, the nature of that experience is not immediately apparent. It is not the result of formal education. Inferences about another person are not taught in the same way that reading or arithmetic is their acquisition is more akin to walking or speaking. Indeed, the sole direct effect of education on these inferences appears to be suppressive. Only a properly trained adult can provide an account of human behavior that does not impute states of mind to the participants. All of this is to argue that this type of theory construction is natural in humans.

Self-Care and Life Stress: A Well-Being Lesson to be Absorbed

Self-care is how we look after our mental, emotional, and physical well-being. It is the things that engage and allows us to remain our best selves as an individual. It is known as positive psychology towards self-attaining the best in life and health. Self-care is an action-oriented approach to showing love, and it can be beneficial. Being self-care is what it sounds like: being in love with oneself. It is a positive and progressive approach to combat life challenges. It entails accepting and loving oneself, including flaws, shortcomings, and the qualities of self that they do not always enjoy. In this way, it is like reconciling oneself positively to correct mistakes. It is also about having high expectations for well-being and happiness for self and others. Many people can be unfamiliar with the notions of self-care and self-love. It has been frequently taught that prioritizing oneself improves performance, particularly in academic life.

On the other hand, a self-centered person has a negative side and devotes time and energy to personal gains without thinking about others. However, practicing self-love does not imply that one is purely selfish or narcissistic. It is just indicated that one is not settling for anything less than themself deserves. Someone's psychological inculcation can understand the difference between narcissism and self-care for well-being. The positive form of self-care and self-love is frequently as simple as providing the same respect and consideration one seek from others as one wants for themself. It is socially known to treat others the way one would like to be treated. However, when contemplating self-love and self-care, it is frequently necessary to examine the opposite. Remember to be friendly and gracious to themselves in the same way they treat their friends, family, and other loved ones. We are far kinder to our family and friends than we are to ourselves most of the time.

Positive or negative self-care is not possible overnight. It is a process that is continual. Positive self-care is a moral practice that can lead to more self-accommodation and love. It gradually enhances independence and welfare. On the other hand, with time and continuous provocative behaviors, self-hatred, severe criticism, perfectionism is miserably the negative form of auto-love. Hence, we can say that it may be gradually induced into ones' life via regular acts.

Self-care can be incorporated into daily routine in tiny, manageable stages to strengthen self-kindness, self-love, and a sense of shared humanity. Mainly when a child is in its developing stage.

Here are five suggestions to keep in mind to embark on a journey to self-care and well-being in youth.

1. Self-Acceptance and Recognition

Self-recognition is essential for students because humans are prone to change. No one can be content all the time. However, it is possible to be optimistic or strive to be the best version of themselves every day. One of the most crucial aspects of self-love is holding youth to a decent standard of behavior. One must accept and remind himself to realize that learning with time may bring a better version of himself than others. It is perfectly acceptable to have a bad day, week, or even a bad semester. It is critical to recognize the emotional state of youth regularly. They need to become familiar with their moods and learn to accept them, which could be the first step to self-recognition in stress. It could help them express themselves so others know what is not going well. Because when someone claims, "I am OK" or "It is nothing," when they are not, and when it is evident that something is wrong, stress aggravates.

Moreover, it is more difficult to understand and stabilize to engage oneself in this situation. Therefore, the first is to recognize that one should accept a lousy patch if the situation is terrible.

- A self-care behavior should come from self-recognition this way.
- It would help to combat not developing self-into-games in a time of stress.
- It would help in recognizing the emotional condition and personal vulnerabilities gradually.
- It would help to plan and follow their emotional needs.
- Self-recognition would also bring awareness to the emotional condition of youth. Emotions are the most critical aspect of youth development; emotional awareness could help avoid false following towards tempting behavior.

Students only need to be aware of their emotional conditions to accept the situation. One of the most critical aspects of an emotional state is to modify their plans according to the situation. The ability to recognize and respond to the current emotional state needs the foundation of any practical self-care mind.

It is also learning and determining that a slump period would last excessively if no remedy has been prepared. Suppose the aim is to make them aware of the crucial ability to think critically and take the right measure or proper time. In that case, it is good to give them some hope that their positive action would help them overcome the situation quickly. It is crucial to recognize that their planned actions, habits, and routines can significantly impact their mood. If experiencing a big slump, like situations beyond human control, they could think about making positive changes in their daily routine with the swing of things. Most of the time, self-care is a delicate balance between offering oneself kindness and forgiving while also keeping healthy practices that actively boost mood.

2. Dietary Consciousness

It is essential to know that not feeling exceptionally good; would never help present the best version in front of others. Stress often affects dietary habits. Self-care and well-being must be educated in young minds about the importance of the dietary concept and health, and food balance could positively help. Mental and physical awareness comes together as far as dietary consciousness plans are concerned. Children are often attracted to junk food and other consumer products that could quickly affect their minds and body at a young age. It can only be tackled through meaningful education and proper awareness. A conscious dietary mind would feel good about their physical and mental health in early life.

Additionally, eating well can make it easy to understand and absorb the reality of health and food balance. It is a self-introspection process that a child could learn at an early age, and thus it should be cared for. There is no need to engage an expert; however, a continuous consciousness development about dietary care balance at an early age can be effective and thus employed. Making dietary plans could be a crucial element of self-care since its practice may impact how one feels and how much energy one have. There are few real-life examples in old age family members; neighbors could be exemplified to learn a lesson. Often a child is inclined to rapid growth; hence this could serve as natural motivation for their dietary consciousness plan.

3. Self-Reconciliation

Developing the ability to engage in positive self-talk is an essential component of the self-care journey of youth. Self-talk is the internal monologue that one always has to go on in thoughts during the day. Talking to oneself often remains unnoticed or an unconscious act. Self-doubt is the feeling of self-doubts, self-judgment, and even self-loathing. It is frequently symptomatic of subconscious thoughts and sentiments that are an occasional internal monologue. Particularly at a young age, where conscious development is in progress, negative self-reconciliation could be dangerous and impactful. One should be alarmed by discovering inner dialogue if it is overwhelmingly negative. It could be encountered by mindfulness practices employed to transform inner dialogue into a more positive tone. However, how to build a reconciliation habit and to use positive psychology could be challenging for children and hence should be inculcated through hypothetical training first. Giving oneself positive affirmations is an actionable and straightforward method of accomplishing this. For example, often, a child uses heroic characteristics abstract to apply on self to imagine and admires themself is repeatedly imagined for gaining inner power. A deliberate act or habit of this crucial aspect of using self-talk advantages could be recognized to engage and combat negative self-talk. It could consider whether this is developing a self-care pattern or inviting blind following aimlessly. This could be taken care of by developing new challenges and games to be observed by a caretaker (parents or teachers) - whether the caretakers are parents or teachers.

4. Challenging Negatives and Forgiving Self-Mistakes and Aim Not to Repeat Them

When negative self-talk is allowed to continue for an extended period, it can lead to negative narratives highly detrimental to self-esteem. It internalizes negative narratives before knowing them; these stories affect attitudes and actions. The first step in identifying and addressing the source of the problem is discovering the negative stories one knows about self. Primarily, one should determine the source of these stories and the outcome of a single occurrence. Afterward, it would be possible to determine why they continue to trust these false stories. Finding out why one is telling themselves these stories would help break the negative thought cycle, creating negative self-talk. Contradicting the negative storytelling, one can employ the same positive self-talk strategies as discussed previously. This process involves learning to be kind to oneself as well as others. Humans make mistakes – both big and small – and while they may appear to have life-altering consequences at the time, they are nothing more than those mistakes. Life goes on, and one and it should continue to do so. It is only through being kind, empathizing with others, and supporting others to look back on self-action with kindness, empathy, and support. Thus, therefore, self-forgive occurs. A grudge against oneself may have results that can be detrimental to one's well-being and someone else's in some cases. It is necessary to hold grudges to sustain a significant amount of negative energy, which can be challenging over time. It is possible to get more energy and emotional capacity by forgiving themselves and others for their negative feelings about self-acts to participate in more loving behavior.

5. Commitment to Learning Through Self-Love

Achieving self-acceptance can be a long and arduous process; it is not something that happens quickly. The terms "self-care" and "mindfulness" are everywhere these days, which is excellent as we all learn to be more introspective and accepting of who we are. This agreement is a new trend that suggests that new studies and methodologies are developed regularly. We are committing to trying new avenues of self-care, and continuing to learn as these ideas progress should be an essential part of students' self-care journey. A continued engagement with new resources may provide ever-increasing knowledge about maintaining youth's mental, physical, and emotional well-being. This knowledge can help improve our compassion and love towards ourselves.

ACKNOWLEDGMENT

There is no funding obtained for this study. This study does not report any conflict, financial or commercial interest. All authors contributed positively to preparing this Book Chapter.

This research is an outcome of the coordination of the laboratory at the Doctoral Program in Human Resource Development, Post Graduate School Universitas Airlangga, Surabaya, Indonesia. This lab is currently undergoing the registration procedure. It is slated to start working officially under Prof. Dr. Fendy Suhariadi, the Head of the Doctoral Program in Human Resource Development, Post Graduate School Universitas Airlangga.

Address: Post graduate School, Airlangga, street 4-6, Campus B, Universitas Airlangga, Gubeng, Surabaya, 60286

REFERENCES

Abbas, A., Dian, E., & Suhariadi, F. (2022). Social Perspective: Leadership in Changing Society. In M. I. Hassan, S. S. Roy, U. Chatterjee, S. Chakraborty, & U. Singh (Eds.), *Social Morphology, Human Welfare and Sustainability*. Springer.

Abbas, A., Ekowati, D., & Suhariadi, F. (2021a). Individual psychological distance: A leadership task to assess and cope with invisible change. *Journal of Management Development*, *40*(3), 168–189. doi:10.1108/JMD-09-2020-0304

Abbas, A., Ekowati, D., & Suhariadi, F. (2021b). Managing Individuals, Organizations Through Leadership: Diversity Consciousness Roadmap. In B. Christiansen & H. Chandan (Eds.), *Handbook of Research on Applied Social Psychology in Multiculturalism* (Vol. 1, pp. 47–71). IGI Global. doi:10.4018/978-1-7998-6960-3.ch003

Abbas, A., Ekowati, D., Usman, I., Saud, M., & Setia, S. (2020). Technology and stress: A proposed framework for coping stress in Indonesia higher education: Technology in Education. *International Journal of Innovation. Creativity and Change*, *13*(4), 373–390.

Abbas, A., Eliyana, A., Ekowati, D., Saud, M., Raza, A., & Wardani, R. (2020). Data set on coping strategies in the digital age: The role of psychological well-being and social capital among university students in Java Timor, Surabaya, Indonesia. *Data in Brief*, *30*, 10558. doi:10.1016/j.dib.2020.105583 PMID:32368599

Abbas, A., Saud, M., Ekowati, D., & Suhariadi, F. (2021). Social Psychology and Fabrication: A Synthesis of Individuals, Society, and Organization. In B. Christiansen & H. Chandan (Eds.), *Handbook of Research on Applied Social Psychology in Multiculturalism* (Vol. 1, pp. 89–109). IGI Global. doi:10.4018/978-1-7998-6960-3.ch005

Abbas, A., Saud, M., Ekowati, D., Usman, I., & Suhariadi, F. (2021). Servant leadership: A strategic choice for organisational performance. An empirical discussion from Pakistan. *International Journal of Productivity and Quality Management*, *34*(4), 468–485. doi:10.1504/IJPQM.2021.120599

Abbas, A., Saud, M., Suhariadi, F., Usman, I., & Ekowati, D. (2020). Positive leadership psychology: Authentic and servant leadership in higher education in Pakistan. *Current Psychology (New Brunswick, N.J.)*, •••, 1–11. doi:10.100712144-020-01051-1

Ardalan, G. (2017). Spreading happiness: A preschool classroom in Washington, DC, investigates citizenship and makes a statement—"Be Happy! *YC Young Children*, *72*(2), 64–71.

Arnett, J. J. (2000). Emerging adulthood: A theory of development from the late teens through the twenties. *The American Psychologist*, *55*(5), 469–480. doi:10.1037/0003-066X.55.5.469 PMID:10842426

Arnold, M. B. (1960). *Emotion and personality*. Columbia University Press.

Bachman, J. G., & Schulenberg, J. (1993). How part-time work intensity relates to drug use, problem behavior, time use, and satisfaction among high school seniors: Are these consequences or merely correlates? *Developmental Psychology*, *29*(2), 220–235. doi:10.1037/0012-1649.29.2.220

Badakar, C. M., Thakkar, P. J., Hugar, S. M., Kukreja, P., Assudani, H. G., & Gokhale, N. (2017). Evaluation of the relevance of Piaget's cognitive principles among parented and orphan children in Belagavi City, Karnataka, India: A comparative study. *International Journal of Clinical Pediatric Dentistry*, *10*(4), 346–350. doi:10.5005/jp-journals-10005-1463 PMID:29403227

Bakker, A. B., Schaufeli, W. B., Leiter, M. P., & Taris, T. W. (2008). Work engagement: An emerging concept in occupational health psychology. *Work and Stress*, *22*(3), 187–200. doi:10.1080/02678370802393649

Becker, G. S. (1993). *Human capital: A theoretical and empirical analysis, with special reference to education* (3rd ed.). University of Chicago press. doi:10.7208/chicago/9780226041223.001.0001

Birren, J. E., & Cunningham, W. R. (1985). Research on the psychology of aging: Principles, concepts and theory. In The handbooks of aging. Handbook of the psychology of aging. Van Nostrand Reinhold Co.

Boujut, E., Bruchon-Schweitzer, M., & Dombrowski, S. U. (2012). Coping among students: Development and validation of an exploratory measure. *Psychology (Irvine, Calif.)*, *3*(8), 562–568. doi:10.4236/psych.2012.38084

Callaghan, D. (2006). Basic conditioning factors' influences on adolescents' healthy behaviors, self-efficacy, and self-care. *Issues in Comprehensive Pediatric Nursing*, *29*(4), 191–204. doi:10.1080/01460860601087156 PMID:17190774

Callaghan, D. M. (2005). The influence of spiritual growth on adolescents' initiative and responsibility for self-care. *Pediatric Nursing*, *31*(2), 91–97. PMID:15934561

Chance, M. R. (2015). *Social fabrics of the mind*. Psychology Press. doi:10.4324/9781315728186

Cohen, P. (1997). Rethinking the youth question. In *Rethinking the youth question* (pp. 179–249). Palgrave. doi:10.1007/978-1-349-25390-6_8

Coleman, J. S. (1988). Social Capital in the Creation of Human Capital. *American Journal of Sociology*, *94*, 95–120. doi:10.1086/228943

Costa, A. L. (2001). *Developing Minds: A Resource Book for Teaching Thinking*. Hawker Brownlow Education.

Cunningham, P. M. (1998). The social dimension of transformative learning. *PAACE Journal of Lifelong Learning*, *7*, 15–28.

Dada, J. O., Babatunde, S. O., & Adeleye, R. O. (2019). Assessment of academic stress and coping strategies among built environment undergraduate students in Nigerian higher education. *Journal of Applied Research in Higher Education*, *11*(3), 367–378. doi:10.1108/JARHE-06-2018-0100

Dalky, H. F., & Gharaibeh, A. (2018). *Depression, anxiety, and stress among college students in Jordan and their need for mental health services*. doi:10.1111/nuf.12316 de Oliveira, M. M., Santos, M. C., & Kiker, B. F. (2000). The role of human capital and technological change in overeducation. *Economics of Education Review, 19*(2), 199–206. doi:10.1016/S0272-7757(99)00020-5

Deb, S., Strodl, E., & Sun, H. (2015). Academic stress, parental pressure, anxiety and mental health among Indian high school students. *International Journal of Psychology and Behavioral Sciences, 5*(1), 26–34.

DeMause, L. (1995). *The history of childhood, Master Work*. Rowman & Littlefield Published.

Demerouti, E., Bakker, A. B., Nachreiner, F., & Schaufeli, W. B. (2001). The job demands-resources model of burnout. *The Journal of Applied Psychology, 86*(3), 499–512. doi:10.1037/0021-9010.86.3.499 PMID:11419809

Elder, G. H. (1998). The life course and human development. In W. Damon & R. M. Lerner (Eds.), *Theoretical models of human development* (pp. 939–991). John Wiley & Sons Inc.

Etel, E., & Yagmurlu, B. (2015). Social competence, theory of mind, and executive function in institution-reared Turkish children. *International Journal of Behavioral Development, 39*(6), 519–529. doi:10.1177/0165025414556095

Fitzsimons, P. (1999). *Human capital theory and education*. Macmillan.

Folkman, S., & Lazarus, R. S. (1988). Coping as a mediator of emotion. *Journal of Personality Social Psychology, 54*(3), 466. doi:10.1037/0022-3514.54.3.466

Folkman, S., Lazarus, R. S., Pimley, S., & Novacek, J. (1987). Age differences in stress and coping processes. *Psychology and Aging, 2*(2), 171–184. doi:10.1037/0882-7974.2.2.171 PMID:3268206

Freud, S. (1953). *Three essays on the theory of sexuality (1905)*. Imago Publishing.

Furlong, A. (2013). *Youth studies: An introduction* (Vol. 1). Routledge, Taylor & Francis Group Inc.

Haywoode, A. (2018). City Connects prompts data-driven action in community schools in the Bronx. *Phi Delta Kappan, 99*(5), 44–46. doi:10.1177/0031721718754812

Helliwell, J. F., & Putnam, R. D. (2004). The social context of well–being. *Philosophical Transactions of the Royal Society of London. Series B, Biological Sciences, 359*(1449), 1435–1446. doi:10.1098/rstb.2004.1522 PMID:15347534

Horowitz, A. (2010). Do humans ape? or Do apes human? Imitation and intention in humans and other animals. *Journal of Comparative Psychology, 17*(3), 325–336. doi:10.1037/0735-7036.117.3.325 PMID:14498809

Huan, V. S., See, Y. L., Ang, R. P., & Har, C. W. (2008). The impact of adolescent concerns on their academic stress. *Educational Review, 60*(2), 169–178. doi:10.1080/00131910801934045

Husky, M. M., Kovess-Masfety, V., & Swendsen, J. D. (2020). Stress and anxiety among university students in France during Covid-19 mandatory confinement. *Comprehensive Psychiatry, 102*, 152191. doi:10.1016/j.comppsych.2020.152191 PMID:32688023

Hynes, C. A., Baird, A. A., & Grafton, S. T. (2006). Differential role of the orbital frontal lobe in emotional versus cognitive perspective-taking. *Neuropsychologia*, *44*(3), 374–383. doi:10.1016/j.neuropsychologia.2005.06.011 PMID:16112148

Janis, I. L. (1989). Stress inoculation in health care. In Stress reduction and prevention (pp. 67-99). Springer. doi:10.1007/978-1-4899-0408-9_3

Klepinger, D., Lundberg, S., & Plotnick, R. (1999). How does adolescent fertility affect the human capital and wages of young women? *The Journal of Human Resources*, *34*(3), 421–448. doi:10.2307/146375

Krechevsky, M., Mardell, B., Filippini, T., & Tedeschi, M. (2016). Children are citizens: The everyday and the razzle-dazzle. *Innovations in Early Education: The International Reggio Emilia Exchange*, *23*(4), 4–15.

Krechevsky, M., Mardell, B., & Romans, A. N. (2014). Engaging city hall: Children as citizens. *New Educator*, *10*(1), 10–20. doi:10.1080/1547688X.2014.868212

Laghi, F., Lonigro, A., Levanto, S., Ferraro, M., Baumgartner, E., & Baiocco, R. (2016). The role of nice and nasty theory of mind in teacher-selected peer models for adolescents with autism spectrum disorders. *Measurement & Evaluation in Counseling & Development*, *49*(3), 207–216. doi:10.1177/0748175615596784

Lazarus, R. S. (1966). *Psychological stress and the coping process*. McGraw-Hill.

Lazarus, R. S. (2006). *Stress and emotion: A new synthesis*. Springer Publishing Company.

Lazarus, R. S., & Folkman, S. (1984). *Stress, Appraisal, and Coping*. Springer Publishing, Inc.

Lerner, R. M., & Overton, W. F. (2010). The Handbook of Life-Span Development: Vol. 1. *Cognition, Biology, and Methods*. John Wiley & Sons.

Lin, S.-H., & Huang, Y.-C. (2014). Life stress and academic burnout. *Active Learning in Higher Education*, *15*(1), 77–90. doi:10.1177/1469787413514651

Mardell, B., & Carpenter, B. (2012). Places to Play in Providence Valuing Preschool Children as Citizens. *Young Children*, *67*(5), 76–78.

Maslach, C. (1982). *Burnout: The cost of caring*. Malor Book Publisher, ISHK.

Maslach, C., & Jackson, S. E. (1981). The measurement of experienced burnout. *Journal of Organizational Behavior*, *2*(2), 99–113. doi:10.1002/job.4030020205

Maslach, C., Schaufeli, W. B., & Leiter, M. P. (2001). Job burnout. *Annual Review of Psychology*, *52*(1), 397–422. doi:10.1146/annurev.psych.52.1.397 PMID:11148311

Meltzoff, A. N. (2011). Social cognition and the origins of imitation, empathy, and theory of mind. In U. Goswami (Ed.), *The Wiley-Blackwell handbook of childhood cognitive development* (Vol. 2, pp. 49–75). John Wiley & Sons.

Neuman, S. (1986). Religious observance within a human capital framework: Theory and application. *Applied Economics*, *18*(11), 1193–1202. doi:10.1080/00036848600000072

Panter-Brick, C., & Smith, M. T. (2000). *Abandoned children*. Cambridge University Press.

Pascoe, M. C., Hetrick, S. E., & Parker, A. G. (2020). The impact of stress on students in secondary school and higher education. *International Journal of Adolescence and Youth*, *25*(1), 104–112. doi:10.1080/02673843.2019.1596823

Premack, D., & Woodruff, G. (1978). Does the chimpanzee have a theory of mind? *Behavioral and Brain Sciences*, *1*(4), 515–526. doi:10.1017/S0140525X00076512

Qi, C. (2019). A double-edged sword? Exploring the impact of students' academic usage of mobile devices on technostress and academic performance. *Behaviour & Information Technology*, *38*(12), 1337–1354. doi:10.1080/0144929X.2019.1585476

Sameroff, A. J., & Fiese, B. H. (2000). Transactional regulation: The developmental ecology of early intervention. In J. P. Shonkoff & S. J. Meisels (Eds.), *Handbook of early childhood intervention* (revised edition, Vol. 2, pp. 135–159). Cambridge University Press. doi:10.1017/CBO9780511529320.009

Schultz, T. W. (1961). Investment in human capital. *The American Economic Review*, *51*(1), 1–17.

Schultz, T. W. (1971). *Investment in human capital. The role of education and of research*. The Free Press.

Selye, H. (1976a). The stress of life. McGraw-Hill.

Selye, H. (1976b). Stress without distress. In G. Serban (Ed.), *Psychopathology of human adaptation* (pp. 137–146). Springer. doi:10.1007/978-1-4684-2238-2_9

Staniscia, B., Deravignone, L., González-Martín, B., & Pumares, P. (2021). Youth mobility and the development of human capital: Is there a Southern European model? *Journal of Ethnic and Migration Studies*, *47*(8), 1866–1882. doi:10.1080/1369183X.2019.1679417

Tagurum, Y., Okonoda, K., Miner, C., Bello, D., & Tagurum, D. (2017). Effect of technostress on job performance and coping strategies among academic staff of a tertiary institution in north-central Nigeria. *International Journal of Biomedical Research*, *8*(6), 312–319.

Temple, J. (1999). A positive effect of human capital on growth. *Economics Letters*, *65*(1), 131–134. doi:10.1016/S0165-1765(99)00120-2

Towbes, L. C., & Cohen, L. H. (1996). Chronic stress in the lives of college students: Scale development and prospective prediction of distress. *Journal of Youth and Adolescence*, *25*(2), 199–217. doi:10.1007/BF01537344

Viner, R. (1999). Putting stress in life: Hans Selye and the making of stress theory. *Social Studies of Science*, *29*(3), 391–410. doi:10.1177/030631299029003003

Volberg, R. A., Gupta, R., Griffiths, M. D., Ólason, D. T., & Delfabbro, P. (2011). An international perspective on youth gambling prevalence studies. In Youth Gambling (pp. 21-56). De Gruyter. doi:10.1515/9783110255690.21

Wang, X., Hegde, S., Son, C., Keller, B., Smith, A., & Sasangohar, F. (2020). Investigating mental health of US college students during the COVID-19 pandemic: Cross-sectional survey study. *Journal of Medical Internet Research*, *22*(9), e22817. doi:10.2196/22817 PMID:32897868

White, R., & Wyn, J. (2004). *Youth and society*. Oxford University Press.

Woodhall, M. (1987). Human capital concepts. In G. psacharopoulos (Ed.), Economics of education (pp. 21-24). Elsevier. doi:10.1016/B978-0-08-033379-3.50011-5

Woodman, D. (2003). Responsibility and time for escape: The meaning of wellbeing to young Australians. *Melbourne Journal of Politics*, *29*(2003-2004), 82–94.

Yan, Y.-W., Lin, R.-M., Su, Y.-K., & Liu, M.-Y. (2018). The relationship between adolescent academic stress and sleep quality: A multiple mediation model. *Social Behavior and Personality*, *46*(1), 63–77. doi:10.2224bp.6530

ADDITIONAL READING

Brooks, K., & Nafukho, F. M. (2006). Human resource development, social capital, emotional intelligence: Any link to productivity? *Journal of European Industrial Training*, *30*(2), 117–128. doi:10.1108/03090590610651258

Nerdrum, L., & Erikson, T. (2001). Intellectual capital: A human capital perspective. *Journal of Intellectual Capital*, *2*(2), 127–135. doi:10.1108/14691930110385919

North, D. C. (1995). *Five propositions about institutional change*. University of Michigan Press.

North, D. C. (2018). Institutional change: a framework of analysis. In *Social Rules* (pp. 189–201). Routledge. doi:10.4324/9780429497278-13

Nyberg, A. J., Moliterno, T. P., Hale, D. Jr, & Lepak, D. P. (2014). Resource-based perspectives on unit-level human capital: A review and integration. *Journal of Management*, *40*(1), 316–346. doi:10.1177/0149206312458703

Okun, O. (2022). The positive face of human capital, psychological capital, and well-being. In *Research Anthology on Changing Dynamics of Diversity and Safety in the Workforce* (pp. 203–222). IGI Global. doi:10.4018/978-1-6684-2405-6.ch013

Ployhart, R. E., & Moliterno, T. P. (2011). Emergence of the human capital resource: A multilevel model. *Academy of Management Review*, *36*(1), 127–150. doi:10.5465/amr.2009.0318

Preko, A. K. (2022). Leadership and Human Capital Management in New Public Management. In R. E. Hinson, N. Madichie, O. Adeola, J. Nyigmah Bawole, I. Adisa, & K. Asamoah (Eds.), *New Public Management in Africa* (pp. 105–131). Palgrave Macmillan. doi:10.1007/978-3-030-77181-2_5

Schultz, T. W. (1961). Investment in human capital. *The American Economic Review*, *51*(1), 1–17.

Schultz, T. W. (1971). *Investment in human capital. The role of education and of research*. The Free Press.

KEY TERMS AND DEFINITIONS

Human Capital: The economic value of humans that is accounted for skills, knowledge, and attributes humans possess.

Human Capital Development: An area of study and instruction that prepares people to be compassionate. Dedicated solutions arise capable of identifying unfair, inhumane, and unsustainable systems and creating alternatives.

Stress: A sensation of mental or physical stress. It might come from an occurrence or thought that makes to feel fatigued, upset, or uncomfortable.

Well-Being: The experience of pleasant feelings such as happiness and contentment and developing one's potential.

Youth: Adolescents between the age of 14 to 24 years.

Chapter 7
Coping With Compassion Fatigue Through Self-Care

Trudi Pinnick Wolfe
https://orcid.org/0000-0001-6942-0204
Loper Elementary School, Shelbyville Central Schools, USA

ABSTRACT

This chapter focuses on how the stress of teaching can lead to compassion fatigue. It will examine the general stressors of teaching which have led to the current teacher shortage with a special focus on the unique stress of teaching students who have experienced trauma. In addition, it will offer a snapshot of how trauma presents itself in the classroom and some of the challenges that educators experience. This chapter will share one school's experience with helping their teachers cope with compassion fatigue through a professional development series covering these topics: defining compassion fatigue and its impact, coping strategies, and the importance of self-care. Data will be presented to show the effectiveness of this intervention at this author's school.

INTRODUCTION

At this time, there is a critical shortage of qualified teachers in public K-12 schools. This chapter will explore some of the reasons for the shortage, especially the issues related to teaching students with significant trauma and the cost of caring for them, which often results in compassion fatigue. This chapter will chronicle the journey of this author's school in helping teachers cope with compassion fatigue in the following ways: understanding the syndrome, helping teachers to reconnect with their mission as educators, and providing information on self-care strategies and practices. Information will be provided for the readers to create a professional development (PD) series to deliver to their teachers and other staff. Personal accounts from two teachers at the author's school as well as a principal are also included in this chapter. From these personal accounts, the reader will learn from the teachers' perspectives what it is like to teach children with Adverse Childhood Experiences (ACEs), the personal toll it takes, and how this PD series helped them cope. The objectives are:

DOI: 10.4018/978-1-6684-2334-9.ch007

- To understand compassion fatigue and its impact
- To understand how working with students who have experienced trauma contributes to compassion fatigue, and
- To know how to create a professional development program to help teachers cope.

BACKGROUND

There have been reported teacher shortages in certain subject areas and some school districts since 2008. In recent years, this shortage has increased to a nation-wide teacher shortage, which has been exacerbated by the conditions that the pandemic has brought to the world of education. The demand for teachers has exceeded the supply of teachers for all grades K-12 since 2019 (Edelman, 2021). There are fewer young people enrolling in teacher education programs. From 2009 to 2014, there was a 35% decline in enrollment in teacher preparation programs (Sutcher, Darling-Hammond, & Carver-Thomas, 2016).

The pandemic is also a significant contributor to the shortage of teachers. The National Education Association (NEA) found in their survey of educators in May 2021 that 33% of the respondents said that the pandemic has led them to plan on leaving the profession earlier than expected. (Walker, 2021) The percentage of Black teachers anticipating early retirement is even higher with 43% reporting that they plan to leave the field earlier than expected (Flannery, 2020). Other contributors are fewer young people entering the field, salary and benefits not being competitive with other professions, and unprecedented teacher workload and burnout (Learning Policy Institute, 2021).

Other factors are also cited in the literature as the reason for teacher shortages. Lever et al. (2017) in their article "School Mental Health Is Not Just for Students: Why Teacher and School Staff Wellness Matters," cite the following reasons for teacher shortages:

- "High-stakes tests
- Large class sizes
- Student behavioral challenges
- Inadequate resources
- Poor physical space
- Bureaucracy
- Workload
- High responsibility for others
- Perceived inadequate recognition or advancement
- The gap between preservice training expectations and actual work experience, and
- Lack of autonomy." (Lever, et al. 2017, para. 3).

Another reason often cited in the literature is the low pay for educators compared to other professions (Buttner, 2021).

A newly emerging contributor to the shortage of teachers is the trauma that students have experienced and how the impact of this trauma presents in the classroom. Murphey and Sacks (2019) in their article "Supporting Students with Adverse Childhood Experiences: How Educators and Schools Can Help" report that the National Survey of Children's Health 2011-2012 (NSCH) found that 45% of the children in the US have experienced one or more ACEs and that 10% of children have an ACE score of three or higher. With the publication of the ACE study in 1998, there has been a growing awareness of the impact of trauma in these areas: physical, emotional, and social health. People who have 4 or more ACEs have much higher incidences of substance abuse, suicide attempts, depression, anxiety, high-risk behaviors, health problems, and even early death (Feliti et al., 1998).

As research into the impact of ACEs continues, additional associated problems have been found. The NSCH has found a correlation between ACEs and emotional, developmental, or behavioral problems as well as the degree in which the child can engage with learning. These are the specific findings of the survey:

- 18.6% of children with an ACE score of 2 displayed emotional, developmental, or behavioral problems compared to 4.4% of children with an ACE score of zero.
- 53.1% of children with an ACE score of 2 were engaged with learning while 75.4% of children with an ACE score of zero were engaged with learning (NSCH, 2016).

MAIN FOCUS OF THE CHAPTER

How does a child with trauma present in the classroom? Although each child is different, there are some generalities. Trauma changes the brain architecture and often puts the child into a state of heightened alertness. The child may be constantly scanning his/her environment for possible signs of danger. In addition, the child who has experienced trauma may interpret neutral events as dangerous. Thus, a child who has experienced trauma may be in a constant state of fight-flight-freeze response. This child may also be so hypervigilant that his/her attention is focused on any stimulus in the environment that could be potentially dangerous. Thus, a teacher's frown may be a sign of danger; a classmate whispering to a neighbor may take the child's full attention as something threatening may be said; or the child may be so aware of the tightness in his/her stomach that it is difficult to attend to what the teacher is saying (van der Kolk, 2014). This brain state may present itself with difficulties in these areas:

- "Processing verbal information
- Responding to teacher directions
- Recalling what was heard
- Retaining information
- Focusing" (*The national institute for trauma and loss in children*, 2020, p. 3)

Without understanding trauma, teachers may interpret these behaviors as symptoms of ADHD, defiance, lack of motivation, or inability to learn. When teachers assign negative labels to these behaviors, it creates barriers in developing relationships with students and in finding appropriate solutions to learning problems. Teachers may also see themselves as failing when a traumatized child has difficulty learning or with responding to traditional forms of discipline. Thus, the teacher may begin blaming him/herself for not being able to help the child be successful in the classroom.

In addition, teachers are not prepared to work with students who have experienced trauma. Even recent graduates receive very little information in their teacher preparation classes about the effects of trauma and how to address these issues with their students. Thus, teachers enter the field thinking that their work is all about lesson plans and following Bloom's Taxonomy Theory. Further frustrating is the fact that any classroom management strategies learned in college focus on traditional discipline with a heavy emphasis on rewards, consequences, and behavior charts. Consequently, teachers enter their first classroom thinking that they are well prepared with great lesson plans, an engaging delivery style, and their colorful "clip-down" behavior chart. So, when they encounter their first student who has experienced trauma, they are unprepared when the student doesn't respond to academic plans for success and when the "clip-down" chart often results in "melt-downs," in which the student becomes even more agitated and less focused on what is being taught (Minero, 2017).

Students carry a lot of "baggage" into the classroom each day. It may be trauma that occurred in the past or present. The baggage may also be immediate daily challenges, such as there not being enough food in the home for dinner or breakfast. The issues may be homelessness that resulted in the student's family being doubled up in a household and not having an adequate place to sleep. It may be difficult situations more acute in nature, such as parents fighting in the morning or parents yelling at them in the morning chaos of getting ready for school. Or, perhaps there is a situation at school that is causing the student to be on edge, such as being bullied or not having friends. All of this results in students entering the classroom with anxiety and being in a state of dysregulation.

In her book *Help for Billy: A Beyond Consequences Approach to Helping Challenging Children in the Classroom,* Heather T. Forbes (2013) describes the cup version of the Window of Stress Tolerance. Everyone has a range of emotions and situations that they can handle. When the stress level is low, there are a variety of difficult situations that people can handle before their cup is full and they show dysregulated behavior. With children who experience a lot of adversity, they come into the classroom with their cups already full. So, a small thing, such as the teacher correcting them or another student making a negative comment, might be enough to overfill their "cup," and they become dysregulated or may even explode. Thus, the teacher is totally confused, thinking "What happened here? I just asked him to pick his book bag off of the floor and hang it up." During a typical day, a teacher may have multiple interactions like this with more than one student, leaving him/her exhausted, both physically and mentally.

In addition, both building and district administrators may be lacking in understanding how trauma impacts children. So, unintentionally, they may add to the teacher's stress by holding him/her accountable for the child's difficulties in the school setting. Even in the administrator's attempts to be helpful, the message to the teacher may be that the teacher is doing something wrong in the classroom. As a result, the teacher struggles with daily challenging behavior, a sense of inadequacy, and unrealistic expectations from his/her administrator.

In recent years, with the growing awareness of trauma in the classroom, there has been more attention paid to the impact on the teachers from dealing with the students who have experienced ACEs. Although it has been recognized for many years that mental health providers and first responders can experience secondary traumatic stress or compassion fatigue from the work that they do, it has only been recently that this same concern has been indicated for teachers. Although teachers rarely hear in-depth personal accounts or witness traumatic events as they happen, they, too, are affected by the trauma that their students carry into the classroom. In addition, some students will disclose incidents of abuse and neglect to their teachers, thus, putting the teacher in a situation in which he/she has an emotional response to what he/she has heard. The teacher may replay the disclosure in his/her mind, deal with powerful emotions of fear and anxiety for the student, and feel a sense of helplessness to help the student improve his/her family situation (Minero, 2017).

In the article, "You Can't Lead on Empty: Supporting School Staff with Vicarious Trauma," Paige Tutt (2021) interviewed Dr. Art McCoy, superintendent of Jennings School District in Missouri, about the impact of vicarious trauma for educators. Dr. McCoy accurately described teaching students with trauma this way: “Yet supporting students can literally suck the life out of you, the spirit out of you. And that is my best description of what secondary trauma is. It’s the impact of literally giving your fuel to another soul so that they can go on another day and live in a brighter way.” (para. 13)

Another stressful part of a teacher’s work is dealing with families. Gone are the days in which teachers are automatically respected in their role as educational experts for many parents and guardians. It is now common for families to challenge teachers on decisions in the classroom, to even be hostile to the teacher, and to accuse him/her of treating their child unfairly. Some of the most challenging parents and guardians that teachers interact with have also experienced adverse experiences in their childhood and may also be living in extremely stressful situations, such as exhaustion from working two to three jobs, intimate partner abuse, or struggling to meet the basic needs of their family. Teachers are often unprepared for the responses that they encounter from families, and they may take these episodes of negative interactions personally.

SOLUTIONS AND RECOMMENDATIONS

One solution to this problem is to educate teachers and administrators about compassion fatigue and self-care. This chapter is a description of how this author’s school chose to address the problem of teachers being overwhelmed and exhausted. Although this school was making progress in understanding trauma, the teachers were still feeling inadequate and depleted. Surveys were completed by the staff and principals early in the 18-19 school year. From the survey, it was obvious that teachers were struggling. Although 75% of them indicated that they understood the impact of trauma, there were several areas in which they felt inadequate:

- 45% reported that they could remain calm with students
- 50% reported that they could manage their level of stress adequately
- 50% reported that they felt supported by their building administrator

The survey of the administrators in the building also showed a disconnect in how they perceived how teachers were doing and how teachers thought they were doing. Here are the results of the administrator survey in these same key areas:

- 100% of the principals thought that their teachers remained calm with students
- 100% of the principals thought that their teachers were managing their stress level adequately.
- 100% of the principals thought that they supported their teachers.

From the survey and through discussions with teachers, it became obvious that they needed support on a more personal level. In this author’s search to help her teachers, she wanted to share information on how to take care of oneself. As she reviewed the literature, it became obvious that most of the self-help information available was inadequate to meet the needs of her teachers. Thus began the journey for this one school to support their teachers in understanding the emotional toll that often accompanies educating students, especially those who have experienced trauma.

This author began the journey by enlisting support from her principal. Having principal support is the most important variable in this type of intervention being successful. If the program is to benefit teachers, the building administrator must also grow in his/her knowledge of compassion fatigue, its effects, and how to cope with it. This author provided a proposal for a summer book study and a professional development series of four presentations. The principal not only agreed to the proposal, but she also agreed to participate in all aspects of the program, which is critical for the teachers to feel supported.

The first step was providing professional development for both the teachers and the principals. This author believed that the most important aspect of this program was for teachers to understand compassion fatigue. Being a social worker, compassion fatigue, burnout, and self-care strategies were part of her graduate classes and internship supervision. So, although social workers may not always practice self-care, they are aware of the impact of working with clients who have experienced trauma. Self-care is so important that the National Association of Social Workers recently amended their Code of Ethics to include self-care in their ethical principles (NASW, 2021). Unfortunately, there is not this same focus in teacher preparation classes or in student teaching experiences.

In planning this professional development series, this author wanted each presentation to offer education about compassion fatigue and its impact, to provide inspiration and encouragement, and to give a coping strategy as well as hope. In addition, this author realized that there needed to be a way to gauge the progress that teachers were making in coping with compassion fatigue. So, just like the teachers were doing in the classroom with students at this author's school, teachers were asked to do an emotional check-in and check-out at each meeting. Another part of each presentation was a mindfulness practice. This author provided teachers with different strategies for mindfulness and also demonstrated for the teachers the importance of making mindfulness an integral part of the school day, not only for the students but also for themselves. Another important part of each meeting was to include a time for open discussion so that the teachers could learn from each other and know that they were not alone with their struggles. Thus, each session provided structured discussion times as well as encouragement for open discussion throughout the presentation. At each meeting, an article was also shared with the teachers so that they could further their understanding of the material that was presented. Thus, each presentation followed this format:

- Emotional check-in, which was anonymous
    - I'm great
    - I'm okay
    - I'm holding on
    - I'm struggling
    - I need support
- Mindfulness practice
- Information
- Self-care tip
- Self-care practice
- Abbreviated mindfulness practice
- Sharing an article
- Emotional check-out, which was also anonymous

The mindfulness practices came from a variety of sources. This author's school uses a program called Calm Classroom with the students (calmclassroom.org). Each day teachers lead two to three Calm Classroom practices with the students. Sometimes, the mindfulness practice came from the Calm Classroom manual (Luster & Luster, 2015). At other times, the practice came from other sources. Some examples of practices that were used in the meetings were:

- Hand breathing
(https://myhappymind.org/wp-content/uploads/2017/08/Copy-of-Happy-breathing-script-Finger-Breathing.pdf)
- Five senses practice
(https://positivepsychology.com/wp-content/uploads/2017/01/Five-Senses-Worksheet.pdf)
- Self-kindness meditation
(https://ggia.berkeley.edu/practice/loving_kindness_meditation)

Professional Development Presentation 1

The purpose of the first presentation was to provide teachers with a definition of compassion fatigue, its impact, and how to identify it. This author believed that it was important to put a name to the signs and symptoms of compassion fatigue. This strategy is in alignment with what Dan Siegel has said in working with children who have difficulty regulating their emotions, "If we can name it, we can tame it." (Siegel, 2015, p. 60).

One of the most important parts of this first session was a self-assessment for compassion fatigue. Since the awareness that compassion fatigue occurs in education is relatively new, this author was not able to find a self-assessment tool specific to education. This author also wanted the self-assessment to be short and easy to take so that it could be done during the time allotted to the staff meeting. This author found a short self-assessment for compassion fatigue that was developed for those in the healthcare field, Compassion Fatigue Self Assessment (Pfifferling & Gilley, 2000). Although this author was not certain that this tool would resonate with the teachers at her school, she believed that it might provide some valuable information about how teachers were coping. This assessment was done as a Google form in which the teachers entered only their total score. Again, this was done anonymously.

This information was provided to teachers in the presentation:

- Mindfulness practice: Calm Classroom manual
- Definition of compassion fatigue
  - Known by other names, such as vicarious trauma, secondary trauma, secondary traumatic stress, and empathic distress
  - Recognition that those giving care are impacted by the trauma that those they help have experienced
  - "The cost of caring"
- Explanation of why compassion fatigue happens in education
  - Incidence of students who have ACEs
  - High stress level of educators
  - High number of educators who leave field
  - Educators put in a lot of extra hours that are unpaid (*Teacher Health and Stress*, 2016)

- Signs and symptoms
  - "Cognitive
    - Lowered concentration
    - Apathy
    - Rigid thinking
    - Perfectionism
    - Preoccupation with trauma
  - Emotional
    - Guilt about not doing enough to help the student
    - Persistently worrying about the student, even when not at school
    - Anger and irritability, often unexplained
    - Numbness
    - Sadness
    - Helplessness and hopelessness
    - Feeling isolated, alone, and disconnected from others
    - Feelings of being a failure
  - Behavioral
    - Withdrawal
    - Sleep disturbance
    - Appetite change
    - Hypervigilance
    - Elevated startle response
  - Physical
    - Elevated heart rate
    - Difficulty breathing
    - Muscle and joint pain
    - Impaired immune system
    - Increased severity of existing medical condition
    - Feeling exhausted
  - Other
    - Lack of empathy
    - Cynicism
    - These signs and symptoms often intrude into personal and family life." (*Secondary traumatic stress, n.d., para.* 2).
- Impact on educators
  - Teachers may recognize that they are experiencing these symptoms but do not understand their cause. They may interpret signs and symptoms as a personal flaw.
  - Teachers do not understand that compassion fatigue comes from caring for students.
  - Teachers do not understand that these signs and symptoms are a **normal** reaction to teaching students who have experienced trauma.
- Discussion: What do you think of the signs/symptoms and/or impact of compassion fatigue?
- Explanation of why doing professional development on compassion fatigue and self-care.

  - Survey results were shared with teachers so that they understood that many of them are struggling with managing their stress level and feeling supported by administrators. The disconnect in perceptions of administrators and teachers was also shared.
- Layers of stress for educators
  - Stress filters down from
    - Federal level
    - State level
    - Community
    - District administrators
    - Building administrators
  - Students
  - Families of students
  - Working conditions
    - Low pay
    - Work demand resulting in many unpaid hours beyond the school day
    - Paying for own classroom supplies for students in need
    - Educators often working multiple jobs due to low pay and high student loan debt
    - Educators working in high-poverty areas are at high risk to experience these working conditions.
- Discussion: What do you think of the layers of stress and/or reasons for a PD series on compassion fatigue.
- Self-assessment questions:
  - "Personal concerns commonly intrude on my professional role.
  - My colleagues seem to lack understanding.
  - I find even small changes enormously draining.
  - I can't seem to recover quickly after association with trauma.
  - Association with trauma affects me very deeply.
  - My students' stress affects me deeply.
  - I have lost my sense of hopefulness.
  - I feel vulnerable all the time.
  - I feel overwhelmed by unfinished business" (Pffiffering & Gilley, 2000)
- Discussion: After scores are shared, the teachers were asked to share their thoughts about their collective scores.
- Abbreviated mindfulness practice: Calm Classroom manual (Luster & Luster, 2015)
- Self-care practice: Gratitude journal
  - Each participant was given a gratitude journal and asked to write down at least three things that he/she is grateful for two to three times a week. A basic explanation of this research showing that this practice improves one's sense of well-being was provided.
- Exit ticket
  - Each teacher was asked to write on paper "Three Things that I Wish my Principal Knew." These papers were collected. Again, this sharing was done anonymously. The sharing of "Three Things" comes from the book, *I Wish my Teacher Knew: How One Question Can Change Everything for our Kids* by Kyle Schwartz (2016). This author's school had previously done a book study on this book, and the "Three Things" was an intervention that the

teachers used in the classroom as a part of the community circle time for students to write important personal information to them..

- Emotional check-out
- Article: "Secondary Traumatic Stress for Educators: Understanding and Mitigating the Effects" by Jessica Lander (2018): https://www.kqed.org/mindshift/52281/secondary-traumatic-stress-for-educators-understanding-and-mitigating-the-effects

The Outcome of Professional Development 1

During this meeting, there was a sense of heaviness that grew in the room as we proceeded through the information. One teacher cried quietly throughout the presentation as she saw her own struggles in the information being presented. And the emotional check-out showed that many of the teachers left feeling worse than what they had indicated when they came in. This author did not expect this outcome. In fact, she felt as if she had failed her teachers. However, the principal reframed this observation as the teachers were beginning to deal with their compassion fatigue for the first time and that this experience brought up feelings that they had not previously acknowledged. This reframing seemed to be a realistic explanation for what had happened.

Another outcome for this meeting was that the self-assessment for compassion fatigue showed a high occurrence for the teachers. On this self-assessment, a score of at least 4 indicates a level of compassion fatigue. 70% of the teachers at this author's school scored a 4 or higher. The following was the breakdown in scores:

- Score of 1=0%
- Score of 2= 14%
- Score of 3=14%
- Score of 4=28%
- Score of 5=14%
- Score of 6=24%
- Score of 7=0%
- Score of 8=3%
- Score of 9=3%

A further result of this session was that the teachers poured their hearts into writing the "Three Things that I Wish my Principal Knew." Many of them shared words of appreciation for the principal and their joy in teaching, but many of them shared heart-felt concerns, both from a personal and professional perspective. Some examples of the concerns are:

- "I am so exhausted all the time."
- "I hate going home and having no energy left to give to my own children."
- "I am so emotionally drained that I yell at my own kids because I am so irritable."
- "Sometimes I can't sleep at night."
- "I want you to know that I am doing the best that I can."
- "I need your support."
- "I need you to understand how incredibly hard it is to teach these kids."

- "I am more than the test scores that my students achieve."
- "I need you to remember what it was like when you were in the classroom with 30 students."

This author then entered all the comments, both the ones that were positive and the ones that showed a concern, into a document so that the principal could not tell from the handwriting who had written the statement. The principal then made a written heart-felt response to the teachers. The principal let the teachers know that she appreciated and valued them and that she heard their struggles. She also shared some of her own concerns, such as not being able to support each teacher as he/she needed and her own exhaustion that carried over into her own family life. Many of the teachers expressed appreciation for the principal responding to their concerns (A full response from a principal is included at the end of this chapter).

Professional Development Presentation 2

This presentation focused on understanding stress and identifying coping skills. In addition, it also provided information about finding your mission as an educator again. In the book, *The Burnout Cure: Learning to Love Teaching Again,* by Chase Miekle (2019), he talked about how educators can lose track of the meaning of their work, which can lead to burnout. He also provided several strategies for educators to get back in touch with the meaning of their work. One of the strategies that he discussed was "Craft the Why'' (Mielke, 2019, p. 164). One of the most important parts of this activity is getting back in touch with the service part of being an educator.

This information was provided:

- Emotional check-in
- Mindfulness practice: Hand breathing
  ¡ Hand breathing was chosen for this PD meeting, because it is similar to the waves that were drawn during the activity in the session. For this meeting, hand breathing was renamed wave breathing.
- Following up with a review of PD 1
- "Knowing your Why"
  - Video: "Know your Why" by Michael Jr. https://youtu.be/1ytFB8TrkTo (2017)
    - Michael Jr. is a comedian who combines comedy with life lessons. This video is from his weekly series, called "Break Time."
    - In this video, Michael Jr interacts with E. Daryl Duff, a music teacher in the audience. He asks him to sing the song, "Amazing Grace." Then, he provides a life story with several adverse situations and asks Mr. Duff to sing again. In this second version, Mr. Duff explodes with meaning and depth to his rendition of this song.
  - Discussion: What was the difference in the two versions of the singing? What was his "why" in the second version?
  - Then, the teachers were asked to write their "mission statement" in their gratitude journal or on a piece of paper, answering these questions:
    - What led you here?
    - How did you get here?
    - Why do you do what you do?
    - What keeps you here?

        - What do you want to accomplish?
        - What do you bring to this work?
        - How has this work changed you?
        - What kind of legacy do I want to leave behind?
    - Discussion: Share your mission statement
- Understanding stress
    - Waves of Stress--Step 1--Identifying Stressors
        - The participants were asked to draw a series of waves in their gratitude journal or on a piece of paper to represent the stressors in their lives. It was explained that the waves may be a combination of large and small, depending on the size of the stressor.
        - They were then instructed to label each wave with the stressor that it represented.
    - Waves of Stress--Step 2--Identifying Coping Skills
        - The teachers were asked to write a coping skill or support person in between each wave.
    - Discussion: Share your waves of stress and coping skills/supports
- Self-Care Tip
    - Read the first two paragraphs of the article: "Self Care for Teachers" by Anne Brunett (2004).
    - Discussion: Reflect on the article.
- Self-Care Tip for Others with Emails
    - Schedule send your emails so that you don't burden others during non-work hours.
    - Build in a delay-send into your email, so that if you forget to schedule send during non-work hours, you can undo and then schedule send.
- Finishing up
    - Teachers were asked
        - To keep wave picture and reflect on it weekly
        - To use tips about emails during non-school hours
        - To further read the article by Anne Burnett (2004) and to use one coping skill
- Mindfulness practice: Hand (wave) breathing

Outcome of Professional Development 2: There was a joyfulness observed amongst the teachers in this session as they shared their mission statements with each other and identified their coping skills and supports. In addition, most of them didn't know how to use their emails for schedule send, and they verbalized a commitment to begin using this feature so that they didn't interrupt their colleagues' time with family and friends. Most of them liked the hand (wave) breathing and even used it with their students in the classrooms. Another outcome of this session was that the emotional check-in/check-out showed that teachers were leaving with a better sense of their emotional state than when they entered the room. The emotional check-in and check-out showed at check-out that more teachers were feeling great and that fewer teachers were feeling as if they were struggling or merely holding on as compared to the check-in when they entered the room.

Tip for Success with Professional Development 2: Since teachers are not accustomed to completing these types of activities, it is helpful to have examples completed to show them. So, this author had her own wave picture drawn with stressors and coping skills/supports identified. She also had her own mission statement written in her gratitude journal and shared it before asking the teachers to write their statement. Here is this author's mission statement:

I love school social work. I love doing different things. I love being on the go. I love making a difference for so many children. I love doing lessons. I love providing counseling. I love that the children are happy to see me in the hallway, for small groups, and in the classroom. I want to accomplish so much. My counseling work over the last 34 years has helped me grow not only as a professional, but as a person and as a parent. I feel honored to have worked with so many children and their families. I feel honored to be part of this school family. I learn from all of you everyday. I learn from those whom I serve. I want my legacy to be that I made a difference--that I made lives better--that I offered hope to the hopeless--that I gave a voice to the voiceless--that this school is better because I was here.

Professional Development Presentation 3

This presentation focused on perspective. Two parts of perspective were included in this presentation:

1. Understanding the effects of complaining and how to reduce complaining, and
2. Understanding what one chooses to focus on contributes to a sense of well-being or lack of well-being.

One of the main parts of this session was the video, "A World without Complaining" with Will Bowen (2018) about the impact of complaining and the "Complaint-Free Challenge."

This information was provided in professional development 3:

- Emotional check-in
- Mindfulness practice: 5 Senses
- Review of the first two PDs
- Complaining
    - Video: "A World without Complaining" with Will Bowen: https://youtu.be/-b8KTLzo5-0 (2018)
    - Effects of complaining
        - "Most people complain 15 to 30 times a day.
        - Complaining builds a neural pathway for complaining and negativity.
        - Complaining shrinks the hippocampus, which is critical for memory and learning.
        - Complaining releases the stress hormone, cortisol.
        - Complaining increases heart rate and blood sugar level. Over time, this can place a person at risk for high cholesterol, diabetes, heart disease, and obesity.
        - Complaining is contagious. Mirror neurons pick up on complaining when we spend a lot of time with someone who complains. Our mirror neurons can mimic this person's mood within ourselves.
        - Chronic complaining can eventually create an environment of negativity"(*A World without Complaining* 2018).
    - Discussion: Discuss "the virus of complaining" and its effects on ourselves and others.
- Perspective
    - The classical perspective-taking pictures of the faces/vases and good/evil were shown and discussed.
    - Video: The Money Business Illusion by Daniel J. Simons: https://youtu.be/IGQmdoK_ZfY (2010)

        - After viewing this video, the teachers answered the questions at the end of the video. The video was replayed for greater awareness.
    - Discussion: How can perspective help us with complaining?
- These self-care tips were presented:
    - Set a goal to not complain for one week.
        - Use a bracelet to increase awareness of complaining.
    - Think of gratitude instead of what's wrong
    - Think of ways the situation could be worse to change perspective.
    - Think of someone else's situation.
    - Ask, "Is this really important?"
        - If it is important, work to change the situation.
        - If it is not important, let it go.
    - Remember to breathe!
    - Read the blog of "Spilling Coffee" by Kate Beddow, founder of Calmer Classrooms (Beddow, 2019).
        - This blog describes a situation in which a person is bumped into and spills her coffee on her shirt. The blog describes that the person spilled her coffee because there was coffee in her cup. It further describes that what is in our cup spills out, so it is important to remember what is in our cup.
- The No-Complaint Challenge
    - The teachers were given the opportunity to try out the no-complaint challenge. Wanting to get teachers to participate in this challenge, the number of days was reduced to five and a few options were presented to them:
        - They voted on whether or not they wanted to do the challenge as a whole-school or not.
        - They voted on how they wanted to do the challenge:
- A whole week
- One day a week for five weeks
- For the whole day or only when in one location of the school, such as the teacher's lounge.
    - The teachers voted to do the challenge for a week with it being throughout the day. They were supplied a bracelet to develop their awareness of times that they complain.
- Abbreviated mindfulness practice: 5 Senses
- Exit ticket
    - Emotional check-out
    - Article: "How Complaining Rewires your Brain" by Travis Bradberry (n.d): https://www.talentsmart.com/articles/How-Complaining-Rewires-Your-Brain-for-Negativity-2147446676-p-1.html

Outcome of Professional Development 3: Teachers expressed developing a greater awareness of the negative effects of complaining and recognized that they were complaining too much. Almost 100% of the teachers voted to participate in the challenge. The emotional check-out board again showed that teachers were leaving the PD in a better state of mind than when they came into the room. During the challenge, there was a sense of levity as teachers caught each other complaining and reminded each other to move their bracelet. Teachers reported that the challenge did reduce the number of complaints that they made.

Professional Development 4

This presentation focused on making a vision book. Most of this information came from a webinar with Calvalyn Day, educational coach and consultant, on January 4, 2020 (https://www.calvalynday.com/). Calvalyn Day (2020) recommended making a vision book rather than the popular vision board for these reasons:

- A book is adjustable (add pages, take out pages).
- It is small enough that you can keep it nearby for frequent reference.

The presentation provided this information:

- Emotional check-in
- Mindfulness practice: Loving Kindness (focusing on only sending loving kindness to people who are loved) https://ggia.berkeley.edu/practice/loving_kindness_meditation
- Review of first 3 PDs
- Vision book
    - Is a roadmap for one's dreams
    - Focuses on the future we would like to have with these elements:
        - What one would have
        - What one would be
        - What one would do
    - Discussion: After thinking about these elements of a vision book, the teachers shared the dream lives that they envisioned for themselves.
    - A vision book includes:
        - Experiences one wants to have
        - Activities that one wants to do
        - The people whom one wants in his/her life
        - Feelings that that one experiences while envisioning their dreams
        - Affirmations
- Focus on the positive, which is important since our brains have a negative bias
- Are for one's own actions, not the actions of others
- Need to be said and/or read daily
    - Can be associated with a trigger point to make it easier to remember, such as being said when one is brushing his/her hair
    - Can be written and placed in a location that is seen every day, such as the bathroom mirror
- Can be associated with an anchor. When the affirmation is read or said and the positive feeling is present, the person can touch a part of their body that is not often touched during a normal day to strengthen the effect of the affirmation. For example, one could say the affirmation, feel happy, and then touch the inside of his/her wrist. If this procedure is followed each time, the effect of the affirmation will be stronger.
- Discussion: Participants shared what affirmation they chose, their trigger point, and their anchor.
- Self-Care Tips

    - Quote by Nicole Spector in her article, "What Is Self-Care?": "... self care is a way for us to give back to ourselves and to release everyday pressures." https://www.nbcnews.com/better/lifestyle/what-self-care-how-cut-through-marketing-noise-actually-practice-ncna1134921
    - Quote by Eleanor Brown: "Self care is not selfish. You cannot serve from an empty vessel." https://www.inspiringquotes.us/author/9028-eleanor-brown#:~:text=%E2%80%9CThere%20are%20times%20in%20our,we%20can%20change%20the%20future.%E2%80%9D&text=%E2%80%9CSelf%2Dcare%20is%20not%20selfish,serve%20from%20an%20empty%20vessel.%E2%80%9D
- Next steps
    - Teachers were asked to make their vision book, to share it with someone who supports them and to review it often.
    - Teachers were asked to use their affirmation daily.
- Mindfulness practice--Abbreviated Loving Kindness
- Emotional check-out

Outcome of Professional Development 4: Again, the emotional check-out board showed that teachers were leaving in a better state of mind than when they entered the room. At a follow-up meeting, teachers shared their vision books which were heartfelt and left an impact on all of the staff. Teachers also shared how they were using their affirmations on a daily basis with trigger points and anchors. As for this author, she found that she made progress with every part of her vision book. It was amazing how simply thinking about what one wanted in his/her life, writing about it, and visualizing it could have such a profound impact on one's daily practices.

Tip for Professional Development 4 to Be Successful: It is helpful if teachers can see a completed vision book as an example. So, this author had her vision book prepared to show to teachers during the meeting.

As a last step, the book *The Burnout Cure: Learning to Love Teaching Again* by Chase Mielke (2019) was chosen for a summer book study. Any book that is chosen for a book study with teachers has a much greater impact if it is written by a teacher. Chase Mielke was a teacher. In this book, he shared his path from being an enthusiastic teacher to burnout to renewal. In this book, Chase provides many strategies for growth, changing mindset, and self-care. The book study took place during the summer of 2020. A written discussion through Google docs was held on a weekly basis. Each week during the summer, this author posted questions about a chapter or two and shared her thoughts and feelings about the topics. Teachers then added to the Google doc discussion. Through the Google doc, teachers were able to also read what others had written so that they could gain more information from each other and know that they were not alone in their struggles. Early in the following school year, there was an in-person meeting to discuss the book, focusing on what was learned and how the information applied to the professional development presentations.

Teacher Perspective

Melissa Romo and Chelsea Nullier are teachers at this author's school. Melissa is a third-grade reading teacher, and Chelsea is a second-grade math teacher as well as serving as a mentor teacher. Both Melissa and Chelsea have embraced a trauma-informed approach to teaching, and Melissa has also implemented Whole Brain Teaching strategies in her classroom. Both Melissa and Chelsea have been teaching for ten years. During separate interviews, both teachers shared how exhausting it is to teach children with trauma, the personal and professional toll that it takes, and how this professional development series helped them cope with the compassion fatigue that they were experiencing.

From Melissa Romo

- *About the stress of teaching students who have experienced trauma*: "I have been teaching for ten years, and it seems that each year the number of students who have experienced or who are experiencing trauma is increasing. Teaching is already a stressful occupation, and when we add on the layer of being a trauma-informed teacher, the stress can be elevated. If a student with trauma is having a difficult day and they are showing different behaviors, it can be mentally and emotionally exhausting for me and the other students in the classroom. When I learn about the trauma that some of my students experience, it makes it difficult to send them home each night, knowing what they may experience, and I worry about what the day at school will be like tomorrow. Each year I say a few times a year 'I would take this child home if I could,' because I genuinely worry about their wellbeing for a big portion of the day, every day."
- *About experiencing compassion fatigue*: "The middle of the school year is always when I feel compassion fatigue the most. By this time in the school year, I have built a close relationship with my students and they are comfortable sharing with me what they are experiencing at home. When I begin to feel compassion fatigue come on, I begin to shut down professionally. This is when I start to feel like I am burnt out in all areas of teaching, and I feel like I have no more to give, and I cannot add more to my plate. I am not engaged in school meetings, I feel my patience with others (adult or child) getting shorter and shorter, and mentally I'm exhausted. I often bring this home to my family, and I can often be short with my husband and children, or I am so mentally exhausted that I don't give them the attention that they deserve."
- *About what she needs to cope with compassion fatigue*: "I need a school leader who can recognize compassion fatigue and be willing to listen when I have compassion fatigue so that they understand that I am not at my best. It also has been beneficial when I work with a team of teachers who are willing to help take something off of my plate. At home, I ensure that I am getting proper rest and try to listen to my body and what it needs. This is when I try to increase self-care days, and I ensure that when I am at home, I am only focused on my family, and do not bring any work home with me."
- *About how the PDs on compassion fatigue were helpful*: "It is beneficial to have PDs on compassion fatigue, because I don't feel so alone. It helps to collaborate with other teachers and listen to them share what they are going through. The PDs on self-care is a great reminder of how important it really is to take care of yourself so that you can recharge and not feel that you have spread yourself too thin. Learning about the gratitude journal was beneficial, because it helped me put everything into perspective and taking time each day to list what I am grateful for allowed me to keep a positive attitude" (M. Romo, personal communication, August 1, 2021).

From Chelsea Nullier

- *About the stress of teaching students who have experienced trauma*: "It is very rewarding to teach students who have experienced trauma. They become so happy to be with me as the school year progresses, and I know that I am making a difference for them. But it is also so hard to teach these children. I know that I am not there to fix their trauma, but I want to so much. I put so much into them that it's almost like being their parent figure. Also, when you teach students with ACEs, you have to do so much more. You have to work really hard to connect with their families and you have to work so hard to connect with the child."

- *About what she needs to cope with compassion fatigue*: "Some of these kids have been so hurt that it is difficult for them to form relationships with adults, and sometimes they lash out at you when you start getting close to them. I pour my heart into these kids, and sometimes it hurts when they lash out at me for no apparent reason. It can be heart-wrenching. I need support from someone at school during these times. I need support at home. I try to focus on the positive. I use my gratitude journal, and I try to remember that whatever difficult behavior they show, it is not about me. I try really hard to not take it personally. I am always trying to understand their trauma and trying to keep in mind that the behavior is a result of what has happened to them. Sometimes I just need a break. I need someone to come into my classroom so that I can reset my mind when I am stressed out. Sometimes I also need someone to come into my classroom and supervise my class so that I can talk with a student who has become dysregulated to try to not only get him/her calm but to also repair our relationship if I have become dysregulated along with the child."
- *About how the PDs on compassion fatigue were helpful:* "I think that just becoming aware of compassion fatigue really helped. I also became more aware that our leadership really needs to understand that teachers need time for self-care. The gratitude journal was very helpful. I also became more aware of the need for self-care. The PDs offered me a word to explain what I was experiencing. Being able to share feelings in the PDs also was beneficial. I knew that I was not alone in my struggles. The PDs also helped us build a sense of community amongst the teachers. I think that it is really important that leadership is part of the PDs so that they understand it and they can understand what the teachers are going through. When it comes to coping with stress, it all filters down from the top. Does the principal support the teachers in managing stress? If so, then the teacher can better support the student in managing stress" (C. Nullier, personal communication, August 4, 2021).

Full Principal Response to the "Three Things" Which Teachers Shared

This response comes from Erin Probus, principal at another school in this author's school district. This PD series was implemented at the three elementary schools in this author's school district. Mrs. Probus agreed for her full response to be a part of this chapter. She sent the following response as an email to her teachers.

"I was impacted by last week's session regarding Compassion Fatigue. I believe that what we learned is very real and it describes the reality that comes with caring so deeply and serving so faithfully here at our school and in education. I was very appreciative of your professionalism and your willingness to be personally vulnerable in conversation with one another and in your honest feedback to me in your "I wish my principal knew" sheets.

"Your responses were compiled into a doc so I can see into some of the unspoken thoughts, feelings, needs, and emotions that swirl around the context of what we do here together each day at Hornet Park. My hope is that we can continue to unpack the weight of our work together, to learn techniques to keep our hearts and bodies healthy, and to create such a positive, supportive momentum that we carry one another if times get tough.

"In this sharing, open spirit, I wanted to let you in on a few things I wish you knew. This exercise is hard for me, like "hand me a tissue" hard...but here we go.

"I wish my school family staff knew...

- I put relentless pressure on myself to do my job with excellence. I worry about what you and others think of me and the quality of my work. All the time. When I make mistakes, I'm really really hard on myself. I punishingly play it over & over again in my mind because I never want to disappoint anyone.
- I believe that our school is a *wonderland*, but I know it is not always rainbows and unicorns. Trust me, I absolutely do. I want you to know that I try to field/absorb/protect you from as much of the "crap" that comes along as I possibly can. I share pain alongside you and it hurts me when you're hurting. It is my "normal" to feel generally upbeat, happy, and positive. However, I get down, feel stressed, and get hurt, too. During tough stuff, I try to switch back to being positive - not to minimize our problems. Instead, I just do it as quickly as I can muster it up because I feel like that is what I should do and it is how we get back on track.
- The pace of my day and the range of topics that cross my plate and mind throughout the day is crazy intense and frequently borderline overwhelming. I know that sometimes this might make me seem scattered and like a bit of a forgetful ding-bat. Just know... I've got this, but my mind has to play catch-up from time to time.
- Being a principal is such a gift, but I want you to know a secret...I still miss teaching and savor each opportunity to be in your classrooms because the classroom feels like "home" to me.
- I try to listen to your voices/needs and then be a person of action, but I need your help in that. If you don't tell me something is wrong or you need something, I don't know. If you share something that needs done, I will make every effort to do it.

"Thanks for listening. Thanks for being folks who I can trust with pieces of my heart!" (E. Probus, personal communication, September 2019).

Outcome of Full Professional Development Series

The teachers and principal at this author's school completed the survey again at the end of the PD series. Although the principals' responses stayed the same, the teacher responses showed significant improvement in these key areas at the conclusion of the PD program:

- 89% reported that they could remain calm with students (compared to 45% prior to PD series)
- 67% reported that they could manage their own level of stress adequately (compared to 50% prior to PD series)
- 89% reported that they felt supported by their building administrator (compared to 50% prior to PD series)

FUTURE RESEARCH DIRECTIONS

Although this plan helped the teachers and principals at this author's school, it would strengthen the results if this professional development series could be implemented at other schools to obtain more data. In addition, it would be worthwhile for this program to be used at the secondary level to find out if it was also effective with educators working with older students.

Further, this program relied heavily on qualitative data to validate its effectiveness. Future research with more quantitative data also seems warranted to strengthen its results. It would also be helpful if more information was known about the long-term effectiveness of the program, as well as if periodic revisiting of the topic of compassion fatigue could strengthen the long-term benefits.

CONCLUSION

There are many stressors that teachers face on a daily basis which has contributed to the current teacher shortage. For many of the issues, there is very little that can be done at the school level to change them, such as the federal and state mandates for high-stakes testing, etc. But for the impact of compassion fatigue, there are many strategies that the local school can implement to support teachers in understanding compassion fatigue and the need for self-care. In addition, building administrators can learn better ways to support teachers. Providing professional development about compassion fatigue and self-care is an important intervention in helping teachers to cope with the stress of being an educator and can build a sense of community within the school. In addition, it can help to build the administrator's capacity to better guide their teaching staff in more effective teaching and in creating an emotionally healthier work environment. With the pandemic continuing, the frequency and intensity of stress, anxiety, and depression are continuing to increase. It is expected that the level of trauma and the number of students who are experiencing trauma will continue to rise. Thus, a program like this to help teachers cope is even more valuable given the current situation.

ACKNOWLEDGMENT

This research was supported by the Lilly Endowment Comprehensive School Counseling Grant (grant number 2018 0229).

REFERENCES

Administration for Children & Families. (n.d.). *Secondary traumatic stress.* https://www.acf.hhs.gov/trauma-toolkit/secondary-traumatic-stress

Beddow, K. (2019, July 21). *Spilling coffee.* Calmer Classrooms. https://www.calmerclassrooms.co.uk/coffee/

BrunetteA. (2004). https://www.wcu.edu/WebFiles/PDFs/CEAP-HS-BK_Self-CareForTeachers.pdf

Buttner, A. (2021, April 19). *The state of the teacher shortage in 2021.* Frontline Education. https://www.frontlineeducation.com/blog/teacher-shortage-2021/

Day, C. (2020, January 4). *Making a vision book.* https://www.calvalynday.com/

Edelman, A. (2021, June 6). Biden wants to fix the nation's teacher shortage. Educators say the problem is worsening. *NBC News.*

Felitti, V. J., Anda, R. F., Anda, R. F., Nordenberg, D., Williamson, D. F., Spitz, A. M., Edwards, V., Koss, M. P., & Marks, J. S. (1998, May 1). Relationship of childhood abuse and household dysfunction to many of the leading causes of death in adults. *American Journal of Preventive Medicine, 14*(4), 245–258. https://www.ajpmonline.org/article/S0749-3797(98)00017-8/fulltext

Flannery, M. E. (2020, August 14). *Safety concerns over covid-19 driving some educators out of the profession.* NEA. https://www.nea.org/advocating-for-change/new-from-nea/safety-concerns-over-covid-19-driving-some-educators-out

Forbes, H. T. (2013). *Help for Billy: A beyond consequences approach to helping children in the classroom.* BookBaby.

Learning Policy Institute. (2021, March 4). *Covid-19 is worsening already critical teacher shortages, potentially jeopardizing school openings.* https://learningpolicyinstitute.org/press-release/covid-19-worsening-already-critical-teacher-shortages-potentially-jeopardizing-school

Lever, N., Mathis, E., & Mayworm, A. (2017). *School mental health is not just for students: Why teacher and school staff wellness matters.* Report on emotional & behavioral disorders in youth. https://www.ncbi.nlm.nih.gov/pmc/articles/PMC6350815/

Luster, J., & Luster, J. (2015). *Calm classroom: In thirty seconds to three minutes, help your students develop self awareness, mental focus, inner calm.* Luster Learning Institute.

Mielke, C. (2019). *The burnout cure: Learning to love teaching again.* ASCD.

Minero, E. (2017, October 4). *When students are traumatized, teachers are too.* Edutopia. https://www.edutopia.org/article/when-students-are-traumatized-teachers-are-too

Murphey, D., & Sacks, V. (2020, September 10). *Supporting students with adverse childhood experiences.* American Federation of Teachers. https://www.aft.org/ae/summer2019/murphey_sacks

National Association of Social Workers. (2021). https://www.socialworkers.org/about/ethics/code-of-ethics

Pffifferling, J. H., & Gilley, K. (2000). *Compassion fatigue self-assessment.* American Academy of Family Physicians. https://www.aafp.org/fpm/2000/0400/fpm20000400p39-rt1.pdf

Schwartz, K. (2016). *I wish my teacher knew: How one question can change everything for our kids.* Da Capo Lifelong Books, a member of the Perseus Books Group.

Siegel, D. J. (2015). *Brainstorm: The power and purpose of the teenage brain.* Penguin Books.

Starr Commonwealth. (2020, February 13). *The national institute for trauma and loss in children (TLC).* https://starr.org/programs/national-institute-for-trauma-and-loss-in-children-tlc/

Surcher, L., Darling-Hammond, L., & Carver-Thomas. (2016, September 15). *A Coming Crisis in Teaching? Teacher supply, demand, and shortages in the U.S.* Learning Policy Institute. https://learningpolicyinstitute.org/product/coming-crisis-teaching

The Pennsylvania State University. (2016, September). *Teacher health and stress.* https://www.prevention.psu.edu/uploads/files/rwjf430428-TeacherStress.pdf

Tutt, P. (2021, August 12). *You Can't Lead on Empty: Supporting School Staff with Vicarious Trauma.* Edutopia. https://www.edutopia.org/ article/ you – cant – lead – empty – supporting – staff – vicarious - trauma? Utm _ content = linkpos9 &utm _ source = edu – newsletter &utm _ medium = email &utm _ campaign = weekly – 2021 – 08 – 18 - A

van der Kolk, B. A. (2014). *The body keeps the score: Brain, mind, and body in the healing of trauma.* Penguin Books.

Walker, T. (2021, June 17). *Educators ready for fall, but a teacher shortage looms.* NEA. https://www.nea.org/advocating-for-change/new-from-nea/educators-ready-fall-teacher-shortage-looms

KEY TERMS AND DEFINITIONS

ACE Study: A longitudinal study by Vincent Felitti and Robert Anda in which the long-term effects of trauma in three major categories were documented.

ACEs: Adverse Child Experiences, a study done by Kaiser Permanente and the CDC. Principal authors were Vincent Felitti and Robert Anda. Documented the long-term effects of trauma in three major categories.

Adverse Childhood Experience: A traumatic event that occurred before the age of 18. Major categories of trauma studied were abuse, neglect, and family dysfunction.

Education: The act of teaching.

Educator: A person who educates.

Principal: The leader of a school.

Professional Development: Providing information to professionals about issues related to their field of work.

Stress: Feeling of being overwhelmed and unable to cope.

Teacher: One who teaches.

Teacher Shortage: The state of not having enough teachers to fill open positions.

Trauma: An event that is overwhelming to an individual, leading to a sense of being unable to cope and/or being fearful of his/her life. Trauma encompasses a variety of experiences and is perceived as being traumatic on an individual basis.

Trauma-Informed School Approach: A systemic approach to working with students that focuses on safety, relationships, and emotional regulation.

Chapter 8
A Critical Conversation About Mindfulness for School Leadership

Adrianne Wilson
University of Tampa, USA

ABSTRACT

The global COVID-19 pandemic has dramatically changed the scope of teaching and leading and has had negative effects on the academic outcomes for students. As a result of stress-induced demands provoked by this pandemic, school leaders are at an increased risk for physical, emotional, and mental health challenges. Recent studies about the pandemic's psychological impact on the general population reveal increased depression and stress levels. This chapter discusses ways university educational leadership programs can integrate self-care using mindfulness practice to effectively prepare aspiring school leaders. Practical approaches and resources for university programs are provided. In addition to suggestions for practical application, this chapter also discusses recommendations for universities and school districts regarding self-care for school leaders.

INTRODUCTION

Over the last decade, the pressures of the principalship have increased due to growing accountability measures associated with teacher and student performance (Wells, 2013; West et al., 2014, Wilson, 2021). Adding to the responsibilities of school administrators is the challenge of improving chronically low-performing schools or maintaining school performance at a satisfactory level. There are millions of students attending thousands of failing schools in the U.S., making it urgent to lessen the achievement gap (Fisher et al., 2011). Even prior to the pandemic, many students of color experienced barriers to educational opportunities; however, such disparities have been exacerbated by the pandemic. The novel COVID-19 global pandemic has magnified the racial, social, and economic inequities amongst students throughout the United States (Wilson, 2021).

DOI: 10.4018/978-1-6684-2334-9.ch008

Adding to the implications of the pandemic is the role of school administrators. School leaders' roles have dramatically morphed due to the COVID-19 crisis. Sudden shifts in response to this crisis have left school leaders in "triage-like" conditions, with either no playbook or a minimal one, to mitigate the challenges of leading schools. As seen across the United States, the pandemic resulted in abrupt school closures coupled with expedited transitions to online learning. Discussions in emerging literature indicate that such abrupt conversions from brick-and-mortar schooling to solely online modalities of learning will negatively impact educational outcomes. A recent study by the Annenburg Institute for School Reform projected that learning loss due to COVID-19 would "result in students likely returning in fall 2020 with approximately 63-68% of the learning gains in reading and with 37-50% of the learning gains in math relative to a typical school year (Wilson, 2021)."

In addition to the unfinished learning during the 2019 – 2020 school year, mental health challenges experienced by children and adolescents also increased. According to a 2020 Gallup poll, nearly three in ten parents surveyed indicated that their child was experiencing a level of "harm to their emotional or mental health, with 45% citing the separation from teachers and classmates as a major concern" (Calderon, 2020). Although most schools across the nation reopened their doors the following academic year, the impact of mental health challenges continues to linger. Unfortunately, due to logistical constraints, a workforce shortage, and uncertain budgets, resource disparities have left some districts unable to provide students with the needed mental health services. According to a 2021 survey conducted by the National Association of Elementary School Principals (NAESP), approximately 70% of school leaders indicated that they could not meet their students' mental health needs due to staff shortages (NAESP, 2021).

School leadership comes with a great deal of responsibility; however, there are limitations in educational leadership literature and research regarding how school leadership programs can adequately prepare candidates and current leaders on how to effectively manage the strains of work-related emotional weight and mental stress. School leaders are often faced with making significant decisions impacting the livelihood and educational outcomes of students. With such elevated levels of stress, leaders are often placed in emotionally demanding situations that can ultimately create a sense of secondary trauma and mental strain if not properly managed (Wilson, 2021). Furthermore, educational leadership literature supports the notion that work-related stress can present emotional, mental, medical, and physical concerns (Boyatzis & McKee, 2005; Murphy, 2011). As a result of the COVID pandemic, organizational management has intensified the stress levels for school administrators. A 2020 study conducted by the Yale Center for Emotional Intelligence (YCEI) and the New York Council of School Supervisors and Administrators (CSA), indicated that 95% of participants experienced unfavorable emotions in response to leading schools during the COVID-19 pandemic (Brackett et al., 2020). The study revealed that anxiety was the most mentioned emotion followed by feelings of being overwhelmed, stressed, sad, frustrated, and worried. In response to these emotions, survey results indicated that most school leaders felt as though they used a range of ineffective strategies to manage their anxiety (Brackett et al., 2020).

The negative emotions reported due to COVID19 have also impacted school principal retention rates, which is exacerbating an already challenging attrition crisis within the profession (Fink & Brayman, 2006; Levin et al., 2020; Pijanowski et al., 2009). For example, a 2020 poll conducted by the National Association of Secondary School Principals revealed that 45% of school administrators planned to accelerate their intentions to leave the profession due to demanding work conditions associated with COVID-19 (Farrace, 2020). The principalship is now regarded as a "job too big for one" and has perpetuated a culture of stress across the United States. Furthermore, a 2018 study indicated that school leaders with higher levels of emotional drain were more likely to experience increased negative emotions, leading to less job satisfaction and an increased likelihood of career change or early retirement (Brackett et al., 2018).

These recent reports on attrition suggests a new need to revisit how educational leadership programs and school districts prepare and support school leaders during times of crisis. Historically, educational leadership programs have been critiqued as needing improvements that reflect the modern-day responsibilities of school leadership. Critics argue that university school leadership programs offer curricula and preparation that are out of touch with modern-day realities associated with the role of school administration (Mahfouz, 2017). To address this need for improvement, the National Policy Board for Educational Administration adopted new professional standards for educational leaders in 2015. These new standards reflect the importance of "promoting each student's academic success and wellbeing;" however, they did not address the wellbeing of school leaders (National Policy Board for Educational Administration, 2018). In addition, prior research on educational reform has rarely considered educators' emotions (Hargreaves, 2001).

Due to such implications, this chapter offers practical strategies to guide educational leadership programs on methods for integrating mindfulness, emotional agility, and self-care practices into their curricula and program design. It is also important to note that for the purpose of this chapter, wellbeing is inclusive of emotional, mental, and physical (health) aspects.

BACKGROUND ON BURNOUT AND RESILIENCE

Due to the high demands of school leadership, most research regarding the profession includes a great deal of discussion and analysis regarding its retention rate. As stated earlier in this chapter, the 2021 NAESP survey reported that approximately 70% of school leaders felt they could not meet their students' mental health needs due to staff shortages because of the COVID-19 pandemic (NAESP, 2021). However, concerns regarding principal retention existed before COVID. According to a 2016-2017 executive summary prepared by the National Association of Secondary Principals (NASSP) and Learning Policy Institute (2019), the national average for principals' tenure in their schools was four years. A more recent national study of public-school administrators indicates nearly 18 percent of school leaders were no longer in the same position one year later (Levin & Bradley, 2019).

Furthermore, high-poverty schools suffered higher turnover rates at approximately 21 percent nationally (Levin & Bradley, 2019). These data indicate that it is challenging to discuss concerns of principalship retention without examining the root causes. Research points to five critical areas as trigger points for loss of retention: Poor working conditions, Insufficient salaries, Lack of decision-making authority, Inadequate preparation and professional development, and high-stakes accountability practices (Levin & Bradley, 2019).

Burnout

Stressors, such as those listed above by Levin and Bradley (2019), have ignited burnout in the educational leadership profession at skyrocketed numbers (DeMatthews et al., 2021). Burnout is often associated with job-related stress and can be an occupational hazard impacting one's personal and professional wellbeing. The American Institute of Stress (AIS) defines burnout as "a cumulative process marked by emotional exhaustion and withdrawal associated with increased workload and institutional stress (American Institute of Stress, 2021)." In their extensive literature review on leadership styles and workplace stress, Erskine and Georgiou (2017) define burnout as "a cluster of psychological factors best represented by emotional exhaustion, depersonalization (seeing others as more like objects than people), and reduced personal accomplishment (p.31).

Literature is robust with defining workplace burnout. However, a new term for burnout has been coined as a result of the heightened challenges exacerbated by the COVID-19 pandemic. Many front-line workers, including those in the education sector, have experienced the stress phenomenon, compassion fatigue. According to the AIS, compassion fatigue is the "emotional residue or strain of exposure to working with those suffering from the consequences of traumatic events and can be experienced through either one single incident or an accumulation of several (American Institute of Stress, 2021)." Compassion fatigue, a form of burnout, is "the gradual lessening of compassion over time" and is compounded due to the negative emotions associated with helping others at work (AIS, 2021). The difference between compassion fatigue and burnout is the origin. More specifically, compassion fatigue originates from dealing with victims of trauma, while burnout originates from occupational stressor associated with being overworked (Rauvola et al., 2019). While the two are similar, one can suffer from one and not the other. For example, someone working in sales with high demands to meet monthly quotas may suffer from burnout. In comparison, a nurse in the ICU unit of a hospital may suffer from compassion fatigue due to the high demands of caring for critically ill patients.

Compassion fatigue is mentioned in this chapter because those in "helping professions", such as teachers and school leaders, are commonly impacted by this type of burnout (Rauvola et al., 2019; AIS, 2021). More importantly, when considering self-care, it is imperative to understand the root cause(s) of work-related stressors and how to go about mitigating its negative impacts. Unfortunately, work-related burnout has severe costs for school leaders. The health of any given school is heavily predicated on the effectiveness of its leaders. The costly effects of burnout can stifle necessary school growth, which ultimately impacts student achievement. Effective leadership requires vision and a level of energy that sets the tone for the organization. It is extremely difficult to maintain a leadership presence when one is plagued with burnout with no end in sight. According to Maslach and Leiter (2004), cynicism and burnout have a strong correlation. Because cynicism is rooted in self-interest and manifests negative thinking, it can lead to dissonance leadership, which is discussed later in this chapter. Additionally, individuals who suffer from chronic burnout often experience emotional exhaustion, stress, mental anguish, and health issues (Maslach & Leiter, 2004). Understanding the correlation between burnout and stress and examining ways to help principals reduce the two is crucial for the profession.

Resilience

Contrary to burnout, resilience refers to one's ability to bounce back from difficult circumstances while becoming personally stronger than before the problem existed (Epstein & Krasner, 2013; Wells & Klocko, 2018). Resilience is cultivated over time and often shapes one's mindset in how they approach problems or difficult people. For example, a resilient mindset can alter an individual's attitude and actions to be more optimistic towards difficult situations that others may perceive negatively. A resilient mindset offers incredible power in being able to shift from negative to positive thought patterns. Understanding the importance and impact of resilience is crucial, not only for personal development but also for organizational leadership. For school leaders, work-related resilience is essential for helping faculty and staff overcome the many challenges of the profession. It is also equally important that school leaders take the time to build their own resilience as a means of self-care, thus reducing the likelihood of work-related burnout or compassion fatigue.

As described previously, resilience is a personal quality that predisposes individuals to bounce back in the face of loss. Resilient leaders, however, do more than bounce back—they bounce forward. Resilient school leaders take action that responds to new and ever-changing realities, even as they maintain the essential operations of the schools they lead (Reeves & Allison, 2009, 2010). Determined leaders remain focused and hopeful of their vision and are able to push through adversity and unexpected challenges. Furthermore, effective leaders maintain a growth mindset and look at challenges as an opportunity to strengthen their leadership capacity. According to the Educational Leadership Disposition Assessment (2010), an assessment used by university principal preparation programs, aspiring school leaders should demonstrate resilience in their professional work by showing persistence (grit), not giving up easily even when confronted with challenging situations, and by demonstrating a strong commitment and consistent follow through on tasks and responsibilities (Wilson et al., 2020).

As school leaders cultivate stronger resilience, they are able to demonstrate alternative responses to challenges that might otherwise derail them. Therefore, in contrast to burnout and compassion fatigue, compassion resilience is the "ability to maintain your physical, emotional and mental wellbeing while responding compassionately to the suffering of others (Beltman et al., 2011)." Compassion resilience is often referred to as a reservoir of wellbeing, based on self-care habits, that can be drawn from during short- and long-term difficult situations. Additionally, compassion resilience is essential in combatting fatigue and burnout.

UNDERSTANDING MINDFULNESS FOR SCHOOL LEADERS

When considering the emotional and mental stress associated with the principalship, mindfulness is one solution to assist in mitigating workplace burnout and compassion fatigue. Mindfulness is not a new concept within certain industries. For example, large corporations such as Nike, Google, General Mills, Target, Ford Motor Company, and Twitter have integrated employee-based mindfulness programs (Hunter, 2013). Although mindfulness-based intervention (MBI) programs may not be as widespread within the educational sector, school leaders can individually use such practices as a means of personal self-care to combat the secondary trauma, stress, and anxiety often associated with the profession. Kabat-Zinn (2003) operationally defines mindfulness as "the awareness that emerges through purposely paying attention, while also remaining in the moment (p.145). McKee et al. (2008) added, "People who deliberately practice mindfulness are consciously self-aware and self-monitoring; they are open and attentive to other people and the world around them (p. 113)." True mindfulness cultivates a state of alertness, allowing individuals to embrace their emotions rather than become stifled by them. In essence, mindfulness is a mental state that does not allow the mind to get caught up in the busyness of one's thoughts and emotions. Boyatzis and McKee (2005) support this understanding of mindfulness in their research by describing it as "the capacity to be fully aware of all that one experiences inside the self, body, mind, heart, spirit, and to pay full attention to what is happening around us (p. 113)." For school leaders, embracing such practices can be crucial for day-to-day decision-making as well as crisis management. Mindful leaders are not constrained by their emotional and mental strongholds but are willing to internally confront, analyze, and self-assess in order to use sound judgment in their leadership.

Fostering mindfulness reduces the likelihood of reactionary behaviors that can often lead to a cycle of "trigger-finger" responses based primarily on emerging thoughts and feelings and can reduce the pitfalls of compassion fatigue. Using mindful practice can interrupt habitual impulses and patterns of thinking, allowing for fresh perspectives and an uncluttered worldview. For example, instead of getting overwhelmed with anxiety, practicing mindfulness cultivates opportunities to self-examine why such emotions exist in the first place. As a result, we can be anxious and notice it without getting lost within it. In addition to strengthening leadership capacity, mindfulness is also proven to have physiological health benefits. In a study conducted by Dr. Richard Davidson at the University of Wisconsin, scientists used imaging devices to study how meditation practices cultivate compassion and equanimity. Study results indicated that mindfulness meditation positively impacted the brain by strengthening the neurological circuits that calm the part of the brain that triggers fear and anger. After eight weeks, the scientists concluded that parts of the brain that help form positive emotions became increasingly active (Davidson et al., 2003).

According to Stuart Shanker (2013), author of *Calm, alert and learning: Classroom strategies for self-regulation*, mindfulness practices include implementing and using self-regulatory methods to manage workplace stress, reframing stress-induced behaviors, recognizing and reducing stressors, and being responsive to the needs of those within the schooling environment.

The benefits of mindfulness are far too great to ignore. According to Boyatzis and McKee (2005), "people who deliberately practice mindfulness are consciously self-aware and self-monitor; they are attentive and open to other people and the world around them." In addition, mindfulness practices have shown to yield many physical, emotional, and psychological benefits, including improved health, decreased stress, stronger mental flexibility, better emotional regulation, and increased attention, which are all key factors influencing teacher performance and student academic success (Baer, 2015; Grossman et al., 2004; Jha et al., 2007).

Resonant Leadership

Similar to mindfulness, resonant leadership is a common leadership style that refers to individuals who are able to manage their own emotions, as well as those they are leading, in ways that promote successful outcomes (Boyatzis & McKee, 2005). Resonant leaders have an intuitive level of self-awareness and are conscious of how their actions can impact others. Resonant leadership serves as a conceptual framework for examining mindfulness as a form of self-care.

According to Boyatziz & McKee (2005), resonant leaders "are inspiring; demonstrate a positive, emotional tone of hope; are in touch with others and demonstrate compassionate understanding (p. 12)." They explain that high-performing leaders should be cautious of the "sacrifice syndrome, " a chronic cycle of giving too much of oneself when dealing with difficult situations (Boyatzis & McKee, 2005). Because education is an altruistic profession, engaging in self-sacrificial tendencies can be the norm. As good-hearted as it may appear, the sacrifice syndrome can be crippling and can lead to many ineffective leadership behaviors such as: blaming others, overreacting to problems, and acting out of character (Boyatzis & McKee, 2005). Furthermore, an uncentered leader can slip into dissonance if their emotional and mental capacities are left unchecked when responding to chronic stressors at work. Unlike resonant leadership, dissonant leaders (often referred to as authoritative or autocratic) tend to be emotionally distant from others, leading to a stressful work environment with heightened disengagement from employees (Erskine & Georgiou, 2017).

With surmounting responsibilities of school leaders, it is understandable how some principals fall susceptible to dissonant leadership. However, as this chapter suggests, university principal preparation programs should heavily consider their role in preparing aspiring leaders to care for their own social-emotional wellbeing.

Emotional Agility

Another critical attribute associated with mindfulness is emotional agility. Emotional agility, first introduced in the Harvard Business Review, is closely aligned to emotional intelligence, although they are not the same (David & Congleton, 2013). Popularized by Daniel Goleman in 1995, emotional intelligence focuses on self-awareness, motivation, self-regulation, and social skills. Essentially, "emotional intelligence refers to one's ability to recognize and manage one's emotions, as well as the emotions of others (Phipps and Prieto 2017, p. 57)." Like emotional intelligence, emotional agility focuses on approaching experiences mindfully and productively, which is paramount for the emotional resilience needed by school leaders.

In her book, "Emotional Agility: Get Unstuck, Embrace Change, and Thrive in Work and Life" (2016), Susan David describes emotional agility as having the capacity to distinguish environmental cues using the needed emotional response at a given time and then responding in a manner that alignments with an individual's values. Essentially, emotional agility is the ability to use accurate emotions during situations in a timely manner to receive the best outcome (Wilson, 2021). Similar to resilience, emotional agility helps individuals steer clear of negative and self-destructive thought patterns so that they can show up as their authentic selves. Understanding how to utilize such agility is also an important deterrent for compassion fatigue, which often incites feelings of helplessness during emotionally challenging times.

School leaders should consider using mindfulness practices to strengthen their emotional agility. Not only does it serve as a form of self-care, but it is also a mechanism for fostering a sense of care and concern for the workplace stressors teachers face. Key tenants of emotional agility include identifying negative emotions and thoughts; taking the necessary time to address and acknowledge the power and impact of such negativity; seeking alignment of one's true personal values; and responding intentionality in a manner that aligns to those values (David, 2016).

Self-Regulation

The last critical attribute of mindfulness mentioned in this chapter is self-regulation. Shanker (2013) refers to self-regulation as "how people manage stress, how much energy is expended due to stress, and how well individuals recover from difficult situations (pg. 5)." Self-regulation also aligns with resilience because both involve bouncing back from difficult situations. Regarding mindfulness, self-regulation is an essential component because it requires one to be self-aware of their emotions and thoughts while also choosing the best emotional and behavioral responses. Historically, stress management approaches for school leaders have primarily focused on reactive strategies instead of proactive methods involving wellness and self-care (Austin et al., 2005; Boyland, 2011; Van der Merwe & Parsotam, 2012; Wilson, 2021). However, current demands exacerbated by the COVID global pandemic have shed light on the deficits in the educational profession surrounding support for the social and emotional wellbeing of educators and school leaders.

Although self-regulation is a personal attribute, educational leadership programs can help to cultivate this characteristic in candidates through coursework and internship experiences. According to the literature, effective self-regulators "pay attention to tasks, persist through difficulties, demonstrate flexibility, and confidently believe that effort leads to positive outcomes (Wilson, 2021)."

PRACTICAL SELF-CARE MODELS FOR EDUCATIONAL LEADERSHIP PREPARATION

When considering self-care and the role of educational leadership preparation programs, there is abundant evidence suggesting that effective school leaders possess compassion, a sense of care, and emotional stability (Berson & Oreg, 2016; Louis & Murphy, 2017; Pijanowski et al., 2009; Tschannen-Moran & Gareis, 2004). For example, Wells (2016) showed how mindfulness promoted experiential learning and related it to leadership. Furthermore, Murphy (2011) suggested that mindfulness practice yields effective leadership by helping leaders gain perspective, be fully present, exercise resilience. Although mindfulness and social-emotional-based intervention programs have demonstrated positive effects on the wellbeing of leaders, this evidence is not yet reflected in state and national educational leadership standards, nor is it a requirement for licensing requirements for school leaders. Although mindfulness and self-care are not blatantly expressed in standards set forth by educational leadership accrediting bodies, there is empirical evidence of this work in literature, which will be discussed in the subsequent sections of this chapter. (Mohouz, 2017; Wells, 2013; Wells, 2015; Wilson, 2021). The remaining discussion of this chapter introduces practical approaches and essential questions for educational leadership university preparation programs and school districts to consider for rising and current school leaders.

Cultivating Awareness and Resilience in Education

The first practical model for discussion is the Cultivating Awareness and Resilience in Education (CARE) program, which has proven to be successful. CARE is a mindfulness-based professional development program initially developed by Patricia Jennings, Christa Turksma, and Richard Brown at the Garrison Institute. CARE was established to support teachers by increasing self-awareness and reflective practices to effectively manage their emotional wellbeing (Mahouz, 2017). CARE, which includes training on mindfulness, awareness, emotional skills, as well as caring and compassion skills, is based on the notion that educators need to be equipped with skills and strategies to facilitate a positive school climate conducive to student achievement (Jennings, 2011; Jennings et al., 2013). CARE includes a variety of practices based on adult learning best practices such as direct instruction, small group discussion, dyadic interaction, reflection, role-playing, experiential exercises, and mindful awareness practices (Jennings et al., 2013; Mahouz, 2017). Pilot studies conducted with approximately 300 participants have proven the CARE program to be effective for teachers in a number of areas such as improvements in teachers' wellbeing, efficacy, burnout, mindfulness, physical symptoms often associated with stress and emotional regulation (Jennings et al., 2013; Mahouz, 2017).

Emerging research surrounding the CARE program recently included a study with principals in a rural school district in central Pennsylvania. CARE for School Leaders involved 20 hours of group training over four weeks with a booster session four weeks after implementation. After completing the program, principals reported improvements in leadership skills, relationships, self-care, increased self-awareness, regulation of emotions, self-management, and self-compassion. Although these findings are promising, further research is needed to investigate the effects of mindfulness programs for school leaders by examining their links to teacher and student wellbeing and school climate (Mahouz, 2017).

Although CARE was initially created for K-12 classroom teachers, its emerging work for school leaders is promising. As stated previously, one method of orienting aspiring school leaders to mindfulness practices and its benefits on effective leadership is through university principal preparation programs. Scholars such as Dr. Caryn Wells, Professor at Oakland University's School of Education and Health Services, has successfully integrated mindfulness training into her university coursework and has publications highlighting her work in this area (Wells, 2013a; Wells, 2015).

Table 1. Components of CARE program

Program Components	Methods
Emotion Skills Instruction (40%)	Introduction to emotions, purpose, universal expressions, relevant brain research How emotions affect teaching/ learning Didactic information about positive and negative emotions Exploring bodily awareness of emotions Exploring individual differences in emotional experiences Mindful practice
Stress Reduction Practices (40%)	Body awareness reflection Mindful practice (breathing, movement, group awareness, role play)
Compassion Practices (20%)	Caring practice Mindful practice (listening partners)

Adapted From: Wilson, 2021

Compassion Resilience Toolkit

The second practical model is the Compassion Resilience Toolkit, which was created through collaborative work between Wisconsin Initiative for Stigma Elimination (WISE, 2021), Rodgers Health, and the Wisconsin Department of Public Instruction. Collective authors of the toolkit included classroom teachers, student services personnel, school leaders, and community mental health professionals. The purpose of the toolkit is to provide information, activities, and resources for school leaders and staff to understand, recognize, and minimize their experiences of compassion fatigue while learning effective strategies for increasing their personal compassion resilience as an educator. Although the toolkit is intended for K-12 school environments, it can also be used as a resource for university educational leadership preparation programs. For university programs, the toolkit can be used twofold. First, it can teach pre-service school leaders how to integrate compassion resilience within their school culture for faculty and staff. Additionally, principal preparation programs can use the toolkit as a resource for educating rising school leaders about mindful strategies that can be adopted into their self-care regiment.

The toolkit includes twelve sections that can each be implemented in 30–60-minute sessions. Sessions can be delivered in various formats such as small group circle conversations, large group presentations with breakouts for application discussions, small online groups, individual activities, and reflection, or a combination of all of these. The toolkit is designed for flexibility and can be customized based on the needs of any school's faculty, staff, and leadership. Each of the twelve sections includes a thorough facilitator guide and an applications activity section comprised of the following: key activity, wellness practice, circle agenda, core content visual, and supplementary activities. Additionally, the following topics are discussed in the twelve sections:

- Compassion in Action
- Wellness, Compassion Fatigue, Resilience, and Self-Compassion
- Compassion Fatigue Awareness, Connection to Trauma, and Assessments
- Systemic Drivers of Compassion Fatigue
- Expectations from Self and Others
- Compassionate Boundary Setting – Personal and Professional
- Contract for Positive Staff Culture
- Strategies – Mind
- Strategies – Spirit
- Strategies – Strength
- Strategies - Heart
- Compassionate Connections with Parents

Research on compassion resilience specifically for school leaders is sparse, indicating an overwhelming need to further explore resilience for administrators from a self-care framework than from a management construct. Although not exclusively for school leaders, the compassion resilience toolkit is a reliable resource that can be used within educational leadership programs to emphasize the importance of self-care as well as instruct candidates on effective strategies.

Educational Leadership Disposition Assessment

The last model for mindfulness that has proven to be instrumental for educational leadership programs is the Educational Leadership Disposition Assessment (EDLDA). Empirical research by Wilson et al. (2020) involved the development of a valid and reliable disposition assessment to assist educational leadership programs in preparing candidates for the interpersonal and intrapersonal aspects of the profession. The EDLDA includes fifteen educational leadership dispositional attributes with a range of descriptors characterizing behaviors at the needs improvement, developing, and meets expectations levels. Currently, this assessment is being utilized in several university educational leadership programs and includes many elements of mindfulness. In addition, most institutions use the EDLDA within their administrative internships and seminars since these two areas yield the most significant opportunities for candidates to demonstrate their dispositional capacity. The table below, which originally appeared in the manuscript, *Emotionally Agile Leadership Amid COVID-19* (2021), illustrates how mindfulness is integrated throughout the EDLDA assessment.

The EDLDA is a practical yet impactful resource for cultivating a healthy and positive habit of mind, which is imperative for school leadership preparation (Roeser et al., 2012; Wilson, 2021). Habits of mind are defined as "those dispositions toward behaving intelligently when confronted with problems, even when the answers to such problems are not immediately known (Costa & Kallinick, 2011, p. 1)." As a school leader, such habits include having a heightened level of awareness, nonjudgmentally reflecting on current, present, and past experiences, demonstrating flexibility and appropriate responsiveness when problem-solving, effective emotional regulation, demonstrating resilience during difficult situations, and demonstrating compassion and empathy towards others, which are all essential for healthy self-regulation and self-care (Jennings & Greenberg, 2009; Roeser, 2012; Wilson, 2021). Furthermore, the EDLDA helps rising school leaders strengthen their emotional agility, resonance, and resilience.

University preparation programs have found success in cultivating such habits by integrating the EDLDA into their programs. Most programs require students to complete an EDLDA self-evaluation upon being accepted into the program and at graduation, with the hopes of seeing growth over a span of time while in the program. Additionally, students receive coaching by the program director and their administrative mentor(s) during their internship experiences. It is through this systemic process that students can self-monitor their dispositional growth and areas of weakness, while also receiving feedback and coaching along the way.

Table 2. Educational leadership dispositions and mindful leadership

Educational Leadership Dispositions in EDLDA	Descriptors Reflecting Mindful Leadership
High Expectations	Demonstrates personal accountability for oneself as evidenced by modeling behaviors of high expectations
Relational	Possesses an ability to create positive and professional relationships with faculty, staff, and students by supporting others within and outside of their presence Demonstrates dedication towards building positive relationships with community stakeholders Creates a climate of respect and rapport amongst faculty, staff, and students
Positive Attitude	Demonstrates a growth mindset towards challenging tasks Anticipates and responds in a positive manner at all times
Conflict Resolution	Listens to understand conflict before acting or offering a resolution
Integrity	Demonstrates accountability for one's own behavior Accepts personal and professional accountability for the educational processes of the school
Possesses Professional Beliefs, Commitment, and Work Ethic	Promotes academic, social, and emotional success for all students
Adaptable	Differentiates leadership based on the different needs of those being led
Self-Aware of Strengths and Weaknesses	Demonstrates a level of maturity to self-reflect on strengths and weaknesses Is able to accurately self-assess to identify weaknesses in order to improve leadership capacity
Determined/Perseverance	Demonstrates persistence (grit) and does not give up easily even when confronted with challenging situations Demonstrates strong commitment and consistent follow through on tasks and responsibilities

Adapted From: Wilson et al., 2020

RECOMMENDATIONS FOR EDUCATIONAL LEADERSHIP SELF-CARE

Cultivating principals' social and emotional wellbeing is paramount to effective school leadership and impacts a leader's ability to achieve and maintain a positive school climate. Educational leadership preparation programs can increase effectiveness by including social-emotional competencies that prepare future school leaders. School leaders usually do not take the necessary time for self-care, nor is it heavily promoted within the profession. For this reason, the following recommendations are provided based on recommendations from research on school leadership burnout and self-care.

- Preparation programs and school districts can emphasize and develop a culture of self-care for school administrators. For example, set aside time during the workday and afterwork hours for principals to engage in peer support. Leaders should not be made to feel guilty for taking time to invest in their own wellbeing (Barnet & Cooper, 2009; DeMatthews et al., 2021; Sogunro, 2012; Wilson, 2021).
- School districts should consider investing in training for all school leaders (assistant principals, principals, coaches, etc.) on topics related to burnout and self-care strategies (DeMatthews et al., 2021; Oplatka, I. 2017).
- State and national accrediting bodies should consider including the wellbeing of school leaders in state and national educational leadership standards. Doing so will create momentum for university coursework for educational leadership programs (Bamonti et al., 2014; Murphy et al., 2017; Wilson, 2021).
- University preparation programs should integrate social-emotional practices into coursework where candidates can learn mindfulness and stress management techniques such as mindful walking, mindful listening, centering, wait time, breathing, and self-compassion practices (Klocko & Wells, 2015).
- University preparation programs should also establish networks for collaboration with local school districts that include coaching and mentoring for aspiring school leaders (Gordon et al.,2016; Green, 2013).
- To support the importance of work-life balance, preparation programs and school districts should support leaders by encouraging annual planning, where leaders are able to effectively map out their schedules and commitments for the school year (DeMatthews et al., 2021; Etzion, D. 2003).
- Lastly, university preparation programs should consider facilitating collaborative learning models using the suggested resources (CARE program, compassion resilience toolkit, EDLDA) in this chapter to allow candidates to study real-life and situational dilemmas where they can engage in mindful practice (Mahfouz, 2017; Wilson, 2021).

Essential Questions to Consider

The implications discussed in this chapter raise questions about the modernization of university programs and measures of effectiveness in preparing future school leaders for the realities of the profession. The following essential questions can serve as a guide for educational leadership programs looking to improve their curriculum.

- How has the principalship role changed within the past five to seven years? Does your program's curriculum reflect those changes?
- What work demands do principals currently face in their professional roles? How does your program address these challenges to prepare aspiring school leaders?
- In what ways does your program address the social-emotional needs of school leaders?
- What resources are used in your program to address the importance of self-care?
- What percentage of your graduates have exited the profession due to stress-related issues?
- How does your program's curriculum reflect opportunities for candidates to demonstrate mindfulness, resilience, emotional agility, and compassion?

- What partnerships does your program have with local school districts and professional organizations to create support networks for current and aspiring school leaders?
- How does your program's internship provide opportunities for candidates to understand, experience, and demonstrate stress management?

CONCLUSION

As a result of the COVID-19 pandemic and associated stressors, adverse outcomes regarding the emotional wellbeing and retention for school leaders are concerning (Boyatzis & McKee, 2005; Brackett et al., 2018; Brackett et al., 2020; Farrace, 2020; Murphy, 2011). To mitigate these negative outcomes and prepare educators for the realities of the profession, educational leadership programs throughout the U.S. can engage current and aspiring school leaders in professional development that focuses on social-emotional wellbeing through the use of mindfulness practices and mindfulness-based programs. These interventions have proven positive effects on cultivating emotional intelligence, emotional agility, resonant leadership, and social intelligence, (Avolio & Gardner, 2005; Browne et al., 2003; Grubb & Flessa, 2006; Hawk & Martin, 2011; Mahfouz, 2017; Petzko, 2008; Shanker, 2016; Wells, 2015; Wilson, 2021).

To prepare school leaders, coursework in principal prep programs should include a focus on self-regulatory practices to include reframing behaviors, recognizing stressors, reducing stressors, and developing personal strategies to respond to stressors to promote restoration and resilience (Shanker, 2016). A variety of recommendations and resources are provided in this chapter to reduce the impact of stressors that often lead to burnout and compassion fatigue amongst school leaders. In addition, to preserve and strengthen the ranks of school leadership, preparation programs should strongly explore integrating social-emotional leadership competencies within their coursework that includes mindfulness, stress management techniques, networks for mentorship, and collaborative models of learning.

REFERENCES

Avolio, B.J., & Gardner, W.L. (2005). Authentic leadership development: getting to the root of positive forms of leadership. *The Leadership Quarterly*, *16*(3), 315-338.

Bamonti, P. M., Keelan, C. M., Larson, N., Mentrikoski, J. M., Randall, C. L., Sly, S. K., Travers, R. M., & McNeil, D. W. (2014). Promoting ethical behavior by cultivating a culture of self-care during graduate training: A call to action. *Training and Education in Professional Psychology*, *8*(4), 253 - 260. doi:10.1037/tep0000056

Barnett, J., & N. Cooper. (2009). Creating a culture of selfcare. *Clinical Psychology: Science and Practice*, *16*(1), 16 – 20. . doi:10.1111/j.1468-2850.2009.01138.x

Beltman, S., Mansfield, C., & Price, A. (2011). Thriving not just surviving: A review of research on teacher resilience. *Educational Research Review*, *6*(3), 185 – 207. doi:10.1016/j.edurev.2011.09.001

Berson, Y. & Oreg, S. (2016). The role of school principals in shaping children's values. *Psychological Science*, *27*(12), 1539 – 1549.

Boyatzis, R., & McKee, A. (2005). *Resonant leadership*. Harvard Business School Press.

Brackett, M., Cannizarro, M., & Levy, S. (2020). *The pandemic's toll on school leadership is palpable. Here's what is needed for a successful school year*. Retrieved from: https://www.edsurge.com/news/2020-07-16-the-pandemic-s-toll-on-school-leaders-is-palpable-here-s-what-s-needed-for-a-successful-school-year

Brackett, M. A., Floman, J. L., & Bradley, C. (2018). *Emotion revolution for education leaders - survey*. Unpublished data. Yale University.

Brown, K. W., & Ryan, R. M. (2003). The benefits of being present: Mindfulness and its role in psychological wellbeing. *Journal of Personality and Social Psychology*, *84*(4), 822 – 848. doi: . doi:10.1037/0022-351484.4.822

Calderon, V. J. (2020, June 1). *U.S. Parents Say COVID-19 Harming Child's Mental Health*. Gallup. https://news.gallup.com/poll/312605/parents-say-covid-harming-child-mental-health.aspx

Compassion Resilience Toolkit. (2021, May 10). https://compassionresiliencetoolkit.org/

Costa, A. L., & Kallinick, B. (2020, September 12). *Describing 16 habits of mind*. https://www.habitsofmindinstitute.org

David, S., & Congleton, C. (2013, November). Emotional agility. *Harvard Business Review*. https://hbr.org/2013/11/emotional-agility

David, S. A. (2017). *Emotional agility: get unstuck, embrace change, and thrive in work and life*. Penguin Life Publishing.

Davidson, R.J. (2003). Alterations in Brain and Immune Function Produced by Mindfulness Meditation. *Psychosomatic Medicine*, *65*(1), 564 – 570.

DeMatthews, D., Carrola, P., Reyes, P., & Knight, D. (2021). School Leadership Burnout and Job-Related Stress: Recommendations for District Administrators and Principals. *The Clearing House: A Journal of Educational Strategies, Issues and Ideas*, *94*(4), 159–167. doi:10.1080/00098655.2021.1894083

Epstein, R. M., & Krasner, M. S. (2013). Physician resilience: What it means, why it matters, and how to promote it. *Academic Medicine*, *88*, 301 – 303. doi:10.1097/ACM.0b013e31828cff0

Erskine, J. A. K., & Georgiou, G. J. (2017). *Leadership Styles: Employee Stress, Well being, Productivity, Turnover and Absenteeism*. Understanding Stress at Work.

Etzion, D. (2003). Annual vacation: Duration of relief from job stressors and burnout. *Anxiety, Stress, and Coping*, *16*(2), 213 – 26. . doi:10.1080/10615806.2003.10382974

Farrace, B. (2020, June 3). *Principals say pandemic conditions are accelerating their plans to leave the profession*. https://blog.nassp.org/2020/08/21/principals-say-pandemic-conditions-are-accelerating-their-plans-to-leave-the-principalship/

Fink, D., & Brayman, C. (2006). School leadership succession and the challenges of change. *Educational Administration Quarterly*, *42*, 62 – 89. doi:10.1177/0031316

Fisher, Frey, & Lapp. (2011). Focusing on the Participation and Engagement Gap: A Case Study on Closing the Achievement Gap. *Journal of Education for Students Placed at Risk, 16*, 56 – 64.

Glass, T. E., Bjork, L., & Brunner, C. C. (2000). *The study of the American school superintendency, 2000: A look at the superintendent of education in the new millennium*. American Association of School Administrators.

Gordon, S. P., Oliver, J., & Solis, R. (2016). Successful innovations in educational leadership preparation. *International Journal of Educational Leadership Preparation, 11*(2), 51 – 70.

Green, R. L. (2013). A response to the call for effective leadership in today's schools: Three essentials: preparation, competency, and dispositions. *National Forum of Applied Educational Research Journal, 26*(1&2), 3 – 16.

Grubb, W. N., & Flessa, J. J. (2006). A job too big for one: Multiple principals and other nontraditional approaches to school leadership. *Educational Administration Quarterly, 42*(4), 518 – 550. doi:10.1177/0013161X06290641

Gyatso, T. (2021, April 26). The Monk in the Lab. *The New York Times*. https://www.nytimes.com/2003/04/26/opinion/the-monk-in-the-lab.html

Hargreaves, A. (1998). The emotional politics of teaching and teacher development: with implications for educational leadership. *International Journal of Leadership in Education, 1*(4), 315 – 336.

Hargreaves, A. (2001). Emotional geographies of teaching. *Teachers College Record, 103*(6), 1056 – 1080. . doi:10.1111/0161-4681.00142

Hawk, N., & Martin, B. (2011). Understanding and reducing stress in the superintendency. *Educational Management Administration and Leadership, 39*(3), 364 – 389. doi:10.1177/17411432039400

Hunter, J. (2013, April). Is mindfulness good for business? *Mindful Magazine*, 52-59.

Jennings, P. A., Frank, J. L., Snowberg, K. E., Coccia, M. A., & Greenberg, M. T. (2013). Improving Classroom Learning Environments by Cultivating Awareness and Resilience in Education (CARE): Results of a Randomized Controlled Trial. *School Psychology Quarterly, 28*(4), 374–390. . doi:10.1037/spq0000035

Jennings, P. A., & Greenberg, M. (2009). The prosocial classroom: Teacher social and emotional competence in relation to child and classroom outcomes. *Review of Educational Research, 79*, 491–525.

Kabat-Zinn, J. (2003). Mindfulness-based interventions in context: Past, present, and future. *Clinical Psychology: Science and Practice, 10*(2), 144–156. doi:10.1093/clipsy.bpg016

Klocko, B., & Wells, C. (2015). Workload Pressures of Principals: A Focus on Renewal, Support, and Mindfulness. *NASSP Bulletin, 99*(4), 332–355. Advance online publication. doi:10.1177/0192636515619727

Kuhfeld, Soland, Tarasawa, Johnson, Ruzek, & Liu. (2020, June 13). *Projecting the potential impacts of COVID-19 school closures on academic achievement*. . doi:10.26300/cdrv-yw05

Leiter, M. P., & Maslach, C. (2004). *Areas of worklife: A structured approach to organizational predictors of job burnout. In Emotional and Physiological Processes and Positive Intervention Strategies* (Vol. 3). doi:10.1016/S1479-3555(03)03003-8

Levin, S., & Bradley, K. (2019). *Understanding and Addressing Principal Turnover: A Review of the Research.* National Association of Secondary School Principals.

Levin, S., Scott, C., Yang, M., Leung, M., & Bradley, K. (2020, June 13). *Supporting a Strong, Stable Principal Workforce: What Matters and What Can be Done.* Retrieved from: https://www.nassp.org/wordpress/wp-content/uploads/2020/04/LPI-and-NASSP-Research-Agenda-Final-Report.pdf

Louis, K.S. & Murphy, J. (2017). Trust, caring, and organizational learning: the leader's role. *Journal of Educational Administration, 55*(1), 103 – 126.

Mahfouz, J. (2017). Mindfulness Training for School Administrators: effects on wellbeing and leadership. *Journal of Educational Administration, 56*(6), 602 –619.

McKee, A., Boyatzis, R., & Johnston, F. (2008). *Becoming a resonant leader: Develop your emotional intelligence, renew your relationships, sustain your effectiveness.* Harvard Business Press.

Murphy, J., Louis, K. S., & Smylie, M. (2017). Positive school leadership: How the Professional Standards for Educational Leaders can be brought to life. *Phi Delta Kappan, 99*(1), 21 – 24. . doi:10.1177/0031721717728273

Murphy, J. T. (2011). Dancing in the rain: Tips of thriving as a leader in tough times. *Phi Delta Kappan, 93*, 36-41.

NAESP Releases Results of Midyear National Principal Survey on COVID-19 in Schools. (2021, February 20). Retrieved from: https://www.naesp.org/news/naesp-releases-results-of-midyear-national-principal-survey-on-covid-19-in-schools/

Oplatka, I. (2017). Principal workload: Components, determinants and coping strategies in an era of standardization and accountability. *Journal of Educational Administration, 55*(5), 552–68. . doi:10.1108/JEA-06-2016-0071

Petzko, V. (2008). The perceptions of new principals regarding the knowledge and skills important to their initial success. *NASSP Bulletin, 92*(3), 242-250. . doi:10.1177/0192636508322824

Phipps, S. T. A., & Prieto, L.C. (2017). Why Emotional Intelligence Is Necessary For Effective Leadership: Know the four reasons! *Leadership Excellence, 34*(6), 56 – 57.

Pijanowski, J.C., Hewitt, P.M. & Brady, K.P. (2009). Superintendents' perceptions of the principal shortage. *NASSP Bulletin, 93*(2), 85 – 95.

Rauvola, R. S., Vega, D. M., & Lavigne, K. N. (2019). Compassion Fatigue, Secondary Traumatic Stress, and Vicarious Traumatization: A Qualitative Review and Research Agenda. Occupational Health Science, 3, 297–336. doi:10.100741542-019-00045-1

Reeves, D. B., & Allison, E. (2009). *Renewal coaching: Sustainable change for individuals and organizations.* Jossey-Bass.

Reeves, D. B., & Allison, E. (2010). *Renewal coaching workbook*. Jossey-Bass.

Roeser, R., Skinner, E., Beers, J., & Jennings, P. (2012). Mindfulness Training and Teachers' Professional Development: An Emerging Area of Research and Practice Child Development Perspectives. *Child Development Perspectives, 6*(2), 167-173. doi:10.1111/j.1750-8606.2012.00238.x

Shanker, S. (2013). *Calm, alert and learning: Classroom strategies for self-regulation*. Pearson.

Shanker, S. (2020, June 20). *What is Shanker Self-Reg?* www.self-reg.ca/self-reg

Sogunro, O. A. (2012). Stress in school administration: Coping tips for principals. *Journal of School Leadership, 22*, 664 – 700.

Sorenson, R. D. (2007). Stress management in education: Warning signs and coping mechanisms. *Management in Education, 21*(3), 10 – 13. doi:10.1177/089202607077985

Tschannen-Moran, M., & Gareis, C. R. (2004). Principals' Sense of Efficacy. *Journal of Educational Administration, 42*, 573 – 585. . doi:10.1108/09578230410554070

Wells, C. M. (2013a). Educational leaders describe a job too big for one: Stress reduction in the midst of leading. *AASA Journal of Scholarship & Practice, 10*(3), 32 – 45.

Wells, C.M. (2015). Conceptualizing Mindful Leadership in Schools: How the Practice of Mindfulness Informs the Practice of Leading. *Education Leadership Review of Doctoral Research, 2*(1).

West, D. L., Peck, C. M., Reitzug, U. C., & Crane, E. A. (2014). Accountability, autonomy, and stress: Principal responses to superintendent change in a large U.S. urban school district. *School Leadership & Management, 34*, 372 – 39. doi:10.1080/136324.2014.928683

What is Stress. (2021, September 18). *American Institute of Stress*. https://www.stress.org/

Wilson, A.G. (2021). Emotionally Agile Leadership Amid COVID-19. *School Leadership Review, 15*(2).

Wilson, A. G., Almerico, G., Johnston, P., & Ensmann, S. (2020). Examining Educational Leadership Dispositions: A Valid and Reliable Assessment of Leadership Dispositions. *Journal of Educational Leadership Preparation, 15*(1).

Wisconsin Initiative for Stigma Elimination. (2021, September 18). https://compassionresiliencetoolkit.org/schools/compassion-resilience/

ADDITIONAL READING

Boodgen, T. (2018). *Take Time for You: Self-Care Action Plans for Educators*. Solution Tree Press.

Murphy, J. (2018). *Dancing in the Rain: Leading with Compassion, Vitality, and Mindfulness in Education*. Harvard Education Press.

KEY TERMS AND DEFINITIONS

Burnout: A stress-induced occupational hazard due to an accumulation of high work demands over time.

Compassion Fatigue: The lessening of compassion over time due to overexposure to traumatic event(s).

Compassion Resilience: The capacity to act effectively during traumatic events or difficult situations using appropriate strategies and emotional responses.

Disposition: The attitude and personality of an individual based on beliefs, habits of thinking, and experiences.

Emotional Agility: The capacity to respond appropriately emotionally in a manner that aligns with one's values.

Mindful Practice: Active approaches that one can engage in to foster a mental state of being fully aware of thoughts, emotions, and bodily reactions.

Mindfulness: A mental state of being where one is fully aware of thoughts, emotions, and bodily reactions in a manner of being present and in the moment.

Mindfulness-Based Intervention: Programs designed to teach individuals how to use strategies for reducing stress, mental health concerns, and emotional imbalance.

Chapter 9
Spiritual Self-Care for Academic Excellence

Sonika Singh
https://orcid.org/0000-0002-5603-7772
DIT University, India

Gagan Singh
https://orcid.org/0000-0003-1143-8764
DIT University, India

ABSTRACT

Our thoughts decide our personality. Our idea of life arrays the complete quality our life. The off-base idea of life is the root of conflict within the life, wherein the cost of inattention is devastating. All our worries are due to spiritual unawareness which needs to be taken care of for excelling in a field. One can have success, but solace and satisfaction would only come if that success is attained through hard work by a pure mind. Science teaches us physical laws that govern the material world but knowledge of absolute or true understanding comes through discrimination which is a byproduct of leading a spiritual life. Yoga of synthesis in our thoughts, beliefs, and action is the only key for any student to practice upon to bear maximum fruits of his efforts and enjoy a holistic development for his bright career and a peaceful life.

INTRODUCTION

One can have success but solace and satisfaction would only come if that success is attained through hard work by a pure mind. Science teaches us physical laws that govern the material world but knowledge of absolute or true understanding comes through discrimination which is a byproduct of leading a spiritual life. The evacuation of numbness and sign of inward heavenly nature driving to God consciousness are consummate through Yoga. There are four primary Yogas(Complete Works of Swami Vivekananda, 2013):

DOI: 10.4018/978-1-6684-2334-9.ch009

- Yoga of knowledge; it is called Jnana Yoga;
- Yoga of Devotion; it is called Bhakti Yoga
- Yoga of Contemplation; it is called Raja Yoga
- Yoga of Work; it is called Karma Yoga

Each Yoga is a self-directed implies of grasping God. But since each Yoga includes the growth of one of the assets such as motive, feeling or will; a mixture of all the four Yogas is important for the all all round growth and emerging a wholesome character of a student. Now the question arises, how to bring this Yoga of Synthesis into practice in our daily lives? So, the aspirant must prepare himself for the reception of this highest knowledge which is the 'Key' to unlock not only the school or college examination but to crack the hardest of life examination because now he has learnt the life arithmetic, now he can easily balance the left hand side and right hand side of any hard life equations. He has mastered himself and such person can master any life problem or overcome any struggle very easily, not losing his inner peace at any point of time. Yoga of synthesis(Complete Works of Swami Vivekananda, 2013) in our thoughts, beliefs and action is the only key for any student to practice upon to bear maximum fruits of his efforts and enjoy a holistic development for his bright career and a peaceful life. Engineering the outside world can create comfort and convenience only but engineering your interior can create academic well-being and excellence. Our fatigued and exhausted mind driven by various forces like newspapers, e-mails, mobiles and internet demands rest. In fact, there is subtle working of mind in dream also so we do not get rest even during leap. Driven by so many sensual forces are fatigued and exhausted mind needs rest to rejuvenate itself which can only be attained through meditation.

The world is a grand moral gymnasium wherein we have all to take exercise so as to become stronger and stronger spiritually. (Swami Vivekananda (C.W., I: 80).

The youth of any country is the vital force and asset for its growth and development. Until and unless the students of a country are focused in right direction the country cannot grow. To keep them in the right path 'Yoga' which means union with the vital force is ultimately required. Man is a triune being. He has a hand, a heart and a head.

1. The hands are our instruments to practice Karma Yoga and leads which leads us to The Path of Action. Here one uses his body or physical action to reach to the Ultimate.
2. The heart is our instrument to practice Bhakti Yoga which leads us to The Path of Devotion. Here one uses his emotions to reach to the Ultimate.
3. The head is our instrument to practice Jnana Yoga which leads us to The Path of Intelligence. Here one uses his intelligence to reach to the Ultimate.

The three works in unification i.e. what the head says, the heart believes and finally hands do the action and the work is manifested.

Yoga is simply the science of aligning these three dimensions. For most of the people head is saying something else, heart is feeling something else, body is altogether going in a different direction, making every work to be a perfect mess! Unless and until the trio i.e. head, heart and hands work in unification we cannot have a holistic development of the child, there will be only confusion and anxieties resulting if the three don't work in harmony. This is exactly what we see most of the teenagers and even elders are going through these days. But to tune up the body, mind and energies at a later age becomes difficult, because by then all impressions of our habits become strong and it becomes hard to change; as a result every day we are stuck with one or another problem. So, we strongly need to practice to unite these three types of yoga into our daily living, especially at an early age; only then we will be able to touch the zenith of our ultimate nature. *Yoga of synthesis in our thoughts, beliefs and action is the only key for any student to practice upon to bear maximum fruits of his efforts and enjoy a holistic development for his bright career and a peaceful life.*

Now the question arises, how to bring this Yoga of Synthesis into practice in our daily lives? So, the aspirant must prepare himself for the reception of this highest knowledge which is the 'Key' to unlock not only the school or college examination but to crack the hardest of life examination because now he has learnt the life arithmetics, now he can easily balance the left hand side and right hand side of any hard life equations. He has mastered himself and such person can master any life problem or overcome any struggle very easily, not losing his inner peace at any point of time.

A student's head heart and hands not working in agreement leads to non-alignment of his physical make-up; they are either candidly testy or presumptuous due to their scholarly capability or riches. This is the features of an unmanageable mind- a mind that is divided into little pieces of deeds and manner due to the non-aligned character which finally tends to a ominous character and sometimes take ruthless forms. For such students' full expectations don't get settled they are unable to control their thoughts and emotions and start living a secluded life and develop suicidal tendencies too.

Thus to break the ice before it gets very late it is very important to integrate the mind into a gestalt (i.e. organized whole) at an early age of the student. This highest integration of mind is achieved through '*Dhyana*' or meditation(Krishnananda, 2018).

To start meditation a serene in mind is the basic requirement. Goldsmith converts an eighteen carat gold into a pure twenty-four carat gold by adding acids and burning it several times in the crucible. Similarly, we too can purify our census mind through concentration, reflection on the works of spiritual receptor following the teachings of our Guru or Master and Meditation.

"Max Muller writes: one pointedness of mind is impossible for us when our minds are diverted in various directions through newspapers, e-mails, mobiles and internet". We need to remove the oscillations of mind to get one pointedness of mind in order to be in peace and enhance our concentration power. This is the key to success and to lead a peaceful life otherwise we will always be living in pieces and lead and unsatisfactory life.

Fatigue of senses demands rest. Our five senses have their doors outwards, for example eye can see objects outside beautiful or ugly, ears can hear outside good or bad and so on. So there is no scope and time for us to look into ourselves inwards, that is the biggest reason of our fault finding nature and every time putting blame on others. Moreover, the internet and fast communication media has all the more contributed in making our minds busy with the unending stuff of news, movies, advertisements out of which 80% we don't even require to see or know. Our mind continuously moves about in the avenues of the senses through the force of desires.

THE NEED FOR AN ATTITUDINAL CHANGE

There's an overwhelming requirement for an alter in our characters. We got to talk about the overwhelming subject of motivations behind all subjectivity. Some questions which come to our mind as:

'What is the perfect time, when I can do the best work'?
To resolve this, the answer given so unfavorable is:
'At the time when I get enough money.'

But it can be realized easily that money cannot be the only reason to frame out the best work from the individuals. Money is only one thing, which can amend in everyone state of mind, the amend included in one's sense of respect, the pride in doing a specific work within the benefit of the country(Russell, 2016). That's a more prominent and inborn inspiration than only money. Money inspiration, un-supported by other higher inspirations, changes over individuals into hired soldiers which work as it were for cash. Typically, the attitudinal alter is to be accomplished in a huge way. No work is giant or little; individual state of mind makes it so. You'll do an attendant work with an attendant's understanding. But if you do the attendant's work with an officer understanding, then the consequences will be there.

ROLE OF TEACHERS IN INCULCATING SPIRITUALITY AMONG THEIR STUDENTS

An educator must create that vitality in his students and grip it in every student.

A teacher should not only to teach but also should be the source of inspiration for the students; he or she is the role model for the students, hence he should cultivate the ethics and values within the students, so that they may be prepare to be the ideal citizen and be ready to take the responsibilities to take care of their nation at large. The instructor has to tell their students the contrast between a person and an individual. As a person, you're a genetically constrained substance, kept to yours possess likes and disdains, your own wants, your claim aspirations. But as before long as you gotten to be an individual, you grow, you're able to enter into the life of other individuals conjointly or in other words you expand.

That's the contrast between singularity and character. Character may play the greater role than individuality.

ROLE OF VEDANTA TEACHINGS FOR ACADEMIC EXCELLENCE

Vedanta always emphasizes a levelheaded, addressing state of mind. In this manner, our teaching must offer help our children to create such a basic, logical, truth looking for character.

- How to identify the truth?
- How to lead a genuine life?
- How to differentiate between true and untrue life?

Vedanta is able to find the answer of these questions. Vedanta tells us the reality of life, it describes the balance between the life and work. It may be great help for students to develop the most noteworthy qualities within their mind, which may be the great asset to the individual and the nation at last.

The Vedanta, underlines the truth of our fundamental unity. It is one and the same Sakti or Divine Vitality, that courses through each and every being, says Vedanta. Subsequently, love and concern for others becomes a by-product of this spiritual growth from individuality to personality.

An aspirant who follows the path of Vedanta must follow the four "pillars of knowledge" which is uniquely called as 'sadhana chatushtaya(Brahmananda, 2000)',in vedantic terminology and helps in developing the rarest skills of patience and intrinsic intelligence in a student having higher goals for life. These four principles to be acquired as an initial preparation to achieve his goals of excellent academic performance and rising high in his career and spiritual life are:

1. Discrimination (*viveka*) – It gives the power to discriminate between the real and the unreal, permanent and the impermanent and acts like a sieve. It helps the student to reject aall undesired things in his life and select what is desirable for him
2. Dispassion (*vairagya*) – once the student has developed discrimination, it becomes very easy for him to overcome attractions and aversions, helping them to become more dispassionate. It doesn't mean abandoning of one's duties or responsibilities in daily life. It also doesn't mean living a secluded life on the foothills of Himalayas. It means mental detachment from all connections of the world. An individual can perform his best when he is at inner peace with himself.
3. Six virtues (*shatsampat*) - these are six qualities necessary for a student to enter in to learn deeper meanings of life and he rises much higher than his fellow colleagues. These are tranquility, training of the senses, withdrawal, forbearance, faith and focus. n.
4. Longing (*mumukshutva*) -this is the greatest longing for liberation and is above all the superficial desires. When an aspirant rises in his spiritual practices he goes beyond the desires of this mundane world and cannot be bound by the attachments and distractions of this superficial world. Nobody can then stop him realize his goals.

The four pillars of knowledge as mentioned above can easily be practiced and realized by a student if he he starts realizing his own strength. The same ideology is given by Swami Vivekananda which has helped the youth and mankind to realise his own supreme self. Few of his teachings are:

- ***To realise potential divinity of the soul:*** Brahman is innate in all creatures. But owing to ignorance, a man identifies himself with his body and runs after the pleasure of senses. This is the main cause of misery. This ignorance needs to be removed to manifest the potential divinity of oneself.
- ***Any work assigned should be performed with sincerity:*** According to teachings of Vedanta, the physical universe is a manifestation of God known as Virât. and there is *no distinction between the sacred and the secular*. Indeed, modest work such as sweeping the floor or repairing shoes is to be done with same consideration and commitment as work within the sanctum which means is that all work is sacred.
- ***All work is worship to God:*** According to Srimad Bhagwadgita (18.46) all work should be done as service to God, with no desires of fruits of action; this is the essence of Karma Yoga.
- ***All work is to be performed as a spiritual discipline:*** When work, any work, is done as a service to God it *becomes a spiritual discipline*; this selfless service performed without any expectations becomes the real service to lord and an aspirant or knowledge seeker reaches to next level as compared to his fellow beings still stuck in trivial benefits of this mundane world.

ROLE OF DIETARY HABITS FOR ACADEMIC EXCELLENCE

Not as it were being our physical body built and kept up agreeing to the nourishment we eat, but our inward nature is additionally conditioned by it. The net portion of the nourishment produces the vitality for the physical device, whereas the unpretentious portion contributes to our thought energy." It takes time for the impacts of dietary changes to show on the intellect. Changing our count calories may not affect our brain research overnight, but in a period of months can influence it altogether. There is an interesting anecdote in Chandogya Upnishad(Krishnananda, 2009) where Sage Uddalaka instructs his son Svetaketu "Food, when consumed becomes threefold: the gross particles become excrement, the middling ones flesh and the fine ones the mind. My child, when curd is churned, its fine particles which rise upwards, form butter. Thus, my child, when food is consumed, the fine particles which rise upwards form the mind. Hence verily the mind is food."

Nature has introduced different components inside each of us that impact our disposition and contribute to our individual contrasts. At an internal level, the diverse proportions of the three modes of nature in a person— sattva (goodness), rajas (energy) and tamas (darkness)—strongly impact our disposition and what we eat. Whereas the prevalence of sattva in an individual causes health-conscious utilization of nourishment, which is said to move forward life span, judgment skills and joy (Bhagavad Gita 17:8), rajas in prevalence causes taste-conscious utilization which will indeed lead to malady. In contrast, tamas causes utilization of nourishment out of numbness, with small respect to wellbeing or taste.

Sattvic nourishments include natural products, most vegetables, cereals, rice, drain, new breads and lentils. Rajasic nourishments incorporate pointlessly hot nourishments, unreasonably salty nourishments and delicate drinks. Tamasic nourishments are ruined, bland, unclean, and/or destructive nourishment things. This category incorporates most deep-fried or prepared nourishments, difficult alcohol, meat, angle and eggs. It can be said that all sattvic nourishments are veggie lover, but numerous veggie lover eatables may be categorized as rajasic or tamasic. In contrast, tamas causes utilization of nourishment out of obliviousness, with small respect to wellbeing or taste.

Irrespective of the yogic path we choose to progress towards our academic or spiritual excellence – bhakti yoga, karma yoga, jnana yoga, or raja yoga; a sattvic diet makes our academic or spiritual progress easier being light and easily digestible.

Effect of Food on Our Thoughts and Subconscious Mind

There could be a two-way association between nourishment and disposition (Krishnananda, 2018): Whereas sattvic individuals incline toward to eat sattvic nourishment, eating sattvic food can make a individual more sattvic. Performing sattvic karma in one range of life increments sattva in all other ranges of life. Within the setting of mien, since the sattva mode of nature implies vision and includes goodness in all its forms—like truth, genuineness, teach, tirelessness, respectfulness and eagerness in work—eating sattvic nourishment leads to the improvement of such excellences. A sattvic count calories impels our mien towards righteousness—including how we think and act. Additionally, by expanding the components of sattva inside us, sattvic nourishment can rouse us to take an interest in bhakti and contemplation and move towards God. Sattvic nourishment impact us to stay candidly adjusted in victory and disappointment which is very difficult for a student. In contrast, eating rajasic nourishments may thrust us towards covetousness, self-centeredness and performing work exclusively for financial benefit. Tamasic nourishments can actuate the most noticeably awful qualities in an individual, like apathy, languor, pomposity and trickery, which are all tamasic characteristics. As non-vegetarianism falls underneath the tamasic category, eating non-vegetarian food escalate negative *samskaras* or karmic impressions inside the judgment skills of a otherworldly competitor. Since karma incorporates all the thought forms utilized to reach at a choice to do or not do something, the eagerly included in planning our menu can be imperative in labeling nourishment as sattvic vs. tamasic.

It is often said "We are what we eat!" The diet can be used as a means of developing self-control and discipline. Not just the right type of food but it is important to eat the proper quantity at the right time. Consistent and dedicated attention to these aspects and forces discipline which increases mindfulness and awareness that soon permeates into every action and slowly translates into a way of life.

Simple Steps to Choose Fit Diet for an Aspirant

1. Avoid junk food.
2. Eat your food while seating, avoid to take food while standing.
3. Eat food silently while thinking anything and try to close all senses while eating.
4. Take small quantity of food, may be you require to take more than one, but it will help go prevent the wastage of food, which is one of the biggest sin on this earth.
5. Chew the food sufficiently and thoroughly.
6. Keep distance from all appliances which may divert your mind while taking food including TV, phone, computer etc.
7. Try to be vegetarian.
8. Before start eating offer prayer to God, who make us eligible to take the food.
9. After taking food conclude with gratitude to the God for giving us with food.

SURRENDER TO FEET OF GURU

Worship of the feet of Guru speaks to lowliness or humility. When we touch the feet of the Guru, we bow down the most elevated portion of our body i.e., head towards the most reduced portion i.e., feet. The student then only becomes humble, is prepared to do what it takes to know the Truth. When we worship the Guru's feet every day, we surrender the ego which is the most important prerequisite to acquire any kind of knowledge from a Master. Without gratitude, even if we have everything, life is still empty and we keep complaining. Presence of Guru or Master represents the Grace of the Lord in our lives. It's the Guru who teaches us the ethics of life:

1. how a student should conduct himself in regard to the ultimate goal of his life.
2. how he should conduct himself in relation to people outside and
3. how he should conduct himself in regard to his ownself.

The real Guru thus sums of the whole reality to his students and then a student is clear about the goals of his life in terms of ethical needs('dharma'), material needs(ártha'), emotional needs('kama') and finally the spiritual needs('moksha').

ROLE OF PUNCTUALITY IN ACADEMIC EXCELLENCE

Promptness is the capacity or a quality in us to total an assignment on time or be display on time.
Simple steps to be punctual:

Recognize and recognize merely have a reliability problem

Often one clears this aside beneath the guise that one has as well numerous errands so it is satisfactory to be a small late. A prevalence of Tamoguna is the reason for dormancy and procrastination.

1. Make it a Priority:

Decide you need to alter this propensity and make it a priority.

2. Ask the WHY behind it:

To alter any propensity, it is very important to know the reason for the change - what is the advantage. One should be persuaded of the reason because it isn't simple overcoming any conditioning over a period of time. Without conviction continuously the ancient propensity will return and one will slip into the same ancient apathy. Ask yourself what you will gain by overcoming your tardiness.

3. **Make a need list:** – To Do list The issue most of us have is that we are terrible troughs of time. We regularly don't spend time in prioritizing the assignments and squander a part of time on doing the superfluous and insignificant ones first.
4. **Be ruthless along with your To Do List**:

One reason why one may have a propensity to be late is since there's essentially as well much to do. It's superior to say "no" to something one doesn't have time for than to say "yes" and after that be an hour late. Take out the To Do list and re-order anything that's not a need. Make beyond any doubt that the list has as it were number of things which can reasonably get done, and which can practically be on time. Prompt individuals acknowledge that they can't do it all.

5. Preparation:

This can be one of the foremost vital steps to guarantee promptness. Eg on the off chance that you have got to go out for a assembly tomorrow early within the morning, press and keep the dress, shoes, embellishments prepared night some time recently. Collect and orchestrate all the documents, pack, and any other fundamentals like car keys, house keys etc together at one put. Put a caution figuring the right time required to urge prepared and to induce the named put keeping in intellect the activity conditions and separate involved. Factor in time for contingencies. Always be arranged to be on time.

6. Learn to Wait:

Generally, individuals don't like to be on time because they ought to wait for others. Be arranged – carry a book or articles or records that you just have not ahd the time to capture up on. Or utilize the time to go to to pending phone calls, emails or indeed interfacing with companions. Utilize the downtime to shut your eyes for a whereas and ponder.8. Fashionably late – a myth

7. Being late- a status symbol?

A few individuals are beneath a fancy that to be late may be a status image which tobe late is to "be cool". Those who are vital keep others holding up. In this manner, being early may be a sign that they're not that vital. And no one needs to feel unimportant. However, being on time or fair a small early is truly a sign of being organized, having regard for others, and having great time administration abilities. Perused approximately effective individuals and you'll take note a common characteristic is punctuality.

ROLE OF SLEEP IN ACADEMIC EXCELLENCE

Rest is the natural pause or rest period for our bodies. In this state the body naturally unwinds, repairs and rejuvenates (Tathagatananda, 2008). In any case anything in abundance indeed rest isn't great. So also intemperate rest or long hours of rest make the body lazy and dull. It could be a common encounter that those who rest for more than10 hours wake up feeling more tired. Another critical calculate is the timing of our sleep. The 3 gunas: sattva, rajas and tamas, are show within the whole creation, in everything. We as well are a combination of these 3 gunas. Prevalence of a guna is there in not only in different stages of our life, but also during different times of the day. Nature as well has its stages - early morning is when sattva guna is overwhelming and thus considered most favorable. Old science has known this and subsequently isolated the 24 hours of a day into 8 prahars of 3 hrs each agreeing to the predominance of the guna. Our digestion system is concurring to the developments of the sun. The sun is the source of our vitality. When it "rises" the environment around us within the mornings is exceptionally unadulterated, and sattva gunna is transcendent. At night, the sun has "set" and the environment is more tamasic, gloomy, we are too exceptionally tired at the conclusion of the day. When we break this run the show, and remain alert late into the night and wake up late within the mornings, the body gets wiped out.

SELF-INTROSPECTION FOR ACADEMIC EXCELLENCE

Each thought, word and deed ought to develop from us bearing the seal of our disposition and acknowledgment. Post a parcel of your consideration as a sentry on the watchtower of your judgment skills. Let it be a quiet eyewitness of the plots of the intellect: the thought processes, the eagerly and purposes that lie behind each thought, word and deed. We are ever wakeful to the going-on in your intellect. Reflection ought to not be befuddled with blame finding or self-condemnation. It is to get it our considerations, sentiments and actions so that we are able coordinated them. In straightforward words, it is to be completely mindful of our eagerly and contemplations whereas acting.

Simple Steps to do Introspection

- Introspection should be practiced at the end of the day just before going to sleep.
- Sit discreetly and take 5 profound breaths.
- Order a parade of your day's exercises (past day's in case worn out the morning) inside your intellect: all considerations, words, activities and feelings that unfolded. Stand separated from them all and fair-mindedly audit your day's occasions as a noiseless witness. Don't halt at any occasion to think around it. Simply witness the event and move on. • It is exceptionally critical to keep in mind that amid contemplation one needs to simply watch the exercises not criticize, analyze or rectify oneself. Such feedback day-after-day may lead to criticism or disappointment in life.
- Observation will lead to mindfulness of one's qualities, goodness, accomplishments as well as one's flaws, shortcoming and animalistic propensities in every day exchanges. This organize is called location. This handle will consequently happen when contemplation is done every day and sincerely.
- Feel great for the goodness in you and fortify your qualities. Conjure Appreciation in your heart and thank the Master for giving you such goodness. • Accept the negativities without self-judgement or condemnation. Fair as you'd acknowledge a tooth throb equitably without mental judgements(Sorenson, 2007).
- The minute one is mindful of the negative thought processes, acknowledges them without advocating and feels embarrassed of these characteristics, that minute they ended up frail.
- This way half the battle is won. As before long as a shortcoming is recognized and nullified, substitute it with its inverse ethicalness and watch your exchanges soaking up this ideal. This organize is called substitution. Very sure it will soon become a personality trait.

ROLE OF EXERCISE FOR ACADEMIC EXCELLENCE

Everyone says that healthy mind lives only in healthy body and healthy body can be obtained only by proper diet and work out or exercise. So keeping body in movement and leaving the lethargic attitude can lead to healthy body. The role of yoga is also important to obtain the healthy body simultaneously with the healthy mind.

It is suggested to do the exercise daily for taking out some time out of your busy schedule. This healthy body along with the healthy mind can be obtained by:

- Workout
- Yoga
- Mediation

These exercise will boost the cardiovascular health, improve the blood circulation, helps fight stress, improves digestion, helps detox the body, improves flexibility, reinforces the spine, helps in weight loss and increments mental sharpness.

ROLE OF PRANAYAMA FOR ACADEMIC EXCELLENCE

From time astute men, rishis and sages have instructed their devotees that life has radiated through a drive. This is Prana or the life force. The incapacity of an individual or the powerlessness we feel is due to the isolation of our individual Prana from the Cosmic Prana or what we call as Divine Energy. We mainly encounter Prana through breathing. All plants, animals, human beings etc. breathe this Prana in, with the air. But we don't realise Pranic vitality is in everything; sullight, food, water, etc. The little space tat is inside a room is same as that is outside and the same exists with Prana also. The Prana that is within us is same as the Cosmic Prana or Divine Energy outside us, we just have to become conscious and aware of this fact and the very moment we'll be able to realise our potential divinity. However, due to arrogance, ego, self-assertion and false prestige we begin to identify ourselves only with the limited gross body. We then have false impressions of our ownself by developing 'mineness' and 'Í'ness. This becomes the major cause of all suffering as we cut ourselves away from the Divine Energy which is everywhere and start feeling weak not only vitally but psychologically also. Pranayama is a Sanskrit word meaning "control of the life force". It is composed from two Sanskrit words: *Prana* implies life force and *ayama*, to draw out. Our gross and subtle bodies are connected through different sheaths or '*kosha*'. Accoerding to Yoga our life span on earth is decided by the number of breaths we take which is predetermined by our Karma. The lighter one breathes, the shorter is one's life. The more intense one breathes, longer is one's life. Birds breathes exceptionally quick and have a shorter life while animals breathes a bit profound and live longer. For great wellbeing, one must breathe profoundly. Practicing pranayama in our daily lives can have enormous effects in improving our wellness. For a growing child who is focusing on his studies, regular practice of pranayama can bring tremendous improvement not only in his physical health but also in his mental health.

The vitality within the body is because of existence of Prana. Prana communicates within an individual through 5 physiological functions (Krishnananda, 2018):

1. Prana Vayu (workforce of Respiration)– consists of what we take in through nourishment, breath, water, etc.
2. Apana (workforce of excretion) – consists of what we toss out ie water, waste, exhale etc.
3. Vyana (workforce of circulation) – consists of circulation of blood
4. Udana (faculty of reverse processes) – vomiting, hiccups, sweating. It is also responsible for the movement of the subtle body out of the gross body at the time of death. It is also responsible for the amount of creativity in an individual, all artists have a strong udana.
5. Samana (workforce of assimilation) – it is responsible for digestion and assimilation of food.

Through Pranayama all the physiological systems of the body can be controlled by practicinge of breath control & self-control. Through regular pranayama we can control the Prana that is vibrating inside. It is the easiest and fastest way to control the mind because the mind is fastened to the Prana. On the otherhand we can also say, if the mind is controlled the prana too can be regulated. Pranayama helps in building a strong digestive system, calms the intellect, increases concentration. Thus it is the easiest way to have a control over oneself and should be essentially carried out by a student to achieve par excellence in academics.

Simple Steps to do Pranayam

1. Sit erect. The head, the neck and spine in a straight line. Come to a comfortable posture.
2. Exhale(Rechak) with both nostrils and after that, take after the method given below:
    a. Inhale with the correct nostril (Purak)
    b. Hold the breath (Antah Kumbhak)
    c. Exhale with the cleared out nostril (Rechak)
    d. Hold the breath (Bahish kumbhak)
    e. Inhale with the cleared out nostril (Purak)
    f. Hold the breath (Antah Kumbhak)
    g. Exhale with the proper nostril (Rechak)
    h. Hold the breath (Bahish Kumbhak)
    i. Follow this prepare. It is called Anuloma-Viloma Pranayama.
3. People with hypertension should kip the step of Kumbhak.

ROLE OF MEDITATION FOR ACADEMIC EXCELLENCE

The inadequacy of the person, the frailty, the impotency that we feel is due to the segregation of a person self from enormous energies. The small space interior a corridor is the same as the space that's outside and all over within the same way vitality inside us is same as enormous vitality. But due to recapture vanity self-assertion we disengage exterior from the Incomparable Control and cut our self from the stream of vitality that's all over and makes a difference keep enduring each presently and after that feeling frail crucially and mentally. Basically talking it is like putting on a switch, interfacing our house light bulb with the control house, in spite of the fact that both are physically exceptionally distant from each other. Usually the craftsmanship of reflection. Hence, contemplation makes a difference us in getting associated with the infinite energies and for this we need to turn our five faculties (i.e, eyes ears nose throat and skin) inwards and center them to be centered in mind. The mind has to be centered in the intellect, the intellect has to be entered into the cosmic intellect which is finally centered to the absolute.

"Meditation is the path in which the ego learns to withdraw Its false evaluations of life and itself and Comes to the final experience of its own Divine nature," Swami Chinmayananda.

Simple Steps for Meditation

1. Take a bath and Ideally chant.
2. Be sure that your head, neck and spine are in a straight line. Make yourself easy in seating pose and try to concentrate avoiding any type of movement.
3. Leave all type of positive or negative thoughts. Do not put your mind into any thinking.
4. Try to concentrate on your inner soul by internally observing your body from head to toe and consume some time about five minutes to observe the changes taking place near to you.
5. Breathe in and breathe out gradually, consistently and profoundly. Do this for 10 breaths atleast.
6. Feel that you are beyond the Body, Mind, Intellect and ego. You are Pure Consciousness. Let the words sink in.
7. Sit unobtrusively for sometime

8. Offer your appreciation and prostrations to the Ruler or Satguru for being able to mull over on the Self.
9. Rub your palms, put them on the confront, delicately open your eyes and get up gradually.
10. Attempt and keep in mind through the day that you simply are not a body but Immaculate Awareness playing diverse parts.

Stable Mind – Master Key to Happiness

- Are we perfectly free from anxiety?
- Are we satisfying in the self or do we require external things to make us happy?

The above two questions truly decide our mental health. 'Thirst' is the pesson who believe in the existence of GOD, but the new definition say a thirst is not only in the existence of GOD, rather he is person, who believe in the disposition or arrangement set up by GOD.

If he has such a kind of faith that whatever is happening in life with him and around him is for his well-being, nothing in life can disturb him. Even the biggest sorrow won't be able to shake him and he will easily cross this ocean of life.

In this Universe man is one of the many spices, but only he is heavily disturbed due to his greed and non-acceptance of reality. Due to our vested interests we react subjectively to circumstances and tends to fix over them.

The main cause of our misery is our self-deception (Tathagatananda, 2008). We add to our misery when,

- We compare ourselves with others and get envious without any reason.
- We become irritated towards life's principles.
- We get egoistic and don't resolve trivial issues and make a mountain out of a molehill.
- We try to fulfill not our needs but greed.
- We broad always over past issues rather than enjoying the fruits of present.

To have a peaceful life that we can focus on our academic excellence we must accept the following unavoidable facts:

- We reap the fruit of our thoughts and actions, both good and bad.
- Everything dear to us is subjected to change, Lord Krishna has loudly stated in Shrimad Bhagwat Gita that change is the law of Nature.
- Disease will come and death is in evitable, so we must not waste even a single moment of our life on this earth, rather make every second worth living making it.
- Honorable and every minute be thankful to God for this precious gift of life in human form. The biggest difference between an animal and human is that we human can think and make society a better place to live in, otherwise eating, sleeping and reproducing even insects, birds and animals are doing.

CONCLUSION

The greatest strength of our religion or individual is this inner stability and the great wisdom acharyas of humanity all attained this inner stability through the knowledge of the self, which says, the kingdom of God is within us. The less we are depending on external things for our happiness, the more we enjoy the blessings of spiritual life.

A disciplined spiritual life combats the weakness of negative thoughts. It brings stability to the mind and a calm and serene mind can confront and resolve every adversity in life through clear thinking and righteous action.

Thus we conclude from shaloka of Srimad Bhagwadgita (Krishnananda, 2018), Yatra yogeśvaraḥ kṛṣṇo yatra pārtho dhanurdharaḥ, tatra śrīr vijayo bhūtir dhruvā nītir matir mama (18.78). Wherever is Sri Krishna, and wherever is Arjuna—Sri Krishna, the Master of yoga, and Arjuna, the wielder of the bow—wherever these are seated in one chariot, there is prosperity, victory, happiness, and firm qualities. Lord Krishna represents divine grace, cosmic power, eternity operating in all temporality; and Arjuna represents humanity, the essence of mankind, the essence of human effort, the essence of aspiration, the essence of movement towards God.

During the legendry war of Mahabharata, whenever Bhishma was accosted and asked who will win finally, he used to say *yataḥ kṛṣṇas tato jayaḥ*: "Wherever is Krishna, there is victory." *Yato dharmas tataḥ kṛṣṇo yataḥ kṛṣṇas tato jayaḥ*, or in another way, *yataḥ kṛṣṇas tato dharmo yato dharma tato jayaḥ*: "Wherever is dharma, there is Krishna; and wherever is Krishna, there is dharma; and wherever is Krishna, and hence dharma, there is victory certainly." For achieving excellence in any field merely human effort will not work. There is a necessity for its being backed by Universal Grace.

ACKNOWLEDGMENT

We would like to express our deepest gratitude to our Spiritual Guru Swami Nirvikalpananda, Ramakrishma Math & Mission, Kankhal Ashram, Uttarakhand, India for sharing his pearls of wisdom and giving a deep insight in writing of this book chapter. Our work also deeply acknowledges true support from our mother and our loving daughter Jhalak singh for motivating us throughout to write something constructive for academic excellence of students under the light of spirituality.

REFERENCES

Brahmananda. (2000). *Supreme Knowledge revealed through Upanishads*. The Divine Life Society.

Complete Works of Swami Vivekananda. (2013). Ramakrishna Math and Ramakrishna Mission, Belur Math.

Krishnananda. (2009). Upanishad. The Divine Life Society.

Krishnananda. (2018). Commentary on the Bhagwadgita. The Divine Life Society.

Russell, B. (2016). *Impact of Science on Society*. Routledge Classics.

Sorenson, R. D. (2007). Stress management in education: Warning signs and coping mechanisms. *Management in Education*, *21*(3), 10–13. doi:10.1177/0892020607079985

Tathagatananda. (2008). Relief of Tension, Depression, and Anxiety Through Spiritual Living. Advaita Ashram.

Chapter 10
Self-Care and Stress Management for Educators in Public Universities

Nurul Naimah Rose
https://orcid.org/0000-0003-3195-0685
Universiti Malaysia Perlis, Malaysia

Aida Shakila Ishak
https://orcid.org/0000-0002-8961-9154
Universiti Malaysia Perlis, Malaysia

Fauziah Ismail
Universiti Malaysia Perlis, Malaysia

Siti Norayu Mohd Basir
Universiti Malaysia Perlis, Malaysia

Nur Qurratul' Aini Ismail
Universiti Malaysia Perlis, Malaysia

ABSTRACT

The role of educators in public university is more than teaching in the classroom. An educator is responsible for teaching students and contributes to their learning development. In fulfilling the job responsibilities, many educators often ignore the practice of self-care and stress management. The lack of awareness to take care of the emotional aspects can lead to high levels of stress that affect educators' health and well-being, causing burnout, lack of engagement, job dissatisfaction, and poor performance. Having a good self-care and effective stress management may result in an excellent work performance and increases motivation in teaching and learning. Educators need to understand the stress phenomenon including the causes and effects as well as the coping strategy.

DOI: 10.4018/978-1-6684-2334-9.ch010

INTRODUCTION

Since the COVID-19 outbreak that began in early 2020, the world community has begun to adapt to a new normal life. Malaysians have also begun to adjust to life in this pandemic era. This includes teaching and learning at the university through the concept of online distance learning that has been practiced throughout university campuses in Malaysia. Lecturers as educators and researchers also need to adapt quickly and agilely in facing current challenges. Flexibility in achieving research objectives needs to be implemented. Various ways can be creatively implemented such as modifying the research objectives to suit if it can still achieve the main goal of the study. Educators should also improve skills in information technology, pedagogy, and online assessment. They should be familiar with the use of technology and software platforms. Not only implementing classes virtually but also uploading quizzes, making assessments, giving assignments and others that are usually given in a conventional way that is face-to-face classes.

This chapter will discuss about the stress and well-being among educators specifically lectures in Malaysian public university. The discussion will follow sequences such as the role of educators in public university, then understanding of stress phenomenon among educators, factors, and effects of stress to educators in higher education as a whole and lastly will touch on the self-care and stress management for educators. However, in this chapter, the term lecturer mostly uses and it referring to educators in public university. Stress is an important phenomenon and is often associated with job performance, health, and productivity level of an individual or employee. Stress can affect the productivity as well as the quality of employees otherwise handled well and effectively. Thus, work stress can have an impact negatively to the health of the employee and hence the well -being of the individual himself. Stress can be regard as a natural feeling, it designed to help you cope in challenging situations. In small amounts it can be good, because it pushes individual to work hard and do the best in anything they pursue.

THE ROLE OF EDUCATORS IN PUBLIC UNIVERSITIES

The Malaysian Education Development Plan 2015-2025, often known as the MEDP, was started in 2013 by the Ministry of Education. As a result, Malaysia today has a higher education policy that was designed by Malaysians for Malaysians, hastening the country's transition to a developed, high-income nation (Pelan Pembangunan Pendidikan Malaysia 2015-2025). Back in 2012, Malaysia had a 48 percent higher education enrollment rate than the United States. 1.2 million students enrolled in public universities, polytechnics, community colleges, private universities, private university institutions, and private colleges during a decade. Bachelor's enrolment climbed sixfold between 1990 and 2010, while undergraduate and PhD enrollment increased tenfold. Malaysia is now ranked third in terms of undergraduate and PhD enrollment among ASEAN countries, behind Singapore and Thailand.

By looking at the number, education is very important in ensuring the civilization of a country. The development of a country's civilization is developed by a good and comprehensive education system. Comprehensive education needs to keep pace with current changes. The transformation process is to ensure that the status of the country's education system is not outdated, relevant and ready to provide a competitive society both in the country and in the eyes of the world. The process of empowering education in Malaysia in general and higher education was introduced through the Malaysian Education Development Plan (MEDP) launched on 6 September 2013. Educational transformation efforts need to be supported by educators, especially in public institutions of higher learning. Educators have a great responsibility in supporting and realizing Malaysia's education plan for sustainable development. The aspiration attribute of students in higher education is to make them equipped with ethical values and spirituality and leadership skills.

Educators at the tertiary level are responsible for exposing students to ethical and moral values, have steady spirituality, loving and concerned; appreciate development sustainable and stylish healthy life. In terms of leadership skills, students need to be educated to be good communicators effective, emotionally intelligent, and able to interact across cultures; responsible, competitive, resilient, and confident. The duties and roles of Educators at the tertiary level are not just focused on teaching alone. In the context of educators, their roles are larger and more comprehensive, including as lecturers who carry out responsibilities to students, researchers who are responsible for solving community and industry problems, and consultants who are responsible for expertise in a field (Pelan Pembangunan Pendidikan Malaysia 2015-2025 (2014), Azreen, Norudin & Zuraida (2016).

According to the Malaysian Education Development Plan, lecturers are responsible for producing students with high ethical and moral values as well as good leadership skills by 2025. As a result, lecturers must push themselves to improve their knowledge, expertise, and personality to be role models for their students (Sharmaa, Laura, Wangc & Loreman, 2021). Educators must cultivate admirable attitudes, high morals, and ethics in their professional lives. Being a lecturer at a university is a serious job that requires a dedicated educator. Teaching is a huge act of faith because it is a cornerstone of the knowledge that students will gain after graduation. Teaching is an important task that needs to be given attention by every lecturer and moderator. Lecturers are usually given formal instruction per week is limited to no more than 18 hours contacts for academic staff to focus on and implement scholarly activities/research/ consulting services, as well as other administrative duties (Garis Panduan Beban Staf Akademik, 2015). Preparation for teaching and learning took place during the semester break. Typically, the lecturer or moderator will be directly involved in planning the teaching and learning activities in the classroom, preparing notes and questions as well as making the assessment and examination process for their students (Azreen, Norudin & Zuraida, 2016).

The role of educators in universities goes beyond simply providing teaching materials (Azreen, Norudin & Zuraida, 2016). Teaching students from various backgrounds is difficult therefore lecturers must identify and develop effective learning approaches to effectively communicate knowledge. Teaching approaches that are skilled, such as dealing with students' emotions, controlling classes, and engaging educational procedures, all have an impact on the success of teaching delivery. Professors, on the other hand, face a significant challenge. The next challenge for Professors is to always be aware of current events. For example, the Industry 4.0 Revolution has influenced developments in the classroom in terms of teaching and learning. Changes requires them to adapt for teaching and learning to run smoothly and effectively without becoming obsolete. The use of technology in the classroom is a modern challenge that must be addressed by an educator. Psychological readiness, such as motivational attributes, self-ideas, and beliefs about technology and its application, influence one's ability to move in line with the digital world (Scherer & Teo, 2019).

Beside teaching, the duty of an educator is to be a supervisor for prospective students for both the undergraduate and postgraduate students (Garis Panduan Beban Staf Akademik,2015). For a lecturer, this supervision activities will be counted as one of the performance indicators. The purpose of supervision is to guide a postgraduate student through the process of research, writing, presentation, and thesis or dissertation examination. The quality of supervision is determined by the interaction between supervisors and students, as well as the extent to which supervisors and students understand their respective roles and responsibilities. They are also fully accountable for student research management and direction, as well as administrative matters (Garis Panduan Amalan Baik: Staf Akademik, 2014).

Postgraduate student supervision necessitates a high level of expertise and skills on the part of the educator. Meng and Zhao (2018) discovered that academic supervisor leadership influenced postgraduate creativity via self-motivation, innovative thinking, and expert knowledge in their study. The ability of a postgraduate student supervisor to guide, motivate, and complete the student's studies is an indicator of his or her success as a supervisor (Meng, Tan & Li, 2017). Since supervision is not the only task supported by an educator, it necessitates continuous effort to be effective and efficient. Supervisors' determination to ensure that students graduate is a lengthy process that requires at least two years of supervision for master's students and three years for doctoral students (UniMAP Academic Regulations for Postgraduate Research Programs, 2021). It is a process that should not be taken lightly because students rely heavily on a supervisor's guidance as one of the driving factors for their success. Besides, the University aspires to produce postgraduate students who can serve as the backbone of their respective fields and build expertise. In this context, supervisors must align with the university's goals by instilling in their students the importance of critical and creative thinking. It is consistent with the findings of Meng and Zhao (2018), in which both the supervisor and the student seek to develop, become, and possess critical and creative thinking.

An educator must carry out research as part of their job (Azreen, Norudin & Zuraida, 2016). Malaysian public universities actively participate in research and contribute to community and industrial problem-solving organisations. Through research experiences, educators will gain more knowledge and skills particularly in their expertise area. According to Morgan, Gliner and Harmon (1999) by involving in research activities, it can help developing one's knowledge of the field as well as one's awareness of oneself as a professional research consumer to evaluate and comprehend new breakthroughs in the discipline. In the long run, it is a factor in determining educators' proficiency in their profession. Being a researcher is a difficult and challenging process that should not be underestimated. Researchers must prepare themselves with the necessary skills, which include the use of proper research methods and meeting the objectives and questions of the study, the skills of reading, thinking, and arguing, and the skills of clear and accurate scientific writing (Ghazali & Sufean,2016).

All the skills are required because research is a process that requires meticulous planning. A study that is carried out arbitrarily is not considered scientific. A research proposal, a systematic literature review, procedural data collection, thorough data analysis, and subsequent critical discussion all contribute to good research. Good research should be able to contribute to the development of methods for assessing important conceptual frameworks, describe themes and their relationships, or provide evidence to support the discipline's theoretical foundation (Morgan, Gliner & Harmon, 1999, Ghazali & Sufean, 2016).

Time, energy, and money are frequently expended in research. When beginning a research project, researchers must plan carefully. It adheres to the following Good Practice Guidelines: Academic Staff (2014) research responsibilities include developing study suggestions, monitoring, and supervising staff research, collecting and analyzing data, writing and submitting publishing papers, and attending national and international conferences and seminars, including paper presentations. Journal publication, research, and consultancy services have all increased because of this. As of 2012, the number of patents submitted by Malaysian universities had climbed by 11% per year, putting the country in 28th place in the world (Ringkasan Eksekutif Pelan Pembangunan Pendidikan Malaysia 2015-2025).

A university is an institution that brings together expertise in various fields, and they are a university's asset. Recognizing this, the university fulfils its role as an institution that promotes development collectively. The university's role is not only to produce quality graduates, but also to maintain relationships with the local community, government and private organizations, and industry. An educator's knowledge and experience qualify them to provide consulting services. These consulting services are available not only to the institution, but also to the community and industry. Educators' knowledge is universal in scope, encompassing not just domestic but also international issues (Garis Panduan Amalan Baik: Staf Akademik,2014). Cooperation between universities and industries is the primary means of transferring scientific and technological achievements, and it is a critical component of the national innovation system (He, 2020). Collaborations between university and industry researchers allow for the transfer of knowledge and expertise.

Industry collaboration may strengthen academic contributions to establish scientific knowledge by providing opportunities for specialization and more productive assignment of tasks on lines of research with both scientific and industrial prospects (Bikard, Vakili & Teodoridis, 2018). Through concentrating work, academic researchers can supply solutions to problems while industry concentrates on commercialization, this combination creates a more effective and efficient workplace. In addition, it becomes a bridge connecting research, practice, and norms (Czarnitzki, Grimpe & Toole, 2014). Educators at the university also have a responsibility to the local community. Universities as centers of knowledge must play a role in supporting the aspirations of developing the country collectively (Albulescu & Albulescu, 2014). By connecting with the local community, the institution, through its academic staff, carries out the national mission. This relationship exposes students to good leadership values, effective communication skills, and the holistic development of good personalities (Donesky, Norton, Fisher & Bunker-Alberts, 2021). In the meantime, knowledge transfer and local development help the community. Universities in Europe, for example, are urged to give back to their communities by giving training and practical for lifelong learning. Universities are encouraged to contribute to the formation and development of a knowledge-based society and economy; continuous education strategies are required to meet the challenges of competitiveness and the use of new digital era, to improve social cohesion, and to provide equal opportunities and high quality of life (Albulescu & Albulescu, 2014)

STRESS PHENOMENON AMONG EDUCATORS

The educational landscape, particularly in terms of learning and teaching, has changed dramatically following the Covid-19 pandemic. Teaching and learning which was previously based on face-to-face learning in the classroom, has now been completely replaced by an entirely online method. This is because the education development agenda cannot be stopped and must be ensured to continue building knowledgeable in accordance with the national education philosophy. Most higher education institutions, particularly local universities, both public and private, as well as schools throughout Malaysia, have no other choice but to use virtual teaching and learning methods to ensure that the teaching syllabus and information delivery are as effective as possible (Abdul Aziz, 2020).

During the pandemic, the new teaching method had been imposed to teaching and learning as well as other work-related matter. This sudden change requires students' adjustment to the new system of learning, particularly in the new norm of education. However, when compared to other professions, educators' responsibilities and roles are extremely challenging and demanding. Workload has increased over time, causing work stress problems for all educators (Wong, Shahlan & Salleh, 2022). Similarly, Nor Haslina (2020) claims that changes in the online education system during the pandemic have caused concern not only among students but also among lecturers. Furthermore, this condition not only strains the emotions but also interferes with mental and physical functioning.

By definition, a state of stress is a state of bearing, a difficult-to-bear load, (Kamus Dewan Edisi Ke-4, 2005). A stressed person represents an individual who is physically, mentally, and emotionally burdened by heavy and disturbing things. According to Islamic psychologists, stress is defined as mental anxiety or human emotional disorders (Fariza, 2005). Stress, according to Hans (1974), the founder of the Theory of Stress, is a non-specific reaction by a person to a burden that befalls him. According to him, stress can result in either a good and positive reaction or feeling known as "eustress" or a bad and negative reaction known as "distress" (Shazarina et al.). Stress is generally divided into two categories: positive stress and negative stress (Nur Izzaty, Azman, Mohamad Shahril Azwan & Sholihien, 2015). Positive stress is beneficial when it causes one person to put pressure in achieving something or accomplishing task. While negative stress, it refers to a stress related to pressure in terms of physiological health, physical health and psychology or mental health aspect.

In most cases, the negative pressures that everyone faces in daily life are beneficial, such as disagreements between spouses, financial problems, family, friends, and even the work environment. Most people's stress can be caused by factors of stress in the workplace, such as regular scenarios involving excessive workloads. The reason for this is that most of the information pertaining to the tasks is not provided clearly, and there is a situation of role conflict. Furthermore, Haryati (2013) asserts that, in addition to overworked aspects of the relationship and organisation, work characteristics, organisational environment, work management, and others can all be sources of stress in the workplace. Workplace stress is always associated with negative consequences. Many previous studies, according to Marimuthu (2019), have shown that work stress has a negative impact on one's mental health while also drawing risks to the organisation and lowering one's work productivity if not immediately resolved. Aside from police, prisons officers, firefighters, nurses, doctors, and pharmacy assistants, one of the organisations that constantly puts pressure on individuals in employment is education institution (Baker & Hazril Izwar, 2014).

A study reviewed by the American Institute of Stress in 2019, the teaching profession is the most stressful professional, and now facing a variety of challenges and potentially causing serious health problems. Since work stress primarily affect behavioural patterns, such as low performance and quality of work, job satisfaction, skipping issues, negative performance, and physical effects when neglecting tasks. In the long run, stress like this will have an impact on mental health issues like depression, anxiety, and mental disorders. Meanwhile, a study conducted in Malaysia, found that the level of stress among Johor Vocational College lecturers is moderate (Normarina, 2015). However, findings also show that system changes are the main contributing factors followed by workload, student frustration, interpersonal relationships and time and resource constraints. Another study conducted in Malaysian Islamic College University on lecturers' emotions level. The level of negative emotions among the lecturers are moderate but they are showing symptoms such as stress, worry and depressed. The main contributing factors include the Key Performance Indicators (KPIs) and employee perceptions of employer behaviour, followed by excessive workload, interpersonal relationships and communication as well as time and resource constraints (Maizan, 2018)

During the pandemic era, Aulia Riska 2020) in her study on the challenges that occur in dealing with online teaching-learning in the pandemic era, emotions of lecturers are affected to some extent. These struggles can be positive stressors that improve work productivity. In this pandemic era, online teaching-learning requires lecturers to be more creative and innovative to create teaching materials that stimulate students' interest and enthusiasm. Furthermore, Syaharuddin and Mutiani (2020) stated that teachers must be skilled in science and technology. This challenge places a high priority on improving lecturers' abilities and renovating teaching patterns to meet the learning needs of the millennial generation. Mohan (2020) argues that some lecturers feel the paradigm shift of practice is difficult when dealing with online teaching-learning. Disruption to routine practices or cessation of existing routines is also one of the causes of stress among lecturers.

A survey conducted by Bani Hidayat (2020) on lecturers at the Institute of Teacher Education, Islamic Education Campus regarding the implementation of online teaching-learning during Movement Control Order (MCO) Phases 1 and 2 discovered that all lecturers and students are fully engaged in online teaching-learning. According to the findings, the main platforms used are WhatsApp, Google Classroom, and Telegram, which are supported by other social media applications. These findings indicate that lecturers respond positively to this challenge by exploring various sources to ensure that online teaching-learning continues. However, the study's findings revealed that the internet network and student data capacity are the two main issues that arise when implementing online teaching-learning. This is because lecturers are more likely to use synchronous interaction methods to replace face-to-face interaction, and this method necessitates excellent access between lecturers and students as well as high costs. Meanwhile, asynchronous online teaching-learning usually requires limited access, but it is commonly used when direct time flexibility and facility constraints, as well as the presence of lecturers and students, are required.

Excessive exposure to the screen can also be a source of negative emotional stress. The use of computers and mobile phones is necessary as the main medium and tool in the online teaching-learning process. Lecturers not only have to face the screen during the lecture, but more time is required to prepare for the lecture. The International Clinical Psychologist of the University of Malaya-Wales stated that when a person is unable to balance computer use, then it will not be able to help them see the learning phenomenon as something positive and will contribute to health problems (Raja Nur Faznie Aida, 2020). Meanwhile, Elizabeth (2020) who studied the impact of technology use on learning in the United Nations during the pandemic era among lecturers found the need to check mobile phones higher when working from home. The mode of working from home also has an impact on lecturers. Unconducive learning environments such as noisy environments, cramped spaces and inappropriate infrastructure affect the effectiveness of delivery and teaching. Lecturers who have families face difficulties in managing the needs of the family, especially children who also need guidance from parents through online learning at home. The increased workload also increases the risk of lecturers experiencing emotional stress.

FACTORS ASSOCIATED WITH STRESS AMONG EDUCATORS

There are numerous factors that can cause significant stress among Malaysian public university educators. Organizational or university factors, individual factors, and family factors will all be discussed as stress factors. Teaching load, career goals, work environment, the leader's style of leadership, communication, and other factors were identified as organizational factors. (Zahrul et. al., 2020; Muhammad Firdaus et. al., 2020; Noordeyana & Siti Zulaikha, 2019; Khairunesa et. al., 2021, Nazli et. al., 2021 & Muhamad Reduan et. al., 2020).

The role of educators in a university is not only to teach, but also to publish, conduct research, supervise students, write papers, consult, and provide social services to the community (Zaini, 2012). These tasks will be evaluated using the lecturers' annual performance targets to determine whether the lecturers' KPIs can be met. These annual performance targets were identified as causing emotional distress among university staff as they were forced to perform (Zahrul, Khairunesa, Lutfan, Zulida & Abdul Halim, 2020, Norzaini & Faridah, 2016). This is because some educators agreed that the universities setting a very high standard of the key performance indicators to be achieved every year. With a limited resources and facilities provided by the university, it seems impossible for all educators to achieve the target.

The requirement made by the university implicitly contributes to the excessive workload among the lecturers. According to Gahlann, V. S. (2014), workload is defined as the amount of work given by an employer to an employee in a given period of time and can be performed by the employee perfectly without risking their health and safety or others related. In a study conducted by Nazli, Noraida and Norhazimah (2021), there are 5 questions related to workload factors, among them are "I have many other side tasks in addition to teaching tasks", "I am stressed with the due date of each task given", "I have to stay up at night to complete essential tasks such as marking tests, assignments and quizzes", "I often have to postpone classes because of having a commitment to other side tasks", "my daily activities are affected due to the workload". The findings of the study showed that "I often had to postpone classes because I have a commitment to other side tasks" obtained a high mean score of 4.3529 compared to other statements. The study conducted on 162 female lecturers showed that there is an excessive workload among female lecturers, especially the side tasks in addition to the actual tasks that need to be performed.

Meanwhile, a study conducted by Muhammad Reduan, Nor Azrizal and Muhammad Masri (2020), they studied the level of work stress among lecturers at Tuanku Syed Sirajuddin Polytechnic (PTSS) in the state of Perlis. A total of 5 dimensions were studied, namely workload, student motivation, appreciation, time constraints and interpersonal relationships. Of these 5 dimensions, workload is the main cause of stress among PTSS Perlis lecturers compared to other dimensions. The mean values obtained for workload were (M = 3.2686), appreciation (M = 3.1500), because of students (M = 3.1071), time constraints (M = 3.0657) and interpersonal relationships (M = 2.8957). This high workload or task contributes to stress and depression if left for a long time and not given attention (Nazli, Noraida and Norhazimah, 2021).

Furthermore, leaders with unfavourable leadership styles, such as agitated leaders, leaders who are not open for discussion, leaders who have no tolerance, and leaders who like to oppress, contribute to stress among university staff (Zahrul Akmal, Khairunesa, Lutfan, Zulida and Abdul Halim, 2020). This tends to happen because a leader is also under stress, which causes the leader to have a negative attitude toward their staff (Hairul Akmal, 2014). Educators work performance and motivations strongly related to leadership styles. Educators is a profession that grows throughout times and experiences. Young lecturers for instance need a mentor among their leaders in the university to learn and build an excellent characteristic as a great educator. If the leaders are not giving their full support but only to put pressure in them, they will end up feels demotivated, loss of confidence, loss of interest and eventually suffer a very high mental and emotional stress.

Environmental factors are also considered to be a source of stress among lecturers (Zahrul, Khairunesa, Lutfan, Zulida and Abdul Halim, 2020). Economic and political instability, as well as technological change, are examples of environmental factors. The organization's operations and performance were also impacted by the economic and political insecurity. While technological advancements encourage employees to master technology skills despite the challenges of learning them. For Schuldt, digital work is a source of stress contributors among academics in higher learning institutions. Other elements in this environmental factor include an unconducive workplace environment, a lack of Teaching and Learning (T&L) equipment, traffic congestion, a lack of building cleaning workers, and air conditioner damage. According to a study (Zahrul et al., 2020), university employees that face a non-optimal work environment and it became a to stress factors in the workplace.

Muhammad Firdaus & Abu Yazid (2020) explained that environmental factors consist of communication elements covering aspects of relationships with leaders and colleagues. This aspect is also supported by Tajudeen (2004) and Cooper & Marshall (1978) in Khairunesa Isa, Wan Hanim Nadrah Wan Muda, Laily Paim, Khadijah Alavi, Jalihah Md. Shah & Nor Aisah Jamil (2021) who explained that stress in the workplace caused by environmental factors in the workplace such as relationships with colleagues, working alone, organizational structure and climate. The relationship element in the organization refers to the aspect of relationship with staff especially with colleagues while the structure and climate of the organization can be referred to as lack of involvement between members of the organization, poor communication, and lack of sense of belonging to the organization.

Individual factors are among the contributing stress factors to educators. Individual factors include personal problems, lack of personal appreciation, financial problem, work environment, lack of encouragement and trust issue (Zahrul et. Al, 2020). Employee personal problems, according to Mohd Akmal Firdaus (2017), become a barrier to excellence performance among employer and employee. Personal issues can be related to financial, health, and attitude problem of the employees. In terms of personal finance, Nuraini (2015) demonstrated that the rising cost of living contributes to employee stress. According to Chong, Muhammad Faizal, and Zuraidah (2018), very little motivation or career guidelines leads to stress in workplace. It's very concerning because if the organisation does not take preventive measures, employees will lose motivation to work.

Family issues, long distance relationship, and lack of family time are all factors that contribute to stress among lecturers. Based on a study conducted by Nor Azimah (2016), the issue of family problems on work occurs when there is a need to takes care of family responsibilities during working hours. For example, in a study conducted by Zahrul et. al., (2020), there are a small number of employees who need to manage family related matters such need to bring their family members for hospital treatment during working hours. In addition, there are staff who do not spend enough time with their families because they allocate more working hours even though the working hours in the office have ended. Meanwhile for staff who lives separately from their families, this will interfere with the execution of work. A study conducted by Tengku Sarina Aini and Fatimah Sahida (2018) found that staff who live far away from their families will in carrying out their responsibilities in the workplace. This is because the tend to get distracted and lose focus.

IMPACTS OF STRESS TO EDUCATORS

Educators are important resources in the teaching and learning process. Educators, particularly lecturers in higher education institutions such as universities, colleges, and other academic institutions or skill centres, have a primary responsibility to ensure that students are prepared to meet market labour demands. Lecturers are responsible for preparing and guiding students to be competitive to take advantage of this opportunity. Educators have a high level of competence in addition to excellent soft skills, and they are involved in more than just teaching and learning. Writing, publishing, research, and community service are all mandatory activities which educators need to be involved. In addition, lecturers should set a good example for their students.

Students are drawn to educators who set a positive example for them by showing good behaviour. By any chance, lecturers must find ways to advance their careers, such as attending courses, gaining new knowledge, upgrading their skills, and remaining compliant with university and government regulations. Despite being an academician, lecturers must devote a significant amount of time and effort to achieve the goals. Struggling to fulfil all these responsibilities can cause stress to lecturers, which can lead to strain in psychology, physiology, and behaviour (Deepti and Hemant, 2018).

A person's stress is an interpersonal conflict that they are going through. When the work required does not match the skills, resources, or requirements of employees, workplace stress may occur. Workers in any organization who are stressed will demonstrate a shift in behaviour, as well as negative consequences on their own health and productivity (Okeke et al., 2016). Long-term stress can have a negative impact on an individual's physical health, depending on how the person reacts to the stress. Individuals in crisis, according to Sweeny et al. (2020), will create stress if they continue to worry about the circumstances, which will eventually cause the individual to lose focus in their life. Individuals who struggle to cope with stress are more likely to get cardiovascular illness such as heart disease, and other physical illness.

According to Rahim and Yatim (2017), there are several other factors that can affect the emotional levels, affecting psychological and physical aspects among educators, such as not being recognised for accomplishments, and salary rates that are not in line with the workload of duties assigned by employers. As a result, Lyubomirsky et al. (2005) and Pressman & Cohen (2005) believed that the workers in organization were dissatisfied while executing their jobs and it leads them to suffer from depression, mental illness, inferiority complex, and social aversion. According to Parent-Lamarche et al. (2020), depression causes stress, which has an impact on an individual's well-being and organisational performance. They will easily feel sad, apprehensive, empty, desperate, and invaluable if they are not happy at work. They will also become agitated and anxious if they are not pleased. Furthermore, if employees lose interest in their jobs, they will lose focus, lose their appetite, and even worst might attempt suicide (Aziz, 2014).

Excessive workload, bad employee roles, inefficient organisational management, auto efficiency leadership, poor communication system, obstacles while working, and lifestyle pressure are all factors that contribute to workplace stress (Yurtkorub, 2013). Workplace stress can be worsened by the physical surroundings of non-ergonomic labour and unbalanced workload (Zafir & Fazilah, 2010). Employee stress levels are closely linked to the working environment because employees spend most of their time at their desk. According to Tajudeen (2004) and Cooper & Marshall (1978), workplace stress is caused by environmental factors such as relationships, essential work, organisational structure, and climate change. There are some misbehaviours among educators that experiencing stress at workplace such as frequent sick leave, high medical expenses, being frequently late to work, skipping work, schizophrenia, working part-time, and taking excessive annual leave.

The interaction between university's top management and educators is addressed in the relationship component. A lack of participation, inadequate communication, and a lack of a sense of belonging are among the managerial dysfunction and work environment factors. The academic staffs will be put under strain if they do not manage their own stress. As a result of the prolonged stress, physical and mental health problems will arise. Physical health issues include increased of pulse rate, high blood pressure, high cholesterol levels, and heart disease. Mental illness manifests itself as a lack of motivation, emotional depression, job dissatisfaction, and a lack of aspiration.

The work environment has a significant impact on employee stress levels. Factors such as ventilation, lighting, overcrowding, sound system, and high temperatures can all have an impact on workers' stress levels (Sunarsi, 2020 & Bao et al, 2009). Employees are also stressed because of the organization's structure and climate, which limit their autonomy. Employees in this situation believe they have little control over their responsibilities and that their employers do not trust them to complete their tasks. As a result, employees take longer to complete the same task and believe that learning a new one will be easy. They also suffer from pain, humiliation, and a loss of identity as an employee, all of which contribute to job dissatisfaction (Haryati & Rahardjo, 2013).

Comparable to other organization, similar situation happens in university, educators experiencing the same circumstances that affected their wellbeing. Thus, affects their job performance and lowering the motivation to perform their duties as an academician. The better educators control their own stress emotions, the more they can be mindful of their stakeholders and effectively manage their jobs and responsibilities. Emotions, in general, have an impact on the wellbeing of psychology, physical, emotion and cognitive. To achieve wellbeing, it is essential for educators to have self-care and stress management. Next, is about the meaning of self-care for educators and some strategy for stress management to help reducing the level of stress among the educators.

SELF-CARE AND STRESS MANAGEMENT FOR EDUCATORS

Self -care is very important to ensure that the level of mental well -being of the individual is in good condition and under control. Therefore, emotional management is needed among lecturers to help control stress better. This is not an easy thing to do. Sometimes we see someone is emotionally strong, yet we don't know what they are going through. Human life is different from each other. Everyone has their own problems and not everyone wants to share the problems with people around them. Some prefer to keep and hide problems until they end up experiencing depression. Every human being is not the same in terms of character and self -resilience. Self-care and stress management among lecturers is very important and should be given attention by the relevant parties (Ismail, N. H., & Noor, A, 2016). Aspects related to mental well -being should not be taken lightly as they are closely related to the work performance and quality of life as a lecturer. Certain parties should take this issue more seriously because if many lecturers are depressed, it must put a strain on the world of education. We do not want the world of education to be filled with depressed people who are unable to carry out their noble responsibilities as educators. If this occurs, students will suffer, and if not addressed, the country will be unable to produce a quality and excellent society.

Working people spend most of their time at work. Workplace roles are a priority for some people, while household or family life takes a back seat. The importance of employment for a person, not just economic factors, but work determines an individual's social status. As a result, a person's success at work is frequently regarded as a predictor of success in life. Failure in one's career, on the other hand, is considered failure in one's life. Individuals will experience stress because of workplace problems. Every job has certain challenges and stresses that can cause depression, moreover the career has certain risks such as journalists, doctors, nurses, and engineers (Park, S. G., Min, K. B., Chang, S. J., Kim, H. C., & Min, J. Y., 2009). In this case, many people think that working as a lecturer is not much stressful compared to other fields. In fact, a lecturer's career is considered the least stressful. In fact, few people are aware of the reality of a job as a lecturer at a university, which would seem simple on the surface but is only felt by the lecturer himself. Today's lecturers must deal with a wide range of responsibilities. They are not only responsible for teaching, but also for tasks outside the scope of their work as lecturers, such as community service and nationwide contributions. Lecturers have a wide range of responsibilities.

In addition to the actual work including teaching, publication writing supervision and consulting, lecturers need to ensure key performance indicators (KPIs) are always achieved. Lecturers must also be members of certain committees within the faculty and work regardless of time. Sometimes until late at night and working on weekends. These are all among the factors contributing to stress and at risk of causing depression. A lecturer can become depressed for various reasons such as work stress factors due to excessive workload and high expectations or personal factors such as family problems, relationship conflicts or interpersonal crises. However, not everyone experiences the same stress as a lecturer. Some are very happy with a career as a lecturer. Some never mind having to do work outside the scope of their work because of their passion. This situation can be relating to job satisfaction where some employees actually loves their job (Kelloway, E. K., Inness, M., Barling, J., Francis, L., & Turner, N., 2010). Lecturers who experience an adaptive response because of stress are typically unable to function effectively. This is because depression makes one irrational, anxious, tense, unable to give full attention to work, and unable to enjoy a sense of happiness or contentment heart for the work done. Failure to control oneself due to stress will have an impact on the lecturer's relationship with students as well as the quality of teaching and learning. As a result, the quality of lecturers will be impacted and efforts to bring Malaysia to the level of excellence and quality excellence education will be hampered.

Any action you take to improve your health and well-being is considered self-care. Self-care is defined by the National Institute of Mental Illness (NAMI) as having six components: physical, psychological, emotional, spiritual, social, and professional (Shepherd, M. A., & Newell, J. M., 2020). Dorothea Orem developed the Self-Care Deficit Theory between 1959 and 2001 to improve the quality of nursing in general hospitals in her state (Berbiglia, V. A., & Banfield, B. (2013). It is regarded as a noble nursing theory because it contains a wide range of general concepts that are applicable to all cases of nursing. According to Dorothea Orem's Self-Care Deficit Theory, nursing is the act of assisting others through the provision and management of self-care to care for or improve human working at the house level of effectiveness. It focuses on everyone's ability to care for themselves. Self-care, according to Orem, is the execution of activities that people trigger and act on to maintain life, health, and well-being. The Self-Care Deficit Theory's assumptions include staying healthy and useful. People must communicate constantly to connect with one another and with the environment.

Self-care is the ability that humans must meet the physical and psychosocial demands that keep life going. Self-care, according to Orem (2013), is the practise of activities that people initiate and participate in on their own to maintain their life, health, and well-being. The ability to act deliberately in meeting one's own needs is referred to as self-care agency. Humans are born with the ability to make decisions and make decisions on their own behalf. Essential conditioning factors influence self-care agency. The need to actively participate in meeting one's health care needs is referred to as therapeutic self-care demand. It is the collection of self-care actions and activities that are required to maintain and promote optimal health and well-being. It is determined by evaluating one's overall situation. This demand is influenced by social, cultural, and political factors.

Educators, like nurses, endure a great deal of responsibility in caring for students, as teaching and supervising are acts of caring and nurturing. According to the Orem Theory of Self Care, nurses must first take care of their own needs and well-being before they can care for their patients. Educators should do the same, they must take care of themselves before they can care for their students and other stakeholders. Educators were frequently preoccupied with duties and responsibilities, so they did not pay much attention to self-care. According to positive psychology, self-compassion is a component of the foundation for human growth and development. The experience of positive emotions aids in the development of a broader mindset that contributes to the development of a great personality. A solid behavioural and psychological foundation leads to resilience and psychological flexibility. Young educators in universities should be exposed to and educated on the importance of self-care for their well-being in the early stages of their careers.

One way to practise self-care is by having an effective stress management. Managing stress is crucial for educators to stay productive and maintain a good psychological health. Stress is a pressure that pushes human being to move, act, change, adapt and response to any stimulating factors. Human being can refuse to response to stress but they will have to bear the consequences. Stress is not always bad for human being but stress functioning to help human being survive then achieve success. In any organizations, stress is so common where every individual who work in organizations will experiencing stress at many levels. Educators should be well taught in managing their stress so that it can become a pushing factor or motivation for them to be more productive. An individual's ability to manage stress well is depends on their personal resources and coping strategies.

The concept of personal resources in managing stress is referring to one's own personal support from internal and external. The most efficient way to manage stress is by understanding and identifying symptoms of stress. The experiences of stress may be different for everyone in terms of causes and effects. Thus, educators need to understand their stress symptoms as an indicator that they need to do something to reduce the stress level as early as possible. By understanding themselves and able to read their own body symptom it helps them to take a break from busy schedule to get some fresh air. It is important to be able to identify the symptoms earlier as a preventive method. Personal resources include social support, self-esteem and self-efficacy, sense of coherence, level of optimism, ability to act assertively and locus of control. Social support is important for educators in managing stress in workplace. Social support can be from family, friends, work colleague and university management. By receiving strong social support, it can help educators especially young lecturers to grow in career as well as personality. Educators need to be given opportunity to learn more so they can have the freedom to grow and go further to contribute to society and the country. Apart from that, aspects of interpersonal such as self-esteem, self-efficacy, optimism, assertiveness, and locus of control serves as great support in coping with stress and maintaining well-being.

Every person must develop their own stress coping strategy. Coping entails adapting to unexpected demands or stressors. This necessitates a greater effort and use of energy than is required in daily life routines. Coping is typically defined as adjusting to or tolerating negative events or realities while maintaining a positive self-image and emotional balance. Stress coping is a process rather than an event. To deal with a stressful event, a combination of the several coping strategies might be helpful. People have different coping styles or prefer to use certain coping strategies over others. These differences in coping styles are usually a reflection of personality differences. Flexibility in coping is referring to being the ability to fit with the most appropriate coping strategy based on the different situations is more likely to help than rigidity in coping.

Educators who experience personal and work stress may try some coping strategies such as lower your expectations in any matters whether personal or work related. Some educators put a high expectation to themselves in achieving success or they put high expectations from other people. Whenever they fail to meet the expectation, frustration will often lead to stress. In doing work, you can ask others to assist you or work in a team. Do not push yourselves to do work that beyond your limit. Always take responsibility for any situation especially in problem solving situation, this will help to increase self-confidences, self-esteem, and resilience. The key to achieve psychologically well-being is to maintain emotionally supportive relationships. The best way to cope with stress is trying to change the source of stress or at least distance yourself from the source of stress. By changing the source of stress, it can change the effects of stress from negative to positive. Educators need to view the problem through different perspectives such as take it as opportunity to grow and change for a betterment in terms of career and personality.

CONCLUSION

Because of the widespread of Covid 19, every human being's life conditions have changed to new norms. The pattern of teaching and learning is the same. The previous traditional methods of teaching and learning have been completely replaced by online teaching and learning. Although online teaching-learning is widely known in universities and colleges, the difficulty in fully implementing it placing an emotional stress for lecturers. The effects of this pandemic have had two distinct effects, positive and negative. However, it is more to the negative effects that involve workload, due to students, interaction, time constraints, KPIs, internet network, unpleasant learning environment, and constant phone monitoring to put pressure on lecturers. As a result, it is possible to conclude that the stress experienced by lecturers manifests itself in a variety of ways, including emotional, physical, mental, and behavioural symptoms. Through this chapter it is hoped that they can help the university management by making this writing a source of reference and information in shaping and planning the activities of the university more effective and productive. In addition, this will help the university in identifying stress experienced among their educators as well as the level of job satisfaction in maintaining service quality. Therefore, it is hoped that the work environment and work process will be better and more effective in the future. It will be able to reduce the problem of deterioration in the quality of work and motivation among lecturers.

REFERENCES

Abdullah, N. H., Ismail, N., & Ismail, N. (2021). A Study of the Work-Life Balance among the Female Academics at Polytechnics. *BITARA International Journal of Civilizational Studies and Human Sciences*, *4*(1), 130–145.

Abu Bakar, M. R., Norazmi, N. A., & Ahmad, M. M. (2020). Level of Job Stress, Job Satisfaction and Organizational Commitment amongst Polytechnic Tuanku Syed Sirajuddin Lecturers. *Jurnal Dunia Pengurusan*, *2*(3), 94–100.

Albulescu, I., & Albulescu, M. University's Contribution to Local and Regional Development by Providing Educational Services for Adults. (2014). The University in the Community. The University's Contribution to Local and Regional Development by Providing Educational Services for Adults. *Procedia: Social and Behavioral Sciences*, *142*, 5–11. doi:10.1016/j.sbspro.2014.07.578

Aziz, A. R. A. (2014). *Happiness Sustainable among Lecturers at the Malaysian Research University. Universiti Teknologi Malaysia*. Skudai. doi:10.1016/j.sbspro.2014.01.918

Azman & Kutty. (2016). Imposing global university rankings on local academic culture. In The global academic rankings game. New York: Routledge Taylor & Francis Group.

Azreen, H.A., Norudin, M., & Zuraida, M. (2016). Impak Beban Kerja Terhadap Prestasi Kerja Pensyarah: Kes Kajian Di Politeknik Sultan Mizan Zainal Abidin (Psmza). *e-Academia Journal UiTMT, 5*(1), 1-12.

Baker, R., & Ibrahim, H. I. (2014). Work Stress in Police Organizations: A Review in the perspective of emotional intelligence. *Journal of the Humanities*, (23), 1–24.

Bani Hidayat Mohd Shafie. (2020). Pelaksanaan PdPc Dalam Talian (OLL) Semasa Perintah Kawalan Pergerakan (PKP) Fasa 1 Dan 2 Covid-19. *Jurnal Dunia Pendidikan*, 2(2), 213-221. doi:10.1287/orsc.2018.1235

Berbiglia, V. A., & Banfield, B. (2013). Self-care deficit theory of nursing. *Nursing Theorists and Their Work-E-Book, 30*(1), 240.

Chee Keong, C., Muhammad Faizal, A. G., & Abdullah, Z. (2018). Cabaran amalan komuniti pembelajaran dalam kalangan guru sekolah rendah berprestasi tinggi Malaysia. *Jurnal Kurikulum & Pengajaran Asia Pasifik, 6*(3), 1–14.

Cooper, C. L., & Marshall, J. (1978). *Understanding executive stress*. Springer. doi:10.1007/978-1-349-03030-9

Czarnitzki, D., Grimpe, C., & Toole, A. A. (2014). Delay and secrecy: Does industry sponsorship jeopardize disclosure of academic research? *Industrial and Corporate Change, 24*(1), 251–279. doi:10.1093/icc/dtu011

Damin, Z. A., Isa, K., Jaes, L., Kadir, Z. A., & Abdul, H. A. R. (2020). Analysis of Stress Contributing Factors in Work Organizations in Public Institutions of Higher Learning. *Journal of Social Transformation and Regional Development.*, 2(3), 11–23. doi:10.30880/jstard.2020.02.03.002

Deepti, B., & Hemant, T. (2018). A Study of Causes of Stress and Stress Management among Youth. *International Journal of Management and Social Sciences, 11*(3), 108–117. doi:10.21013/jmss.v11.n3.p1

Kamus Dewan. (Edisi Ke-4). (2005). Kuala Lumpur: Dewan Bahasa dan Pustaka.

Donesky, D., Norton, L., Fisher, E., & Bunker-Alberts, M. (2021). Health services and the Project RoomKey COVID-19 initiative for the unhoused: A university and community partnership. *Journal of Professional Nursing, 37*(6), 1175–1179. doi:10.1016/j.profnurs.2021.10.008 PMID:34887037

Elizabeth, S. (2020). *How to handle the stress of working from home*. Access from https://www.verywellmind.com/the-stress-of-working-fromhome-4141174

Gahlann, V. S. (2014). The Effect of Role Overload and Role Ambiguity on Job Performance of IT Professionals in India. *The IUP Journal of Management Research, 13*(3), 37–49.

Garis Panduan Amalan Baik. Staf Akademik. (2014). Retrieved on 14 March 2022. https://www2.mqa.gov.my/qad/garispanduan/2017/GGP%20Academic%20Staff(BM).upload%20website%2013.10.17.pdf

Garis Panduan Beban Staf Akademik. (n.d.). Retrieved on 14 March 2022. https://www2.mqa.gov.my/qad/garispanduan/2015/Garis%20Panduan%20Beban%20Staf%20Akademik.pdf

Ghazali, D., & Sufean, H. (2016). *Metodologi Penyelidikan Dalam Pendidikan: Amalan dan Analisis Kajian*. Penerbit Universiti Malaya.

Hairul Akmal Mohd Halim. (2014). *Stres sebagai moderator ke atas hubungan antara gaya kepimpinan ketua dengan tingkah laku buli* (Master Dissertation). Universiti Teknologi Malaysia, Skudai.

Haryati, R., & Rahardjo, S. N. (2013). *Influence of Corporate social responsibility, Environmental Performance and Corpor*. Fakultas Ekonomika dan Bisnis.

He, J. (2020). Progress and Prospect of Research on University-Industry Cooperation: From the Perspective of Researchers. *American Journal of Industrial and Business Management, 10*(05), 920–934. doi:10.4236/ajibm.2020.105062

Isa, Muda, Paim, Alavi, Shah, & Jamil. (2021). Kelaziman Punca Tekanan Pensyarah Di Universiti Awam Malaysia. *Journal of Social Sciences and Humanities, 18*(2), 84-97.

Ishak, A. A., & Talaat, A. Z. M. A. (2020). Online learning: A survey of readiness and motivation among logistics and supply chain management diploma students. *World Journal of Education, 2*(4), 68–82.

Ismail, N. H., & Noor, A. (2016). Occupational stress and its associated factors among academician in a research university, Malaysia. *Malaysian Journal of Public Health Medicine, 16*(1), 81–91.

Kamarudin, H. (2013). Work stress factors among Mains Holdings Sdn. Bhd. Research Project. Kuala Lumpur: Open University Malaysia.

Kelloway, E. K., Inness, M., Barling, J., Francis, L., & Turner, N. (2010). Loving one's job: Construct development and implications for individual well-being. In *New developments in theoretical and conceptual approaches to job stress*. Emerald Group Publishing Limited. doi:10.1108/S1479-3555(2010)0000008006

Maizan Mat @ Muhammad. (2018). Profile of negative emotional levels among lecturers of Selangor International Islamic University College. *Proceeding International Research Management & Innovation Conference (5th IRMIC)*.

Marimuthu, K. (2019). *Demographic factors and work stress of Kedah PDRM Traffic Investigating Officer* (Master Thesis). Sintok: Universiti Utara Malaysia.

Meng, Y., Tan, J., & Li, J. (2017). Abusive supervision by academic supervisors and postgraduate research students' creativity: The mediating role of leader-member exchange and intrinsic motivation. *International Journal of Leadership in Education, 20*(5), 605–617. doi:10.1080/13603124.2017.1304576

Meng, Y., & Zhao, C. (2018). Academic supervisor leadership and its influencing mechanism on postgraduate creativity in China. *Thinking Skills and Creativity, 29*, 32–44. doi:10.1016/j.tsc.2018.05.006

Mohamad, N. I., Ismail, A., Rozi, M. S. A. M., & Ahmad, S. (2015). Work stress and its relation to employee health: An empirical study of a police contingent in Peninsular Malaysia. *Malaysian Journal of Society and Space, 11*(10), 63–75.

Mohd Akmal Firdaus Mohamad Hamim. (2017). *Kompetensi guru reka cipta dalam bidang elektrik di sekolah menengah harian di Johor (Disertasi Sarjana)*. Universiti Tun Hussein Onn Malaysia.

Morgan, G. A., Gliner, J. A., & Harmon, R. (1999). Definition, Purposes, and Dimensions of Research. *Journal of the American Academy of Child and Adolescent Psychiatry*, *38*(2), 217–219. doi:10.1097/00004583-199902000-00023 PMID:9951223

Muhammad, F. M. R., & Abu Bakar, A. Y. (2020). Stress and Job Satisfaction Among Polytechnic Lecturers in Malaysia: A Need Analysis Study. *Bisma The Journal of Counseling*, *4*(1), 1–6. doi:10.23887/bisma.v4i1.24708

Nor Azimah Chew Abdullah. (2016). Konflik Kerja-Keluarga Dalam Kalangan Pensyarah: Satu Tinjauan. *Sains Humanika, 8*(4-2), 131-135.

Nugraheny, A. R. (2020). *Peran teknologi, guru dan orang tua dalam pembelajaran daring di masa pandemi*. https://osf.io/preprints/lissa/hz57r/

Okeke, M. N., Echo, O., & Oboreh, J. C. (2016). Effects of stress on employee productivity. *International Journal of Accounting Research*, *42*(3495), 1–12.

Parent-Lamarche, A., Marchand, A., & Saade, S. (2020). Does Depression Mediate the Effect of Work Organization Conditions on Job Performance? *Journal of Occupational and Environmental Medicine*, *62*(4), 296–302. doi:10.1097/JOM.0000000000001822 PMID:31977926

Park, S. G., Min, K. B., Chang, S. J., Kim, H. C., & Min, J. Y. (2009). Job stress and depressive symptoms among Korean employees: The effects of culture on work. *International Archives of Occupational and Environmental Health*, *82*(3), 397–405. doi:10.100700420-008-0347-8 PMID:18622624

Rahim, N. A., & Yatim, N. M. (2017). *Hubungan Kepuasan Kerja Terhadap Prestasi Kerja Dalam Kalangan Pensyarah: Satu Kajian Di Kolej Komuniti Bukit Beruang Melaka*. Academic Press.

Ramlee, N. (2015). *Tahap Stress dalam Kalangan Pensyarah Kolej Vokasional di Johor*. Tesis Sarjana. Universiti Tun Husseion Onn Malaysia.

Rathakrishnan, M. (2020). Covid -19 Ubah Pengajaran dan Pembelajaran dari Rumah. *BH Online*. https://www.bharian.com.my/rencana/komentar/2020/07/710464/covid-19

Ringkasan Eksekutif Pelan Pembangunan Pendidikan Malaysia 2015-2025 (Pendidikan Tinggi). (n.d.). *Kementerian Pendidikan Malaysia*. Retrieved on 16 March 2022 https://www.mohe.gov.my/muat-turun/penerbitan-jurnal-dan-laporan/pppm-2015-2025pt/104-ringkasan-eksekutif-pppm-2015-2025/file

Scherer, R., & Teo, T. (2019). Unpacking teachers' intentions to integrate technology: A meta-analysis. *Educational Research Review*, *27*, 90–109. doi:10.1016/j.edurev.2019.03.001

Schuldt, B., & Totten, J. (2008). An exploratory study: Business faculty and the faculty stress index. *Proceedings of the Allied Academies*, *13*(2), 128–133.

Sham, F. M. (2005). Tekanan emosi remaja Islam. *Jurnal Islamiyat*, *27*(1), 3–24.

Sharmaa, U., Sokalb, L., Wangc, M., & Loreman, T. (2021). Measuring the use of inclusive practices among pre-service educators:A multi-national study. *Teaching and Teacher Education*, *107*, 2–9. doi:10.1016/j.tate.2021.103506

Shepherd, M. A., & Newell, J. M. (2020). Stress and health in social workers: Implications for self-care practice. *Best Practices in Mental Health, 16*(1), 46–65.

Sunarsi, D. (2020). The Analysis of The Work Environmental and Organizational Cultural Impact on The Performance and Implication of The Work Satisfaction. *Jurnal Ilmiah Ilmu Administrasi Publik, 9*(2), 237-246. doi:10.26858/jiap.v9i2.11761

Sweeny, K., Howell, J. L., & Kwan, V. W. (2020). Losing control: Comparing the role of personality during two types of stressful life experiences. *Personality and Individual Differences, 156*, 109771. doi:10.1016/j.paid.2019.109771

Sze, W. Y., Surat, S., & Amat, S. (2022). Teacher pressures and challenges towards new norms during the covid-19 pandemic in a Sarawak State District. *Malaysian Journal of Social Sciences and Humanities, 7*(1), 230–239.

Tajudeen, A. B. A. (2004). *Kepuasan kerja dan tekanan yang dihadapi oleh guru sekolah menengah.* Retrieved from http://psasir.upm.edu.my/6399/1/FPP_2004_20(1-%0A24).pdf%0A

Tambi & Awang. (2019). Hubungan Antara Tekanan Kerja Dan Kecerdasan Emosi Terhadap Kepuasan Kerja Dalam Kalangan Pensyarah Fakulti Sains Sosial Dan Kemanusiaan, Universiti Kebangsaan Malaysia. *Journal of Social Sciences and Humanities, 16*(5), 1-19.

Tengku Sarina Aini Tengku Kasim & Fatimah Sahida AbduRajak. (2018). Pengalaman pengajaran guru novis Pendidikan Islam: Implikasi terhadap reka bentuk kurikulum latihan pendidikan guru. *Jurnal Pendidikan Malaysia, 43*(1), 59–66.

Unimap Academic Regulations for Postgraduate Research Programs. (2021). Retrieved on 14 March 2022. https://cgs.unimap.edu.my/images/REGULATIONS/R.pdf

Yurtkorub, S. (2013). Job stress and job performance among employees in public sector in Istanbul: Examining the moderating role of emotional intelligence. *Procedia: Social and Behavioral Sciences, 75*, 518–524. doi:10.1016/j.sbspro.2013.04.056

Zafir, M. M., & Fazilah, M. H. (2010). Stress at the Workplace: How the Ergonomic Factors Minimize it? *The 5th National Human Resource Management Conference 2010*, 642–657. 10.1080/00140130400029282

Zaini, U. (2012). *Akademia Baru: Memartabat UTM Berjenama Global 2012-2020.* Penerbit UTM Press.

Chapter 11
Occupational Health and Well-Being in Higher Education Institutions in Mexico:
Self-Care During Pandemic-Induced Remote Work

Cynthia Maria Montaudon- Tomas
https://orcid.org/0000-0002-2595-6960
UPAEP Universidad, Mexico

Ingrid N. Pinto-López
https://orcid.org/0000-0002-1580-1375
UPAEP Universidad, Mexico

Anna Amsler
https://orcid.org/0000-0003-3183-0878
Independent Researcher, Mexico

ABSTRACT

This chapter presents an overview of occupational health in remote work from the self-care perspective. A literature review regarding remote working conditions and their effects on health and well-being is included, along with an analysis of the most relevant self-care and practices that have been developed for working at the distance. The study focuses on faculty, specifically at a private university in Puebla, Mexico, and the effects of the pandemic-induced remote work schemes on their well-being, along with the most common ailments that emerged from remote working conditions and self-care practices that can be adopted to prevent or reduce them. A survey was conducted among faculty members to understand the health implications of remote work and what people have been doing to deal with them. The concept of health circles is introduced to help explain specific actions taken to promote self-care and group care.

DOI: 10.4018/978-1-6684-2334-9.ch011

INTRODUCTION

The health crisis took the world by surprise, affecting every aspect of human life with restrictions such as quarantines, confinement, and social distancing measures. Higher Education Institutions were no exception and had to adapt to comply with the limitations imposed by the pandemic. Initially, universities worldwide had to decide whether to suspend courses until the situation started to fade, which would have produced significant disruptions to educational calendars considering the uncertainty surrounding the crisis, or developing and implementing strategies that would allow courses to continue on their traditional time frames. Initially, there were expectations that the crisis would subside in a matter of months. However, what started as an emergency response continued for more than a year and a half.

Before the COVID-19 pandemic, the effects of remote work had been analyzed in terms of positive effects on mental health, general well-being, and increased productivity. Remote work was an ideal form of work in which employees would relax, manage their own time under flexible conditions, and possibly working in an idyllic paradise. However, the health crisis imposed remote employment under utterly different working conditions, not as a choice for most workers, but a decision to maintain jobs for some. Changes did not occur in the expected conditions of freedom and independence but were restricted by safe distancing measures in less-than-optimal conditions at home. Under this scenario, the effects of remote work started to be analyzed in negative terms based on the adverse impact it had on mental health and general well-being, as well as productivity.

Because of a lack of preparation time to move to remote work, most homes were ill-prepared, lacking the primary conditions such as internet connectivity, privacy, soundproofing, and even ergonomic furniture to provide a good working environment (International Labor Organization, 2020). These conditions resulted in various health-related problems, accidents, and injuries that were not traditionally considered work-related because they happened in the privacy of the home but are now taken into account as part of workplace safety risks.

As remote work extended in different sectors, concerns for self-care grew due to the underlying challenges of not working in an office environment, the extended working hours facing a computer or other digital devices, frequent interruptions, and the need to tend to specific family or home issues during working hours.

In Higher Education Institutions (HEIs), the transition to remote work was done virtually overnight. Universities and students expected courses to continue seamlessly; therefore, everything had to move online in a matter of days without proper training about the tools required to teach in a virtual format. Initial difficulties faced by faculty resulted in increased stress and excess working hours. Pandemic burnout became rampant in academia due to working conditions that demanded continuous long-term physical, cognitive, or emotional efforts (Gewin, 2021). Workplace stress in academia has become a global issue that can lead to anxiety and depression and other problems. A study developed by the Chronicle of Higher Education (2020) determined that most faculty are experiencing elevated levels of frustration, anxiety, and stress and are struggling with increased workloads and deterioration of work-life balance. Many are even considering retiring or changing careers and leaving higher education.

The abrupt and, later on, prolonged changes to the work routine of professors also exacerbated existing inequalities in HEIs. Therefore, it is essential to analyze the effects on remote workers' health and general well-being in the education sector. This chapter aims to present the results of a survey about the effects of remote work on the health and well-being of faculty in a private university in Puebla, Mexico, and their coping mechanisms and self-care strategies. This will help shed some light on the leading health and well-being challenges that employees and employers faced during the COVID-19 pandemic, including the most common ailments that emerged from remote working conditions.

Because of social restrictions, traditional business practices to promote occupational health and well-being were left in the hands of the employees. Online courses and virtual well-being check-ups increased, but it became up to the employees to care for themselves. Implementing self-care measures minimizes health risks and other downsides of working remotely. It is also essential to maintain positive feelings and boost confidence and self-esteem, which correlates directly to productivity at work. Some relevant questions that emerged include: how did faculty members cope with remote work? In which ways did they take care of themselves? Did they manage stress properly? How well were they able to balance work and life? What specific self-care practices did they follow, and which practices worked best?

The specific conditions in which academic life occurred during the pandemic are also presented, giving special attention to extended workloads and working hours (International Labor Organization, 2017), working over the weekends (Potratz, 2020), increase in training and development, and changes in numerous actions surrounding the teaching and learning process, which can increase stress levels and can result in burnout of faculty. For some, it has come as a surprise to feel stress once the novelty of working from home wears off, and although stressors may not be comparable to being stuck in traffic during morning commutes, they can still take a toll (Scott, 2021).

Maintaining a healthy lifestyle and establishing clear boundaries between work and personal life is becoming more critical than ever, as well as creating self-care routines. This chapter will include a series of guidelines for the future of remote and hybrid education, emphasizing employee well-being and self-care, targeted explicitly to academic life.

BACKGROUND

Occupational Health and Remote Work

During the Industrial Revolution, working conditions involved significant risks related mainly to accidents and health problems, particularly due to fumes and harmful products to which workers of all ages, including children, were exposed; this resulted in severe diseases and a high mortality rate (Cameron, 2021). Since then, significant progress has been made, including improving lighting and ventilation conditions, providing protective equipment, and incorporating ergonomic principles to reduce health problems and accidents and improve conditions in the workplace.

Occupational health began to increase in importance in the 1970s, with the development of various international regulations to guarantee healthy and safe working conditions for all workers (EHS Insight Resources, 2019). Globalization and rapid technological progress have been regarded as some of the most important forces of change in the world of work, and as economies become more and more integrated, employment patterns shift, which leads to new standards for occupational safety and health being developed and widely adopted (Alli, 2008).

In recent years, occupational health has been a constant concern of companies and governments. The World Health Organization (2021a) has stated that the health of workers is essential, which is why it has established parameters to improve conditions in the workplace. This organization has also determined that occupational health focuses on all aspects of health and safety in the workplace, with emphasis on the prevention of risks that can lead to diseases, accidents, musculoskeletal injuries, respiratory diseases, hearing loss, circulatory diseases, stress-related disorders, and communicable diseases, among others (Ibidem).

The scope of occupational health has continued to evolve and adapt to social, political, and economic changes, as well as technological developments (Alli, 2008). In 2020, the COVID-19 pandemic brought a reconsideration of occupational health due to new worker designations and the fact that, in most cases, employers were not responsible for the physical or mental well-being of employees on remote work schemes. In this sense, the World Economic Forum (2020) established three categories of workers during the health crisis: Essential employees, remote employees, and non-essential employees.

For the purpose of this chapter, the population of the study will be remote employees in the Higher Education sector who became responsible for their own occupational health during the pandemic, transitioning into self-care practices. It has been suggested that remote workers were better able to protect their health by relocating their work (Faller, 2021).

The Principles of Self-Care

Self-care is a practice that grew substantially due to diminishing resources in service settings and an increase in worker burnout (Bressi & Vaden, 2017). Conditions like those have only escalated due to the COVID-19 pandemic, and therefore, self-care acquired even more importance than before.

In literature, self-care has been sometimes used as a synonym with self-management and self-monitoring. While the terms self-care and self-management have been discussed in detail in the literature, it is still unclear what the specific differences between the concepts are and how they are linked to each other (Omisakin & Ncama, 2011).

Definitions of self-care abound. It can refer to the individual responsibilities to achieve and maintain a healthy lifestyle through the behaviors required for human functioning development and the necessary attitudes to deal with health conditions (Ibidem). The World Health Organization defines self-care as "the ability of individuals, families, and communities to promote health, prevent disease, maintain health, and to cope with illness and disability with or without the support of a healthcare provider" (WHO, 2021).

Self-care can be broadly defined as the activities that individuals undertake to promote their own health, preventing diseases, limiting their own illnesses, and monitoring their own health (Levin & Idler, 1983). Also, as the "actions directed toward oneself or the environment to regulate one's functioning in the interest of one's life, integrated functioning, and well-being." (Orem, 1985). It is a purposeful goal or an activity that seeks a specific result (Peters & Templin, 2010), helping improve health and prevent illnesses and disabilities (Lupton, 2013). Self-care involves both the ability to take care of oneself and the actual actions performed in the process of achieving, preserving, or promoting one's health and is sometimes described in terms of a continuum that goes from complete health management independence to absolute reliance on external care (Omisakin & Ncama, 2011).

In this sense, self-care is a broad term that encompasses many aspects of living a healthy life, including hygiene, nutrition, general lifestyle and exercise, and environmental factors such as living conditions (WHO, 2021b). Positive self-care behaviors involve following the path towards optimal health but also being able to recognize possible problems, understand symptoms, and respond to them adequately to maintain or improve one's general well-being both in personal and professional life (Omisakin & Ncama, 2011).

Self-care is based on the theory of planned behavior, which suggests that attitudes, subjective norms, and perceived behavior control predict intention and that intention, along with perceived behavioral control, can predict actual behavior (Peters & Templin, 2010). Self-care behaviors are mostly individual learned behaviors but also relate to community-based practices. The core principles of self-care integrate aspects related to the individual, such as self-reliance, empowerment, autonomy, responsibility, and self-efficacy, as well as those associated with the greater community, like participation and involvement (WHO, 2021b).

Behaviors of self-care are learned, therefore require to be taught or self-taught, and are supported on personal responsibility. Sometimes, self-care practices require specific educational programs, stand-alone courses, or can even be developed based on instructions given by a medical practitioner, for instance, taking medication, and changing lifestyle factors such as non-smoking, exercising, reducing stress, eating healthy, and others (Bressi & Vaden, 2016; Orem, 1985).

El-Osta, Webber, Gnani, Banarsee, Mummery, Mated & Smith (2019) developed a matrix to analyze the different factors that make up self-care, determining that it is constituted of four cardinal dimensions: Self-Care Activities, Self-Care Behaviours, Self-Care Context, and Self-Care Environment. The first dimension is related to individual capacities, knowledge, capabilities, and activities to improve and promote health, as well as monitor and self-manage common quotidian conditions. The second dimension also focuses on the individual but includes generalized behaviors within the social network that motivate individuals to engage in positive actions to take care of themselves. For its part, the third dimension focuses on the extent to which a person relies on external resources, be it professional or not, to take care of themselves; it analyzes the level of autonomy of an individual with regards to their health. Finally, the fourth dimension encompasses the prevailing culture and normative attitudes that influence self-care practices in a community, including culture, narrative, communication, and policies surrounding public and individual health and well-being (El-Osta, Webber, Gnani, Banarsee, Mummery, Mated & Smith, 2019).

Still, there are differences between personal and professional self-care. "Personal self-care is defined as a process of purposeful engagement in practices that promote holistic health and well-being of the self" (Lee & Miller, 2013, 98). "Professional self-care is understood as the process of purposeful engagement in practices that promote effective and appropriate use of self in the professional role within the context of sustaining holistic health and well-being (Lee & Miller, 2013, 98).

MAIN FOCUS OF THE CHAPTER

This chapter presents a literature review on the topic of the different health problems and risks associated with remote work and self-care practices to promote and maintain health while working from home. Publications from various organizations, consulting companies, and service providers for remote work that had developed studies on the effects of remote work during the pandemic were analyzed. Additionally, a study was conducted among faculty members at a private university in Mexico using part of a validated scale to evaluate remote working conditions during the pandemic, which was developed by the authors. From the information obtained, categories of risks and conditions were established, and self-care recommendations were included for each one.

At the university, interest in analyzing health-related problems due to remote work emerged since the beginning of the pandemic when all activities had to be moved online. As the pandemic progressed, it became evident that additional evaluations needed to be carried out frequently to maintain a clear perspective of the situation. Checking-in with employees was established as a care practice, and different activities to promote health were developed. Activities included online sports classes, virtual therapy, instructional webinars, and others. The main concern was that the authorities could not keep up with the health and well-being of every single employee at the distance and that different strategies needed to be established, being the most important, the promotion of self-care. In the second semester of 2021, a new scale was developed to confirm the most common health problems related to remote work in order to create specific strategies for the promotion of self-care.

Issues, Controversies, Problems

Numerous studies have examined the psychological and physiological implications of remote work, obtaining diverse results (Maruyama, Hopkinson & James, 2009). On the one hand, there is talk of greater benefits for employees in terms of freedom to choose where and when to work and how to organize, and the added perks of eliminating commute time. On the other hand, some studies have emphasized the rise of problems related to the inability or impossibility to disconnect from work and other factors that negatively affect the well-being of remote workers.

This section presents information on remote working conditions and the associated issues, controversies, and problems in terms of individual well-being and occupational health that can be addressed through self-care practices. It includes a field study which helps shed light on the magnitude of physical and mental health ailments derived from working from home.

One of the main issues that have emerged in relation to remote work and occupational health is that the employer has a limited ability to monitor working conditions from home and the hours worked, as well as the workloads of its employees (The Center for Occupational Safety, 2020). Self-care becomes an essential strategy to promote the health and well-being of remote and hybrid workers, but it is important to develop targeted strategies based on the most prevalent physical and mental health-related problems, which are presented in the following subsections.

In terms of the general population in Mexico, studies show that there are very high costs involved in unnecessary doctor visits for common non-health conditions that can account for more than 745 million US dollars a year. Millions of people seek treatment for non-serious health conditions in the public healthcare system, despite the wide availability of self-care solutions (Asociación de Fabricantes de Medicamentos de Libre Acceso, 2017). Therefore, promoting self-care is beneficial for individuals, organizations, and society as a whole.

Remote Working Conditions during the COVID-19 Pandemic

Teleworking, or remote work, is a form of employment that considers the home, a coffee shop, coworking spaces, and other public and private spaces as the place of work. Under this scheme, the need for a fixed space to carry out work activities is eliminated, and various technologies are used to perform job-related duties (World Economic Forum, 2020). The conditions imposed by modifying the characteristics of employment have forced the development of policies that allow the application of occupational health rights and obligations, including the necessary precautions for both the employee and the employer in teleworking and hybrid work models (Chandler, 2020).

When remote work practices started to rise, there was a concern that employees would use most of their time to tend to personal and family problems instead of work. Currently, the concern has moved towards the analysis of the lack of limits in remote work. Studies have been carried out that show that people who work from home tend to work longer hours due to the limited control they have over the time they work (International Labor Organization, 2017), sometimes even working on weekends (Potratz, 2020).

An important thing to consider when analyzing occupational health and self-care practices in remote working conditions is that, in the case of the COVID-19 pandemic, the shift to teleworking was abrupt. Initially, not knowing how long this new working scheme would last, people did not have time to adapt or prepare the spaces of the home to carry out office work that, in general, involves sitting in front of a computer for more than eight hours.

Work went from being carried out in a space designed for such activities to being carried out on the kitchen or dining room table, the living room, or even the bedroom. In some cases, people had a desk and chair, but perhaps without the necessary adjustability provided by the furniture and equipment of a suitable work environment (International Labor Organization, 2020).

This context, along with other factors such as added stress, can negatively affect occupational health and well-being, also contributing to a decrease in worker productivity and performance. The main occupational risks of remote work are ergonomic, psychosocial, and those derived from the difficulty of separating family life from work life. In the space of the home, the reduction or management of these risks usually involves the adoption of self-care practices.

Field Study

A brief scale was developed and validated to confirm the most prevalent health-related issues of remote and hybrid working faculty and staff, as identified in previous studies. The study was conducted between December 2020 and March 2021. The occurrence of accidents at home was also included as a suggestion from the area of the university that handles insurance policies and due to the occurrence of a variety of mishaps while working remotely.

In all, 250 employees working remotely (at least part-time) participated in the study. The health conditions attributed to remote work that were identified in the literature were classified into physical and mental health problems. Furthermore, the most important risks that people face when working at home were also included as a separate category. All of these ailments were integrated into the scale to measure the occurrence of each one.

Occurrence of Physical Problems

The so-called tech-neck, or technological neck, is a new term used to describe neck pain caused by repetitive stress and injuries to the muscles and other tissue structures of the cervical spine (Miller, 2020), which are related to factors such as the hunched position when working on a laptop, being in the same position for long periods of time, the reduction of physical activity due to confinement during the pandemic and the lack of ergonomic furniture available in the household (Upham, 2021). It is one of the most prevalent health risks of remote work (UNUM, 2020), and 61% of the participants of the study reported experiencing it.

Various studies have suggested that the most common musculoskeletal issue for remote workers is lower back pain, caused by less-than-optimal working conditions, such as the use of non-ergonomic furniture (Di Donato, Iles, Buchbinder, Xia, and Collie, 2021). According to Moretti, Menna, Bulichino, Aulicino, Paoletta, Liguori, and Iolascon (2020), spinal pain is one of the most common health problems in the working-age population worldwide, as sustained sedentary work in a forced posture is a risk factor for low back pain. The risk of low back pain seems to increase when people sit more than 7 hours a day (Moretti et al., 2020), although the incidence of this condition is also associated with factors such as age, mass index, the position of the body when sitting, the type of backrest and the distance between the person and the computer screen. Results of the study show that 48% people suffered lower back pain as a result of remote work.

In that same line of thought, repetitive physical stress injuries while working from home has become a growing problem (Porter, 2021). The lack of adequate and enabled space for remote work and the use of digital devices such as tablets, laptops, and cell phones to work has caused many teleworkers to experience joint pain (Torres, 2020). Working on the computer requires a position where the wrists are bent at an acute angle for hours. This can lead to discomfort and even carpal tunnel syndrome (DePaul, 2019). Symptoms include numbness, tingling, or pain that can occur in the thumb and fingers, as well as the forearm (Ibidem), and has a 52% prevalence rate in this study.

The increase in body weight during the pandemic has also been a phenomenon recorded around the world in people who worked remotely during confinement, although less common than other with only 21% of people in this study experiencing it. This phenomenon has been called Quarantine-15, to refer to the average weight gain expressed in pounds (Wood and Thomas, 2021); it has also been called Covid-Curves (Katella, 2020). The reasons for weight gain are diverse, such as the disruption of routine and an increase in stress, changes in eating habits, and reduced physical activity (Gutiérrez & Orihuela Quispe, 2021; Wood and Thomas, 2021).

Other ailments related to remote work include computer vision or digital eye strain syndrome. This involves dryness and irritability of the eyes that is aggravated by working long hours on the computer and other electronic devices and by not maintaining an adequate distance between the person and the device (News Center 1, 2020; Cleveland Clinic, 2021). When vision is focused on a nearby object such as a screen, the tiny muscles inside the eyes contract; this contraction changes the shape of the lenses inside the eyes, focusing the image towards the retina (Brown, 2021). Studies carried out worldwide indicate that between 22% and 38% of those who have worked remotely consider that their vision has been affected since the beginning of the pandemic (Ibidem); in the present study, the figure is higher, at 51%. Some symptoms of this type of condition are blurred vision (Leckey, 2021) and red, itchy, dry eyes (Cleveland Clinic, 2021), making eyes more prone to infections (Brown, 2021).

Additionally, changes in the work environment and working hours have contributed to a higher incidence of tension headaches and migraines, with 42% of participants reporting this problem. Ergonomics plays an important role. Sensitivity to blue light is also a major trigger (Upham, 2021), and increased stress levels also contribute to headaches and migraines.

In terms of insomnia, bed-time habits have been affected by the pandemic and remote work (Sánchez, 2020). Sleep deprivation can result in irritability and exhaustion and has been linked to a series of severe health problems, including heart disease, type 2 diabetes, and depression (Walters, 2021). Reports developed even before the pandemic have suggested that working from home, as well as changes in routines (Kiger, 2020), could be causing insomnia (Kekatos, 2017). Results showed 34% of respondents suffer from sleeping problems. Very high rates of insomnia are due to two major factors. First, the low levels of detachment that exist in terms of work in remote employment models are linked to an insufficient quality of sleep at night and fatigue in the morning (Mostafa, 2021). When life becomes repetitive, the lack of dynamism contributes to poor sleep. This condition has been called "coronasomnia", referring to insomnia produced by the coronavirus pandemic (UC Davis Health, 2020). Working after hours is also keeping people up (Sánchez, 2020).

Finally, other related ailments include pandemic fatigue, which has been considered a natural response to the prolonged health crisis and the demotivation derived from restrictions such as confinement conditions and social distancing. This type of fatigue increases gradually over time, and people who suffer from it are affected by a variety of emotions, experiences, and perceptions that generate exhaustion (World Health Organization, 2020). This type of excessive fatigue is linked to dissatisfaction, discomfort, dissonance between mind and body, and an excess of work demands (Zerbe, 2020), and it is the most prevalent issue reported by 64% of participants.

In terms of the issues that affect the mental state of the person, the following section presents the results for the most common problems identified in the literature.

Occurrence of Mental Problems

The effects and implications of isolation in remote work have not been analyzed in detail; however, the health contingency has highlighted the need for its study. Many employees, who had a space for socialization in the workplace, said leaving that environment and moving to their homes has had a significant psychological impact (Zielinska and Kirtzman, 2021), with 30% of respondents reporting feeling lonely and isolated.

It should be noted that loneliness is an emotional response to lack of connection, while isolation is related to access or lack of it. Employees facing isolation at work lack the materials or information they need to carry out their activities or think their achievements are being ignored (Hickman, 2019). Isolation is more of a technical problem than an emotional one, unlike loneliness; however, loneliness can contribute to isolation and vice versa.

The pandemic also increased the levels of stress. This can be related to multiple causes, ranging from fear of contagion to job security, working from home, confinement, forced coexistence, or isolation (Montaudon-Tomas, Pinto-López, Olivera-Pérez, and Amsler, 2021). The health crisis also produced other types of stress related to technology, which have been considered as modern diseases that can occur from the inability to handle new technologies (Ingusci, Signore, Giancespro, Manuti, Molino, Russo, Zito, and Cortese, 2021). Those who experience this type of stress are also usually people who are exposed to information technologies for long periods of time (Bondanini, Giorgi, Ariza-Montes, Vega-Muñoz, and Andreucci-Annunziata, 2020). Stress can lead to numerous health problems, affecting the psychological and physiological state and people's behaviors and cognition (Houtman, Jettinghof, and Cedillo, 2007). In the present study, 41% of people acknowledged feeling more stressed while working from home.

An increase in anxiety levels is also among the consequences of the pandemic and the conditions of remote work, with 29% of participant suffering from it. Uncertainty about the future and the return to normalcy makes people feel more stressed, tense, and even aggressive. Rising fear and anxiety among the world's population are intensified by essential but socially disruptive measures such as quarantines, lockdowns, and social distancing. This can lead to significant psychological and psychiatric disorders, such as post-traumatic stress disorder, depression, anxiety, panic, and behavioral changes (Sood, 2020).

Finally, burnout syndrome has been reported as one of the most damaging consequences of remote work, particularly because it tends to blur the line between professional and personal life. It has been defined as the emotional consequence generated in an individual in relation to the work they perform. It has three main characteristics: high emotional exhaustion, depersonalization, and lack of personal fulfillment (Morales-Cadena, Fonseca-Salazar, and Fonseca-Chávez, 2020). This syndrome occurs when the person is constantly exposed to work situations that lead to a state of emotional overload, long work hours, excessive physical work, high levels of stress, little autonomy, a bad work environment, and feelings of inability to perform the tasks entrusted, among others (World Health Organization, 2019; Martínez-Mejía, Villa-George, Martínez-Guerrero, 2020). In the case of the faculty and staff that participated in the study, burnout syndrome occurs with a prevalence rate of 32%.

Occurrence of Home-Based Accidents

Working from home can have other risks aside from mental and physical problems. Such is the case of home-based accidents. Poisoning by toxic products, including inhalation of gas and carbon monoxide, is the number one cause of accidental death in the home, followed by falls (Sandorf, 2019). Trips, slips, and falls have increased significantly since employees work remotely due to the number of hours they spend in homes and particular conditions such as the use of cables to charge digital devices; results from the study show 16% of participants have suffered this type of accidents. Remote employees often trip over objects such as children's toys or slip due to wearing inappropriate footwear or due to spilled water for coffee or tea (Previsor Insurance, 2020). Although these accidents can be the result of house-related chores and activities, it is relevant to identify them because they occurred when work and home duties converged in the same space.

SOLUTIONS AND RECOMMENDATIONS

Based on the ailments that were identified in the literature and then incorporated into the scale for the study, self-care recommendations were included. The following subsections present an overview of the suggestions by category.

Self-Care Recommendations for Physical Ailments

For people suffering of tech-neck, maintaining good posture is essential, so it is recommended to rethink the workspace at home, especially in terms of ergonomic furniture (Healthline, 2020a). A chair that reclines and leans back slightly at 25° to 30° is recommended (Hansraj, 2014). An alternative is to use folded towels or cushions to support both the neck and the back (Chandler, 2020). Frequent stretching can also help, getting up from the chair at least every half hour and walking at least a few steps (Hansraj, 2014). Certain yoga postures are also helpful (Kassel, 2020).

In terms of lower back pain, the best way to prevent it is to recreate the office workspace at home, using ergonomic furniture (Moretti et al., 2020). This also extends to routines, where remote workers should stick to their work schedules and not spend more time sitting in front of the computer. Working from the bed should be avoided unless people have a special table for that purpose (Hedge, 2020). It is recommended not to work on chairs or soft surfaces that do not offer back support (Chandler, 2020). Additionally, people can place a footrest or some other object to support the feet (Ibidem) when working at a table. As with neck problems, regular exercise and stretching can help prevent lower back problems. Moving around, walking, and stretching frequently can help reduce the problem, alleviate stress, and also increase endorphins (Walters, 2021).

For joint pain, carpal tunnel syndrome, and tendonitis, it is suggested to avoid using any type of wrist support cushioning, as this adds pressure to the tendons and nerves (Hedge, 2020). Performing hand and finger stretches, as well as rotations (Hand & Wrist Center, 2020), can help prevent or decrease joint pain. DePaul (2019) recommends adjusting the keyboard height to reduce the flex required for typing or investing in an ergonomic keyboard that eliminates harsh angles entirely.

With regards to increased body weight, the first recommendation is to avoid having junk food fixes around the house (Stange, 2021). Registering the food consumed throughout the day and reducing the intake of sugary drinks (Healthcare, 2021) have been considered as good strategies to avoid gaining weight. Exercising regularly and eating healthy is important. It is also recommended to deal with associated mental health problems, such as anxiety and isolation, and to try to understand the origin of the need to eat. Seeking socialization with others, even in a virtual way, can serve to channel emotions towards more positive actions (Kelly, 2020). Some remote workers have been able to drop the quarantine weight and even up to 25 pounds by incorporating walking into their routines, including walking during meetings that do not require a camera to be on (Michael, 2021).

In order to avoid computer vision or digital eye strain syndrome, it is recommended to maintaining an adequate distance from the screen is important. It is best to position the computer screen about one arm's length away and adjust the view angle (Cleveland Clinic, 2021; Chandler, 2020). Reducing the glare of the screens can also help relieve some of the symptoms of digital eye (Cleveland Clinic, 2021), as well as resting the eyes every so often and moisturizing them frequently (Forster, 2020). It is important to blink frequently (Greenstein, 2020) in order to prevent the eyes from drying out because if there is no moisture in the eye, the cornea dries out, and vision becomes blurry (Brown, 2021). A humidifier can be placed in the room where work is carried out to help with dry environments (Vision Health, 2020). It is recommended to relax the eye muscles, using the 20/20/20 rule, taking a 20-second break every twenty minutes, closing the eyes, and then directing the vision somewhere 20 feet away (Cleveland Clinic, 2021; Brown, 2021). People can also use glasses that filter blue light from screens (Leckey, 2021) and enlarge the size of the text to avoid eye strain (Brown, 2021). It is not advisable to work with natural light from a front or back window; it is best to have light from the side to reduce harmful reflections and glare (Hedge, 2020).

To prevent headaches, it is recommended to stay hydrated, control caffeine intake and keep it as regular as possible, and limit the amount of sugar. Avoiding or reducing digital eye strain is also applicable to headaches and migraines, as symptoms may be related (McCallum, 2020).

When dealing with insomnia, trying to go to bed at the same time each day to build a routine and maintain healthy sleep patterns is crucial (Walters, 2021). Those who have trouble sleeping should set a regular schedule that matches their internal clocks, develop a relaxing routine before bed, and reduce light intake (especially from electronic devices) for an hour or two before bed. Daytime naps, caffeine, and alcohol can also affect sleep (Kiger, 2020), so avoiding them is essential to reduce sleep problems. Limiting the intake of negative news, especially before sleeping, is also recommended (Walters, 2021).

Some psychologists suggest that the fatigue derived from remote work may result from the need for greater concentration and attention effort. It is recommended that, whenever possible, meetings be audio-only to avoid sensory overload (James, 2021). Also, shortening meetings from one hour to 45-50 minutes allows people to have quick breaks between meetings. When taking these breaks from the screen, it is important not to use that time to check other mobile devices (Ibidem).

Self-Care Recommendations for Mental Ailments

When dealing with isolation from the individual perspective, having a pet or adopting one can be of great help to avoid loneliness from remote working conditions (Shah, 2020). Creating a change of scenery by incorporating plants into the home office also seems to work. In terms of the organization's perspective, Gallup recommends promoting frequent and continuous conversations, using specific language for remote workers (Hickman, 2019). The best strategy is to create opportunities for meaningful connections, such as making formal presentations to colleagues and linking the employee with others for certain projects. Online group chats also allow teams to maintain continuous communication (Ibidem).

For people suffering from stress, exercise can be of great help, experts recommend yoga, but any form of physical activity is beneficial. Getting enough sleep is also important for effective stress management, so developing healthy sleep habits is essential. Furthermore, setting boundaries between work and personal life can help reduce stress; this involves taking time to recharge and disconnect from work (Abrahams, 2019). Some companies have developed useful digital applications such as telemedicine tools through smartphones so that their remote employees can control their stress levels, and these can be monitored by health services (Gleason, 2021).

In terms of anxiety, caffeine tends to induce it, and alcohol changes the levels of serotonin and other neurotransmitters in the brain, so avoiding them is essential for people with these problems (Healthline, 2020b). Similarly, anxiety can be derived from an accumulation of adrenaline; in these cases, exercise can help use that additional adrenaline. Not drinking enough water can make anxiety symptoms worse, as dehydration can cause heart palpitations that lead to feelings of panic and anxiety attacks (Ibidem). Therefore, people should monitor their water intake.

With regards to burnout syndrome, it is essential to replenish physical and emotional energy. Good sleep habits, nutrition, exercise, social ties, and other practices that promote well-being must be prioritized. Finding balance is crucial; if people spend the day in a hectic and noisy environment, a quiet moment alone can be a healthy break (Blaschka, 2020). It is recommended to closely observe the thoughts and emotions in relation to work, reflecting on which aspects of the situation are fixed and which can change; this can help give some perspective and reduce the negative impact of stress related to inflexible aspects (Valcour, 2016).

Self-Care Recommendations for the Prevention of Home-Based Accidents

In order to avoid some of the most common accidents, it is important to keep workspaces orderly and electrical cables in good condition. People should not run cables under mats or leave them in places where they obstruct the way. Always disconnect all devices and cables that are not in use. Likewise, people should not connect many cables in the same contact or extension to avoid electrical overloads (ESFI, 2021).

It is also wise to have a smoke and carbon monoxide detector, an extinguisher for electrical fires, and a first aid kit. It is suggested to avoid loose rugs that could cause tripping and hold on to the handrail and not carry too many things, such as computers and materials while going down the stairs (Previsor Insurance, 2020). For remote workers, avoiding drinks in open containers near electrical sockets (Ibidem), as well as not placing computers or devices near a heat source, and ensuring that they do not overheat are some strategies that can help avoid mishaps.

Good Practices

Because identifying problems and promoting self-care habits was relevant for the university, they decided to implement the strategy of health circles (HC) or small groups of employees who would be responsible for checking in on each other, creating an ambiance of collective care.

These are groups of employees or circles of employees that have been used in various fields. Perhaps the best-known similar structure is quality circles, which are based on a group of employees who meet periodically to solve problems that affect their work area (Lawler & Morhman, 1985). For their part, health circles or healthy circles have been used to empower employees and encourage their participation in organizational health. Employees are considered experts to identify the working conditions that generate problems and stress and therefore are the most appropriate source to determine the best intervention strategies (Munn-Giddings, Hart and Ramos., 2005; Aust and Ducki, 2004; Linos and Kirch, 2008). Developing these types of groups will allow employees to monitor the risks and their own health problems, as well as those of their colleagues, even from a distance, and promote actions that reduce the feeling of isolation, favoring occupational health. These groups must report the state of health and well-being of remote workers to the competent authority, such as human resources or similar areas. These reports will allow generating policies and strategies according to the needs of those who collaborate from a distance, beyond simple compliance with legal precepts, favoring a true culture of care.

HC are participatory processes based on the democracy at work model and other initiatives for the humanization of working, which started in the 1970s in different countries in Europe, particularly Germany, Denmark, and Italy, to contribute to the improvement of working conditions and reduce stress through health-related interventions which started to grow substantially in the 1980s. Originally, they were created to lower costs by reducing absenteeism and motivating employees (Faller, 2021). In the last decade, they have been used to implement comprehensive workplace changes, especially in terms of physical and psychosocial working conditions (European Agency for Safety and Health at Work, 2009). With the COVID-19 pandemic, HC acquired more importance as meetings among peers in which participants could openly discuss work-related health problems and challenges to improve their well-being in remote workplaces.

They provide a safe space in which employees can share their experiences and understand that certain problems they are facing are also being faced by others, creating a sense of a support group. Interesting examples show the way in which HC has been established through support and expert information to improve stress management and physical health, resulting in positive changes (Konradt, Schoom, Wilm & Hertel, 2000). HC has helped develop appropriate coping strategies and can function as an intervention to correct problems and improve remote working conditions. When adequately used, they have been perceived as a successful tool to face certain remote working stressors (Kondradt et al., 2000).

The higher education institution in which the study was performed created HC to provide support for employees. Small groups of 10 to 12 employees, in which participation was voluntary, were created. These groups functioned as teams, and certain activities were developed to "compete" against other teams in practicing self-care. Participants used a digital platform to record all actions taken towards their personal self-care and actions to help others through support or providing valuable knowledge. All individual and group actions received a certain number of points, and at the end of each semester, prizes and awards were given to the team with the most points. Prizes were aligned with self-care, for instance, monitoring bracelets, free yoga and exercise classes, sports gear, meditation sessions, dietitian services, travel and activities that promote health and well-being, small social gatherings respecting social distancing, and others. Because of the interest the program attracted and the results in terms of improving personal health and maintaining cross-check-ins between employees, the program became institutionalized, and it is expected to continue beyond the pandemic.

Another interesting project has been the health application. Every week, employees need to monitor their own mental and physical health through a short questionnaire, and the overall results are shared. It includes awareness of the personal energy levels, sleeping habits, small practices such as minutes for mindfulness, exercise and restoration breaks, decluttering and workspace organization tips, and socialization moments have been introduced as part of the self-care practices using digital technologies.

FUTURE RESEARCH DIRECTIONS

Future studies could focus on the specific actions carried out by individuals and their behaviors towards more sustained self-care practices in remote and hybrid work. Data could help shed light on the gap between recommendations made by health professionals and the actual efforts to guarantee personal well-being. Perhaps one of the main challenges will be to identify changes in health-related issues and self-care practices in hybrid work since some of the work will remain at home, people will have to commute, and also do some of the job at the office. Additional changes to pre-acquired routines will most likely create additional research interests. Modern applications of digital technologies to promote self-care will create new research opportunities.

CONCLUSION

Constant technological innovations and their impact on organizations ensure that the future of business, work, and the economy will be digital. In this context, it is essential to deepen research on the physical and psychological impact of remote work, with the aim of identifying, preventing, and managing the corresponding risks. With the health crisis caused by the COVID-19 pandemic, the number of people who practice telework increased substantially, and many organizations have contemplated maintaining remote work or hybrid work schemes even when activities return to normal. In these conditions, it is especially important to consider self-care because people tend to lose touch with their authentic selves and fall into practices of self-neglect and self-sabotage that affect their health (Su, 2017).

In the study that was conducted, results revealed that participants report more physical problems than mental ones when comparing the data both categories. This might be due to the fact that physical problems are easier to notice and understand, which is why raising awareness on these issues is crucial. In this sense, promoting self-care is extremely important because most of the care that a person requires to prevent and manage physical and mental health problems comes directly from the individual.

The best contribution of self-care has been better individual health because people are able to transform their health significantly, influencing important habits which become the foundation for healthy behaviors later in life (Bayer Consumer health, 2018). There are small tweaks that a person can do to improve his/her health through what have been called micro self-care practices, which include scheduling "me time", being more efficient, moving more than usual, redefining productivity, and seeking out a change of scenery (Michael, 2020). Self-discovery to recognize emotional disturbances and other signs of distress are also essential (Bressi & Vaden, 29016).

Self-care has been the dominant form of medical and health care (Grant, 1990). Recent developments have made health practices that once were in the hands of healthcare professionals available for all, shifting how people engage in self-care. New commodities are encouraging self-awareness of one's health and increasing access to simple information and practices that help individuals take better care of themselves (Chaney & Mechanael, 2020).

During the health crisis, digital health acquired renewed importance, especially for self-monitoring and self-care, through preventive health efforts using technology (Lupton, 2013). This is not new but became more relevant during the health restrictions. Technology is becoming a promise for better self-care. In fact, we are entering self-care in the digital age in which the individual can interact with different health systems and services with any digital device, democratizing self-care through universal phone ownership.

REFERENCES

Abrahams, Z. (2019). *The future of remote work: When it's done right, telework can improve employee productivity, creativity and morale, psychologists' research finds*. American Psychological Association. https://www.apa.org/monitor/2019/10/cover-remote-work

Alli, B. (2008). *Fundamental Principles of Occupational Health and Safety*. International Labour Organziation.

Asociación de Fabricantes de Medicamentos de Libre Acceso AFAMELA. (2017). *The economics of self-care in Mexico*. https://www.selfcarefederation.org/resources/value-otc-self-care-mexico

Aust, B., & Ducki, A. (2004). Comprehensive health promotion interventions at the workplace: Experiences with health circles in Germany. *Journal of Occupational Health Psychology*, *9*(3), 258–270. doi:10.1037/1076-8998.9.3.258 PMID:15279520

Bayer Consumer Health. (2018). *Self-care. Better daily health for individuals and societies. A global policy blueprint*. https://www.bayer.com/sites/default/files/2020-04/self-care-policy-paper-2018-08-16.pdf

Blaschka, A. (2020). This Is The Best Way To Avoid COVID Burnout. *Forbes*. https://www.forbes.com/sites/amyblaschka/2020/07/30/this-is-the-best-way-to-avoid-covid-burnout/?sh=35e055a0509d

Bondanini, G., Giorgi, G., Ariza-Montes, A., Vega-Muñoz, A., & Andreucci-Annunziata, P. (2020). Technostress dark side of technology in the workplace: A scientometric analysis. *International Journal of Environmental Research and Public Health*, *17*(21), 8013. doi:10.3390/ijerph17218013 PMID:33143270

Bressi, S. K., & Vaden, E. R. (2017). Reconsidering self care. *Clinical Social Work Journal*, *45*(1), 33–38. doi:10.100710615-016-0575-4

Brown, D. (2021). *Covid-19: Five ways to avoid lockdown eye strain*. BBC News. https://www.bbc.com/news/uk-55933168

Cameron, D. (2021). *History of Workplace Health and Safety*. Staysafe. https://staysafeapp.com/blog/2020/08/21/history-workplace-health-and-safety

Chandler, C. (2020). *Working from home occupational health and safety implications*. https://www.lexology.com/library/detail.aspx?g=9fbe1053-b59e-4fe9-b6c1-5e45d8489042

Chaney, S. C., & Mechael, P. (2020). *Digital Self-care: A Framework for Design, Implementation & Evaluation.* Self-Care Trailblazer Group. https://www.psi.org/wp-content/uploads/2020/09/Digital-Self-Care.pdf

Cleveland Clinic. (2021). *6 tips to help combat computer vision syndrome.* https://health.clevelandclinic.org/computers-and-blurry-vision-5-fixes-for-your-tech-induced-eyestrain/

DePaul, K. (2019). *Remote Work Health Risks: What You Need to Know.* Remote Co. https://remote.co/remote-work-health-risks-what-need-know/#:~:text=Carpal%20Tunnel%20Syndrome,problem%20called%20Carpal%20Tunnel%20Syndrome

Di Donato, M., Iles, R., Buchbinder, R., Xia, T., & Collie, A. (2021). Prevalence, Predictors and Wage Replacement Duration Associated with Diagnostic Imaging in Australian Workers with Accepted Claims for Low Back Pain: A Retrospective Cohort Study. *Journal of Occupational Rehabilitation*, 1–9. PMID:33913056

EHS Insight Resources. (2019). *A Brief History of Occupational Health and Safety.* https://www.ehsinsight.com/blog/a-brief-history-of-occupational-health-and-safety#:~:text=In%20the%20United%20States%2C%20occupational,of%20their%20job%20or%20industry

El-Osta, Webber, Gnani, Banarsee, Mummery, Mated, & Smith. (2019). The Self-care Matrix: A Unifying Framework for Self-Care. *SelfCare*, *10*(3), 38–56.

ESFI. (2021). *Electrical Safety While Working From Home.* https://www.esfi.org/electrical-safety-while-working-from-home/

European Agency for Safety and Health at Work. (2009). *Heath circles, an effective and enjoyable way to conduct risk assessments.* https://osha.europa.eu/en/publications/health-circles-effective-and-enjoyable-way-conduct-risk-assessment/view

Faller, G. (2021). Future Challenges for Work-Related Health Promotion in Europe: A Data-Based Theoretical Reflection. *International Journal of Environmental Research and Public Health*, *18*(20), 10996. doi:10.3390/ijerph182010996 PMID:34682748

Forster, V. (2020). Are Your Eyes Hurting During The Coronavirus Pandemic? You May Have "Computer Vision Syndrome". *Forbes Magazine.* https://www.forbes.com/sites/victoriaforster/2020/06/01/are-your-eyes-hurting-during-the--coronavirus-pandemic-you-may-have-computer-vision-syndrome/?sh=32dcb8326cf9

Gewin, V. (2021). Pandemic burnout is rampant in academia. *Nature*, *591*(7850), 489–491. doi:10.1038/d41586-021-00663-2 PMID:33723408

Gleason, A. M. (2021). *Remote Monitoring of a Work-From-Home Employee to Identify Stress: A Case Report.* Workplace Health & Safety. https://journals.sagepub.com/doi/abs/10.1177/2165079921997322

Grant, M. (1990). The effect of nursing consultation on anxiety, side effects, and self-care of patients receiving radiation therapy. *Oncology Nursing Forum*, *17*(3), 31–36. PMID:2342981

Greenstein, M. (2020). *Tips for eye health while working from home.* https://www.kshb.com/news/coronavirus/tips-for-eye-health-while-working-from-home

Gutierrez, S. B., & Quispe-Orihuela, K. (2021). Weight gain and physical inactivity during the COVID-19 pandemic. *Revista Panamericana de Salud Pública*, *45*, 1. Advance online publication. doi:10.26633/RPSP.2021.136 PMID:34703462

Hand & Wrist Center. (2020). *4 Hand-Wrist Stretches for Remote Workers During COVID-19*. https://northfloridahandandwrist.com/4-hand-wrist-stretches-for-remote-workers-during-covid-19/

Hansraj, K. K. (2014). Assessment of Stresses in the Cervical Spine Caused by Posture and Position of the Head. *Surgical Technology International*, *25*, 277–279. PMID:25393825

Healthcare. (2021). *Pandemic Weight Gain — It's a Thing*. https://www.muhealth.org/our-stories/pandemic-weight-gain-its-thing

Healthline. (2020a). *4 Simple Tips to Avoid Developing 'Tech Neck' During COVID-19*. https://www.healthline.com/health-news/4-simple-tips-to-avoid-developing-tech-neck-during-covid-19#How-to-treat-tech-neck

Healthline. (2020b). *12 Ways to Calm Your Anxiety*. https://www.healthline.com/health/how-to-calm-anxiety

Hedge, A. (2020). Getting Back Pain While Working From Home? An Ergonomics Expert Offers Advice. *Time Magazine*. https://time.com/5821252/back-pain-work-from-home-tips/

Hickman, A. (2019). *How to Manage the Loneliness and Isolation of Remote Workers*. Gallup. https://www.gallup.com/workplace/268076/manage-loneliness-isolation-remote-workers.aspx

Houtman, I., Jettinghof, K., Cedillo, L., & the World Health Organization. Occupational and Environmental Health Team. (2007). *Raising awareness of stress at work in developing countries: advice to employers and worker representatives*. World Health Organization. https://apps.who.int/iris/handle/10665/42956

Ingusci, E., Signore, F., Giancaspro, M. L., Manuti, A., Molino, M., Russo, V., Zito, M., & Cortese, C. G. (2021). Workload, Techno Overload, and Behavioral Stress During COVID-19 Emergency: The Role of Job Crafting in Remote Workers. *Frontiers in Psychology*, *12*, 12. doi:10.3389/fpsyg.2021.655148 PMID:33912116

International Labor Organization. (2017). *The future of work*. International Labor Organization. https://www.ilo.org/global/topics/future-of-work/langen/index.htm

International Labor Organization. (2020). *Defining and measuring remote work, telework, work at home, and home-based work*. https://www.ilo.org/global/statistics-and- databases/publications/WCMS_747075/lang--en/index.htm

James, J. (2021). *Remote work exhaustion: 13 tips to reduce fatigue*. The Enterprises Project. https://enterprisersproject.com/article/2021/1/remote-work-13-tips-reduce-fatigue

Kassel, J. (2020). *6 Chiropractor-Approved Exercises to Fight Text Neck*. Healthline. https://www.healthline.com/health/fitness-exercise/text-neck-treatment#does-text-neck-really-cause-pain

Katella, K. (2020). *Quarantine 15? What to Do About Weight Gain During the Pandemic*. Yale Medicine. https://www.yalemedicine.org/news/quarantine-15-weight-gain-pandemic

Kekatos, M. (2017). *Work at home? Watch out! You're more likely to suffer insomnia, stress and depression.* Daily Mail. https://www.dailymail.co.uk/health/article-4227786/Work-home-likely-suffer-insomnia.html

Kelly, J. (2020). *Q&A: Why people are 'stress eating' during the pandemic, and how to stop*. https://news.virginia.edu/content/qa-why-people-are-stress-eating-during-pandemic-and-how-stop

Kiger, P. J. (2020). *Pandemic Is Turning Some Older Telecommuters Into Insomniacs*. AARP. https://www.aarp.org/work/working-at-50-plus/info-2020/work-from-home-insomnia.html

Konradt, U., Schmook, R., Wilm, A., & Hertel, G. (2000). Health circles for teleworkers: Selective results on stress, strain and coping styles. *Health Education Research*, *15*(3), 327–338. doi:10.1093/her/15.3.327 PMID:10977380

Lawler, E. E., & Mohrman, S. A. (1985). Quality circles after the fad. *Harvard Business Review*, *63*(1), 65–71. PMID:10269357

Leckey, R. (2021). *A year of screens: How more remote work & virtual learning affects our eye health.* https://www.wnep.com/article/entertainment/television/leckey-live/computer-screens-remote-

Lee, J. J., & Miller, S. E. (2013). A self-care framework for social workers: Building a strong foundation for practice. *Families in Society*, *94*(2), 96–103.

Levin, L. S., & Idler, E. L. (1983). Self-care in health. *Annual Review of Public Health*, *4*(1), 181–201.

Linos, A., & Kirch, W. (Eds.). (2008). *Promoting health for working women*. Springer.

Lupton, D. (2013). The digitally engaged patient: Self-monitoring and self-care in the digital health era. *Social Theory & Health*, *11*(3), 256–270.

Martínez-Mejía, E., Villa-George, F. I., & Martínez-Guerrero, J. I. (2020). Prevalence of Burnout Syndrome in Mexican Employees in Mexico City. *Journal of Basic and Applied Psychology Research*, *2*(3), 23–33.

Maruyama, T., Hopkinson, P. G., & James, P. W. (2009). A multivariate analysis of work– life balance outcomes from a large-scale telework programme. *New Technology, Work and Employment*, *24*(1), 76–88.

McCallum, K. (2020). *Is Excess Screen Time Causing Your Headaches?* Houston Methodist. https://www.houstonmethodist.org/blog/articles/2020/apr/is-extra-screen-time-causing-your-headaches/

Michael, J. (2021). *Remote Work And Mental Health: How To Maximize Your Time For Micro Self-Care.* https://www.forbes.com/sites/forbescoachescouncil/2021/07/19/remote-work-and-mental-health-how-to-maximize-your-time-for-micro-self-care/?sh=122430144a7b

Miller, L. (2020). *How bad is working from home making your tech neck?* EWIWORKS. https://www.ewiworks.com/blog/bad-text-neck/

Montaudon-Tomas, C., Pinto-López, C. M., Olivera-Pérez, E., & Amsler, A. (2021). *Informe: El Estado del Trabajo Remoto en México durante la Pandemia de COVID-19. Observatorio de Competitividad y Nuevas Formas de Trabajo*. UPAEP Universidad.

Morales-Cadena, G. M., Fonseca-Salazar, N. F., & Fonseca-Chávez, M. G. (2020). Prevalence of professional burnout syndrome in postgraduate residents of surgical and non-surgical specialties. *Anales de Otorrinolaringología Mexicana*, *65*(2), 64–70.

Moretti, A., Menna, F., Aulicino, M., Paoletta, M., Liguori, S., & Iolascon, G. (2020). Characterization of Home Working Population during COVID-19 Emergency: A Cross-Sectional Analysis. *International Journal of Environmental Research and Public Health*, *17*(17), 6284.

Mostafa, B. A. (2021). The Effect of Remote Working on Employees Wellbeing and Work-Life Integration during Pandemic in Egypt. *International Business Research*, *14*(3), 41–52.

Munn-Giddings, C., Hart, C., & Ramos, S. (2005). A participatory approach to the promotion of well-being in the workplace: Lessons from empirical research. *International Review of Psychiatry (Abingdon, England)*, *17*(5), 409–417.

News Center 1. (2020). *How to alleviate digital eye strain while working from home*. https://www.newscenter1.tv/how-to-alleviate-digital-eye-strain-while-working-from-home/

Omisakin, F. D., & Ncama, B. P. (2011). Self, self-care and self-management concepts: Implications for self-management education. *Educational Research*, *2*(12), 1733–1737.

Orem, D. E. (1985). *Nursing: Concepts of practice. 3*. McGraw-Hill.

Peters, R. M., & Templin, T. N. (2010). Theory of planned behavior, self-care motivation, and blood pressure self-care. *Research and Theory for Nursing Practice*, *24*(3), 172–186.

Porter, R. (2021). *Is COVID-19 Causing Carpal Tunnel?* Korn Ferry. https://www.kornferry.com/insights/this-week-in-leadership/is-covid-19-causing-carpal-tunnel

Potratz, A. (2020). *Managing remote workers during the COVID-19 Pandemic*. https://ohsonline.com/Articles/2020/08/09/Managing-Remote-Workers-During-the-COVID-19-Pandemic.aspx?Page=7

Potratz, A. (2020). *Managing remote workers during the COVID-19 Pandemi*. https://ohsonline.com/Articles/2020/08/09/Managing-Remote-Workers-During-the-COVID-19-Pandemic.aspx?Page=7

Previsor Insurance. (2020). *Tips to Avoid Work-Related Injuries While Working from Home*. https://previsorinsurance.com/blog/tips-to-avoid-work-related-injuries-while-working-from-home/

Sánchez, B. (2020). *Coronavirus and Sleep: How Work From Home Has Affected Americans' Bedtime Habits*. The Active Times. https://www.theactivetimes.com/coronavirus-work-from-home-sleep

Sandorf, B. (2019). *Home Accident Statistics: Is Your Home as Safe as You Think?* https://www.asecurelife.com/home-accident-statistics/

Scott, E. (2021). *8 Tips to Handle the Stress of Working From Home*. https://www.verywellmind.com/the-stress-of-working-from-home-4141174

Shah, P. F. (2020). *Working Remotely? Here Are 21 Self-Care Tips For Remote Workers Thrive Gobal*. https://thriveglobal.com/stories/working-remotely-here-are-21-self-care-tips-for-remote-workers/

Sood, S. (2020). Psychological effects of the Coronavirus disease-2019 pandemic. *RHiME.*, *7*, 23–26.

Stange, J. (2021). *6 Ways to Support Remote Worker Wellbeing*. Quantum Workplace. https://www.quantumworkplace.com/future-of-work/remote-worker-wellbeing

Su, A. J. (2017). 6 Ways to Weave Self-Care into Your Workday. *Harvard Business Review*. https://hbr.org/2017/06/6-ways-to-weave-self-care-into-your-workday

The Center for Occupational Safety. (2020). *Mobile work and remote work*. Finlandia. https://ttk.fi/en/well-being_at_work_and_occupational_health_and_safety/the_basics_for_occupational_safety_and_health/work_environment/mobile_work_and_remote_work

The Chronicle of Higher Education. (2021). *"On the Verge of Burnout" Covid-19's impact on faculty well-being and career plans*. https://connect.chronicle.com/rs/931-EKA-218/images/Covid%26FacultyCareerPaths_Fidelity_ResearchBrief_v3%20%281%29.pdf

Torres, M. (2020). *This Is What Happens To Your Body When You Work From Home*. Huffpost. https://www.huffpost.com/entry/what-happens-body-work-from-home_l_5e84bfb5c5b6a1bb765185df

UC Davis Health. (2020). *COVID-19 is wrecking our sleep with coronasomnia – tips to fight back*. https://health.ucdavis.edu/health-news/newsroom/covid-19-is-wrecking-our-sleep-with-coronasomnia--tips-to-fight-back-/2020/09#:~:text=And%20a%20report%20from%20the,a%20surprise%20to%20no%20one

UNUM. (2020). *Remote working and the risks to physical health*. https://www.unum.co.uk/resources/remote-working-and-the-risks-to-physical-health

Upham, B. (2021). *The Link Between Migraine Headache and Neck Pain*. Everyday Health. https://www.everydayhealth.com/migraine/the-link-between-migraine-headache-and-neck-pain/

Valcour, M. (2016). Beating Burnout. *Harvard Business Review*. https://hbr.org/2016/11/beating-burnout

Vision Health. (2020). *Tips to Reduce Eye Strain When Working From Home*. https://www.deltadentalia.com/a-healthy-life/vision-health/tips-to-reduce-eye-strain-when-working-from-home/

Walters, R. (2021). *9 self-care strategies for remote workers*. https://www.robertwalters.com.br/en/hiring/hiring-advice/9-self-care-strategies-for-remote-workers.html

Wood, A., & Thomas, N. (2021). *If you've gained weight during the pandemic, you're not alone. Here's what to do about it*. CNN. https://www.cnn.com/2021/03/24/health/weight-gain-during-covid-wellness/index.html

World Economic Forum. (2020). *The Future of Jobs Report 2020*. World Economic Forum. https://www.weforum.org/reports/the-future-of-jobs-report-2020

World Health Organization. (2019). *Burn-out an "occupational phenomenon": International Classification of Diseases*. https://www.who.int/news/item/28-05-2019-burn-out-an-occupational-phenomenon-international-classification-of-diseases

World health Organization. (2020). *Pandemic fatigue. Reinvigorating the public to prevent COVID-19*. https://apps.who.int/iris/bitstream/handle/10665/335820/WHO-EURO-2020-1160-40906-55390-eng.pdf

World Health Organization. (2021a). *Occupational health*. https://www.who.int/health-topics/occupational-health

World Health Organization (WHO). (2021b). *What do we mean by self-care?* https://www.who.int/reproductivehealth/self-care-interventions/definitions/en/

Zerbe, K. J. (2020). Pandemic fatigue: Facing the body's inexorable demands in the time of Covid-19. *Journal of the American Psychoanalytic Association*, *68*(3), 475–478.

Zielinska, M., & Kirtzman, F. (2021). *The Mental Health Toll of Working in Isolation*. Korn Ferry. https://www.kornferry.com/insights/this-week-in-leadership/mental-health-remote-work-coronavirus

ADDITIONAL READING

Allen, T. D., Cho, E., & Meier, L. L. (2014). Work-family boundary dynamics. *Annual Review of Organizational Psychology and Organizational Behavior*, *1*(1), 99–121. doi:10.1146/annurev-org-psych-031413-091330

Freer, C. B. (1980). Self-care: A health diary study. *Medical Care*, *18*(8), 853–861. doi:10.1097/00005650-198008000-00006 PMID:7412429

Gantz, S. B. (1990). Self-care: Perspectives from six disciplines. *Holistic Nursing Practice*, *4*(2), 1–12. doi:10.1097/00004650-199002000-00004 PMID:2404999

Hricova, M., & Lovas, L. (2017). Self-Care-Self-Regulation. *Ad Alta: Journal of Interdisciplinary Research, 7*(2).

KEY TERMS AND DEFINITIONS

Computer Eye: Dryness, itchiness and tiredness of the eyes when using digital devices for a prolonged period of time.

Health: The absence of illnesses or ailments.

Pandemic: An outbreak of a global disease.

Pandemic Fatigue: Extreme fatigue resulting from the prolonged pandemic.

Remote Work: A flexible form of work in which labor is delocalized.

Self: The personal existential being.

Tech-Neck: Strain and pain in the neck due to the excessive use of technology.

Chapter 12

Reflection on Management of Compassion Fatigue Among Psychology Professionals:

Compassion Fatigue Management Through Self-Care Strategies

Kavita Gupta
The Maharaja Sayajirao University of Baroda, India

B. S. Parimal
The Maharaja Sayajirao University of Baroda, India

ABSTRACT

Compassion fatigue is often experienced by helping professionals, especially psychologists and counsellors. The goal of this chapter is to reflect how self-care strategies and techniques can be used to combat compassion fatigue among psychologists/psychology professionals when dealing with different stressors at the workplace front. Psychology professionals/therapists treating trauma patients have been shown to undergo indirect trauma, which can result in changes in emotions, cognitions, and behaviors. The first section of this chapter discusses compassion fatigue, including its causes, symptoms, and progression. It entails the creation of the notion of compassion fatigue, as well as how it is stated in the literature and comprehended by psychologists. The second part explores the resilience skills of the psychology professionals in order to mitigate distress, discomfort, and anxiety caused due to compassion fatigue. Implications for practice as well as future research are discussed in this chapter.

DOI: 10.4018/978-1-6684-2334-9.ch012

INTRODUCTION

Compassion is the emotion that arises while observing another person's suffering and leads one to want to help that person (Goetz et al., 2010). It can also be thought of as a collection of five elements, rather than just an emotion: (1) recognizing suffering, (2) comprehending the universality of human suffering, (3) feeling for the person who is suffering, (4) tolerating unpleasant feelings, and (5) motivation to act to alleviate suffering (Strauss et al., 2016). Compassion can be felt in respect to oneself, which Neff (2003) defines as compassion directed inwards, towards oneself as an object of concern and interest in suffering situations.

Despite the awareness of the importance of minding one's own mental health and armed with the knowledge of how to do so, many psychology professionals appear not to practice what they preach.

COMPASSION SATISFACTION (CS)

The term "compassion satisfaction" is used to describe a phenomenon that is supposed to contribute to the mental, physical, and spiritual well-being of persons who work in caring professions. It could even protect you from compassion fatigue (Harr & Moore, 2011). Compassion satisfaction is about the pleasure you derive from being able to do your work well. For example, you may feel like it is a pleasure to help others through your work.

EMPATHY AND COMPASSION

Empathy and compassion are inextricably linked. Understanding the similarities and distinctions between empathy and compassion may help to explain why self-oriented empathy could be a precursor to compassion fatigue. Empathy is the ability to identify and understand the thoughts and emotions of others, or the ability to put oneself in their shoes, which can trigger emotional responses in caregivers (Davis, 1983). Dealing with clients who are stuck in unpleasant emotional states can be emotionally draining, contributing to burnout and compassion fatigue among professionals (Figley, 2002). The recognition of others' suffering, which is the same as empathy, is the beginning of compassion (Goetz et al., 2010). Compassion, on the other hand, differs from empathy in terms of sentiments and behavioural repercussions (Goetz et al., 2010). When professionals deliver compassionate care, the client/patient is concerned that the professional understands their pain, albeit from a distance.

Empathy is thought to have a significant role in Compassion Fatigue. Compassion fatigue was considered a cost of empathy by Figley (2002), who developed a theoretical framework (i.e., the etiological and multi-factor model) to better understand how other factors (e.g., client exposure, disengagement, and sense of accomplishment) influenced the effect of empathy on Compassion fatigue. Davis (1983) developed a multidimensional construct of empathy to help researchers better comprehend the concept of empathy.

Personal suffering (i.e., self-oriented empathy), empathic concern (i.e., other-oriented empathy), fantasy, and perspective-taking were deemed by Davis (1983) to be four components of empathy. In many prior research, the terms "personal anguish" and "self-oriented empathy" were used interchangeably to describe negative emotional responses evoked by witnessing others' suffering (Batson et al.,

1987; Nagamine et al., 2018; Takamatsu, 2018). Many researchers investigated the relationship between self-oriented empathy and compassion fatigue among nurses (Duarte and Pinto-Gouveia, 2017b), social workers (Thomas, 2013), and healthcare professionals based on their understanding of the multidimensional construct of empathy. They discovered that self-oriented empathy was positively associated with compassion fatigue among nurses (Duarte and Pinto-Gouveia, 2017b), social workers (Thomas, 2013), and healthcare professionals (Hunt et al., 2019). Furthermore, a prior study discovered that, when compared to other types of empathy, social workers' self-oriented empathy had the largest link to compassion fatigue (Thomas, 2013).

Individuals working in the caring professions typically strive to change their clients' actions and emotions by giving emotional support (e.g., empathy), coping strategies, or improved cognitive management abilities (Boscarino, 1997; Francis, 1997; Thoits, 1986). Providing therapy to clients who have endured a traumatic event can be particularly distressing in the setting of formal caregiving (Figley, 1995).

COMPASSION FATIGUE (CF)

Compassion fatigue arises when therapy-related stress reaches acceptable levels; however, individual appropriate levels of stress may differ depending on factors such as motivation. Excessive stress among psychology professionals who work with serious clients can develop to a syndrome known as "compassion fatigue," which can be dangerous for both the professionals and the clients. Figley refined the concept of indirect trauma experienced by therapists by coining the term "Compassion fatigue" (Bride, Radey, Figley, 2007). Professionals in the mental health industry frequently see their clients' traumatic experiences (Showalter, 2010), and repeated exposure to such situations might cause a stress reaction in them (Coetzee & Klopper, 2010). When stress levels are optimal, it can help the professional function better by increasing motivation, mental alertness, and vitality (Craig & Sprang, 2010).

Compassion fatigue is a sympathetic reaction that occurs as a result of constantly experiencing others' emotional or physical suffering or listening to someone who is suffering from mental or physical illness (Figley, 2002; Hamilton et al., 2016; Sinclair et al., 2017). It not only has an impact on the mental and physical well-being of professional helpers, resulting in high turnover and absenteeism, but it also has an impact on the quality of client/patient treatment, resulting in a decline in client/patient trust and confidence (Udipi et al., 2008; Sorenson et al., 2016). Compassion fatigue is a state of stress and preoccupation with traumatized patients caused by re-enacting terrible experiences and avoiding the client and reminders of the trauma, which lowers our interest in and capacity to bear the suffering of others (Figley, 2002a). It's commonly used interchangeably in the literature with terminology like secondary traumatic stress or vicarious traumatization.

According to Craig and Sprang (2010), 5% of clinical psychologists and social workers who work with traumatised people are at high risk of compassion fatigue. Compassion fatigue describes a "state of tension and obsession with traumatised patients caused by re-enacting horrific experiences, avoidance/numbing toward reminders, and continuous arousal (e.g., anxiety) linked with the client" (Figley, 2002, p.1435).

Compassion fatigue can be accompanied by a wide range of symptoms affecting seven different domains. Figley (2002b) divides these into cognitive (e.g. decreased concentration, disorientation, apathy), emotional (e.g. powerlessness, anxiety, numbness), behavioural (e.g. irritability, withdrawal, hypervigilance), spiritual (e.g. loss of purpose, questioning prior beliefs, lack of self-satisfaction), personal relations (e.g. decreased interest in intimacy, isolation from others, increased interpersonal conflicts), somatic (e.g. lowered motivation, absenteeism, exhaustion).

Empathic engagement with traumatised clients frequently necessitates the professional discussing specifics of the traumatic experience, such as role playing and dramatic re-enactment of the events, which are thought to be beneficial to the therapeutic process but can be emotionally draining for the professional (Figley 2002a, 2002b).

A history of trauma, a lack of social support, and an inability to cope with the responsibilities of caregiving, are all thought to raise the risk of developing compassion fatigue. Previous studies have tended to back up the proposed links between these risk variables, Compassion fatigue, and psychological discomfort (Figley, 1995, 2002a; Nelson-Gardell & Harris, 2003; Sabin-Farrell & Turpin, 2003; Salston & Figley, 2003; Schauben & Frazier, 1995). For example, Schauben and Frazier (1995) discovered that female psychologists and violence counsellors who had a higher percentage of sexual violence victims as clients experienced more vicarious trauma, which was linked to more psychiatric disorders.

Compassion Fatigue is common in professional helpers such as Psychologists and Counsellors who are subjected to many pressures (Gleichgerrcht and Decety, 2014; Yu et al., 2016). During the COVID-19 pandemic, India's psychological counsellors promptly formed many service teams and volunteered to provide hotline professional psychiatric assistance to those affected by the virus. When dealing with help-seekers, these hotline psychiatric counsellors suffered Compassion Fatigue from time to time, as the help-seekers had been exposed to psychological stress or traumatic situations. According to studies, delivering such care can be both extremely rewarding and quite stressful (Ohaeri, 2003). Professionals in the caring professions, on the other hand, may be exposed to occupational contexts and caregiving responsibilities that raise the risk of negative psychological effects (Figley, 2002a; Sabin-Farrell, 2002; & Turpin, 2003).

BURNOUT

Another comparable phrase used throughout the chapter is "burnout." From the research perspective, burnout is one of the elements of Compassion Fatigue (CF). Burnout is one element of compassion fatigue, which is related to workplace stressors and associated with feelings of hopelessness and difficulty coping with work; the second element is secondary traumatic stress, which is associated with fear, difficulty sleeping, intrusive thoughts, or avoidance in response to traumatic stressful events (Stamm, 2010). Burnout is the result of a slow loss of resources brought about by continual stress from the work environment. Burnout syndrome is characterised by emotional weariness, depersonalization, and a reduction in personal accomplishment as a result of extended exposure to challenging interpersonal situations (Maslach, Schaufeli, & Leiter, 2001). "Burnout is a psychological syndrome of emotional exhaustion, depersonalization and reduced personal accomplishment" (Maslach & Goldberg, 1998; 2003). High emotional engagement combined with a lack of social support or emotions of personal work accomplishments (i.e., job satisfaction) might lead to burnout in the caring professional.

Even though burnout can exacerbate the symptoms of compassion fatigue, it is fundamentally different. Burnout, unlike compassion fatigue, is frequently the outcome of a conflict between an individual and the needs of the workplace (Deighton, Gurris, & Traue, 2007). It's linked to a lack of job satisfaction, and it usually develops gradually rather than abruptly. Burnout affects people in a variety of professions, not just those who work with trauma victims (Harr & Moore, 2011). Finally, burnout differs from compassion fatigue in that it is not accompanied by the secondary symptoms of Post-traumatic stress disorder (PTSD) (Craig & Sprang, 2010).

It is associated with feelings of hopelessness and difficulties in dealing with work or in doing job effectively. These negative feelings usually have a gradual onset. They can reflect the feeling that professionals' efforts make no difference, or they can be associated with a very high workload or a non-supportive work environment. Higher scores on this scale mean that you are at higher risk for burnout.

SECONDARY TRAUMATIC STRESS

The second component of Compassion Fatigue (CF) is secondary traumatic stress (STS). It is about work related, secondary exposure to extremely or traumatically stressful events. Secondary traumatic stress is defined as the "natural consequences of learning about a traumatic event experienced by a significant other—the stress arising from assisting or trying to assist a hurting person" (Figley, 1995, p.7). In terms of intrusive imagery, avoidance, hyperarousal, uncomfortable emotions, cognitive alterations, and functional impairment, secondary traumatic stress is quite similar to PTSD (Figley, 1995). Developing problems due to exposure to other's trauma is somewhat rare but does happen to psychology professionals who care for those who have experienced extremely or traumatically stressful events. For example, repeatedly hearing stories about the traumatic things that happen to other people, commonly called Vicarious Traumatization. If work puts professional directly in the path of danger, for example, field work in a war or area of civil violence, this is not secondary exposure; the exposure is primary. However, if exposed to others' traumatic events as a result of professional's work, for example, as a therapist or an emergency worker, this is secondary exposure. The symptoms of STS are usually rapid in onset and associated with a particular event. They may include being afraid, having difficulty sleeping, having images of the upsetting event pop into professional's mind, or avoiding things that remind them of the event.

Compassion Fatigue's Clinical and Ethical Consequences

A professional's therapeutic effectiveness and judgement can be harmed by severe compassion fatigue (Bride, Radey, & Figley, 2007). This failure of judgement could result in unethical and inadequate care. Therapists, for example, may experience depersonalization, which may result in unpleasant attitudes toward their clients (Ackerly et al., 1988). These negative emotions may make it difficult for the clinician to strive toward goals that are in the client's best interests (Negash & Sahin, 2011). McCarthy and Frieze (1999) found that therapists who are suffering sentiments of ineffectiveness and worthlessness linked with compassion fatigue are more likely to use maladaptive treatment practises. Clinical social workers with compassion fatigue symptoms are more likely than clinicians without compassion fatigue symptoms to misdiagnose, have poor treatment planning, or abuse clients, according to research (Rudolph, Stamm, & Stamm, 1997). A therapist suffering from compassion fatigue may also document in an insufficient or erroneous manner, documenting biased or misleading facts about a client (Negash & Sahin, 2011). Finally, compassion fatigue can harm the therapeutic connection by causing the therapist to lose their ability to sympathise with and respect the client (Skorupa & Agresti, 1993).

Ethical Standard 2.06 of the Ethical Principles and Code of Conduct for Psychologists states that "psychologists refrain from commencing an activity when they know or should know that their personal issues will prohibit them from completing their work-related activities competently" (American Psychological Association, 2010, pg. 6). "When psychologists become aware of personal problems that may interfere with their ability to perform work-related duties adequately, they take appropriate measures, such as seeking professional consultation or assistance, and determine whether they should limit, suspend, or terminate their work-related duties," according to the same standard (American Psychological Association, 2010, pg. 6). It's possible that a therapist recognises compassion weariness but refuses to acknowledge it. Denial of symptoms can occur for one of two reasons: the therapist is seeking to cope with the stress reaction, or he is afraid of being labelled unprofessional by peers (Munroe, 1999).

Factors contributing to the development of Compassion Fatigue among Psychology professionals include:

1. The client may request a speedy solution, which the professional provides, yet the result is slow.
2. Professionals may be unable to assist since they are not the best person for the job at the time.
3. Professionals who are attempting to assist may be experiencing motivational difficulties.
4. Clients may reflect unpleasant thoughts onto experts at times.
5. The Professional's inability to refuse.
6. Constant empathy, interpersonal sensitivity, and one-way care are all important traits.
7. Boredom and cognitive deprivation
8. Excessive workload
9. Inadequate remuneration
10. Lack of control
11. Significant value divergences

Compassion Fatigue Management in Psychology Professionals: A Theoretical and Conceptual Framework:

THE ACCELERATED RECOVERY PROGRAM (ARP) MODEL

Gentry, Baranowsky, and Dunning (1997) at Florida State University (FSU) under the guidance of Dr. Charles Figley developed the Accelerated Program for Compassion Fatigue (ARP). The ARP is a five-session programme for treating the negative consequences of burnout and compassion fatigue in professionals who are exposed to trauma as a result of their employment (Baranowsky & Gentry, 1999, 1999b; Gentry & Baranowsky, 1999). The ARP is intended to help professionals who work in high-stress, and high-demand jobs.

The ARP was created as a short (five-session) treatment programme to help professionals reduce the severity, frequency, and duration of symptoms associated with Compassion Fatigue. Treatment sessions are structured and focused on achieving all of the primary goals.

The ARP programme consists of symptom identification, recognizing the causes of compassion weariness, Locating and making use of available resources, examining the professional's personal and professional past up to this point. This program utilizes the use of the PATHWAYS for self-care programme to create a helpful aftercare plan.

An Accelerated Recovery Program (ARP) is an interventional package that includes guided imagery, Neuro-Linguistic Programming (NLP), Thought Field Therapy (TFT), self-management plan, and self-analysis which can augment the clinical competencies and enrich the personal well-being of nurses.

ARP is a consecutive 5-week program based on an individualized standard treatment protocol in 5 sessions, each lasting 90–120 min. The program involves didactic and experiential training along with audios. Session 1 focuses on the assessment of condition, life goals, conflicts, followed self-care strategies, stressors. The participants practice the guided imagery with the "retirement party visualization" script for 30 min. Session 2 focuses on developing a personal and professional time-line telling a story in which the participants narrate the achievement have had and hurdles have overcome in their life. Session 3 emphasizes a review of graphic time-line review and constructing the target/trigger list. Based on this, individualized self-management plans were developed and trained. In TFT, the troubling memories of participants were identified and tapping was conducted 5–8 times on the eyebrows, under the eye, beneath the armpit, on the collarbone, and the gamut series point located just above, and between the little and ring finger knuckles. In the NLP, safety and competency anchors were created, the negative anchors I and II were identified, and negative anchors were released through desensitization and reprocessing. Session 4 focuses on supervising the self; the "Letter from the Great Supervisor" is read and reread repeatedly, and then, introspected. Session 5 highlights the evaluation of program goals and addressing pathways for recovery.

PREVENTION OF BURNOUT AND COMPASSION FATIGUE

This section of the chapter focuses on the various techniques that Psychology Professionals can employ to preserve professional vitality in the face of internal and external sources of stressors (Baker, 2003; Freudenberger, 1990; Norcross & Guy, 2007).

A lack of non-reciprocation within the counselling relationship, overwork, difficult client behaviours, discouragement as a result of the slow and uneven pace of the helping process, the professional's existing personal issues that emerge in response to involvement in the counselling process, isolation, and administrative demands from agency and managed care organizations are all factors that contribute to the burnout and compassion fatigue (Dupree & Day, 1995; Farber, 1990; Figley, 2002; Kassam-Adams, 1995). When a professional's energy is continually exhausted as a result of this intense engagement process, burnout happens. Counseling work, according to Farber (1983), can have a significant detrimental impact on professional's self-identity, conduct, and attitudes, both inside and outside of the workplace.

The following are some of the stressors that psychology professionals might face at workplace:

1. Issues testing professionals' competency, particularly in Red Flag cases of suicidal and self-harm reported cases, cause stress. Furthermore, a client's suicide has a significant emotional impact on the professional. Other scenarios include chronically unwell individuals who do not show significant improvement or comes to a standstill due to client resistance. All of these circumstances may contribute to an increase in professional's distress.
2. Professionals' personal life crises and troubles generate difficult conditions in their work roles. Despite the fact that they may have established proactive techniques for dealing with these challenges, they frequently report a profound sensation of discomfort when confronted with such a task. For example, if the professional is sitting with clients and they're discussing anything that even closely resembles, identifies with, or touches on, the anxiety level will skyrocket. Now comes the dilemma of how to handle that degree of anxiousness while also trying to be there for the customers.

The tactics and techniques that professionals can use to promote self-wellbeing and maintain professional vitality are listed below. The Professionals could think of the self as a collection of pieces which can be from ongoing cultivation.

1. **Nurturing the Emotional self**: The Professionals must recognize that what is beneficial for others is also healthy for them through emotional self-care, 'In their book The Psychotherapist's Own Psychotherapy: Patient and Clinician Perspectives, Geller, Norcross, and Orlinsky (2005)'. The ability to forgive oneself and recognize that imperfection is a part of the human experience is enhanced by practising self-compassion. In their studies, Neff, Kirkpatrick, and Rude (2007) and Hall, Row, Wuensch, and Godley (2013) discovered a relationship between self-compassion and psychological well-being. Developing self-compassion techniques can assist professionals in responding more productively to the highs and lows of their jobs.
2. **Nurturing the Financial self**: Moderate salaries or income can be a big source of stress among many professionals. The key to building one's financial self, according to professionals, is to spend less and invest more. Another thing to consider is the counsellor's, or therapist's financial situation. The salary in these positions is normally average, but it is sometimes even mediocre because the professional lacks assertiveness when it comes to money. Professionals must be more proactive and assertive when it comes to financial needs. Because of financial hardship, financially unassailable professionals can feel particularly discouraged. They must devote time to actively planning their financial well-being. The financial self can be tremendously stressed if a professional has bad money skills or is financially unassailable, and has also been attracted by the consuming culture. This can eventually influence the professional to the point where he or she is unable to form the essential emotional bonds with clients or patients. If this occurs, competent work in relationship-focused professions will be impossible.
3. **Nurturing the Humorous self**: Actively laughing, playing, telling jokes, and being amusing are all beneficial coping activities for the professionals who operate in an environment that is frequently packed with serious human issues. Laughter keeps practitioners going. Learning to be playful and have fun can aid in self-sustenance (Stevanovic & Rupert, 2004).
4. **Nurturing the Loving self**: Affection in a professionals' personal life can be a tremendous source of professional vitality, allowing the professional to stay afloat in the face of substantial professional stress. A family is a very rich source of the ideal components for self-care for many professionals. Others experience love and being loved in a different way. However, the overall impact is a feeling of well-being that emanates from the professionals' personal life. It's perhaps crucial to remember that self-care is a sacred responsibility, according to the attachment process mentioned earlier as a key component of professionals' success. For people in the Psychology professions, being loved by another, or others, is a fantastic form of self-care. Being looked after in one's personal life may be incredibly sustaining, and the professionals often appreciates it. Hou (2015) discovered that highly resilient therapists had a strong network of vivid connectedness in his research. Nissen-Lie et al. (2015) discovered that the most successful professionals showed significant positive attachment and love for themselves in their personal life. The point is that in order to give love, they must first receive love!
5. **Nurturing the Nutritious self**: Kate Hays had made eight nutritional recommendations for Psychologists' optimal performance (At a "Taking Care of Yourself" symposium in 1999).

a. **Happiness** is a constant blood glucose level – This concept opposes bingeing and skipping meals, such as "sugar hits," and advocates for regular eating. One strategy for maintaining a stable glucose stream is to eat short meals with snacks (Schafer, 1996).
b. **Establish a regular eating schedule** - Routine offers structure and consistency, as well as encourages planning. Planning helps to avoid the impulsive eating that leads to (low blood sugar) hell, which is paved with good intentions but clogged with traffic.
c. **Breakfast** is the one meal of the day that should not be skipped – This one is constantly suggested in a world of inconsistent, contradicting, and confusing nutrition messages. Breakfast appears to be used as fuel to get the body moving. Without eating early in the day, the body runs out of gas and screams for food later in the day. Food consumed late in the day tends to be stored in large quantities, maybe indefinitely.
d. Body requires **Water** - One of the main nutritional secrets appears to be enough of water because water makes up more than 70% of the human body. "To keep the body working properly, it is vital to consume at least eight 8-ounce glasses of excellent water each day," Balch and Balch (1997) write (p. 30). Caffeine-containing products, such as cola and coffee should be avoided since caffeine serves as a diuretic, causing the body to lose water.
e. **Befriend food** and be flexible - It is preferable to enjoy the friendship of food in the same way that one enjoys, but does not abuse, the friendship of other friends. The failure of fad diets is due to their inflexibility, which causes them to stop rather than continue. Small indulgences can be accepted for long-term success because of flexibility.
f. **Figure out how to tell the difference between actual hunger signals and other physical or emotional signals** – Many professionals eat in response to negative emotions such as worry, loneliness, anger, fear, bewilderment, sorrow, and grief. They grab for food even when they aren't hungry, and they often reach for the most nutritionally devoid foods and beverages, resulting in their eating not only too many calories but also too little nutrients.
g. **Recognize when the body is hungry or thirsty** — Self-awareness is an important social skill. Listening to oneself can reveal a wealth of information. Knowing the language of hunger and thirst can lead to more efficient reactions to the body's messages rather than responses in another language, such as emotional hunger, which may lead to overeating.

6. **Take a long-term approach to eating habits** – Eating lasts an eternity, which is a long period for most individuals. This means that all types of quick fixes (like losing 20 pounds before the reunion) aren't going to cut it. It takes more than a little gloss to transform a negative relationship with food into a good one. It's sometimes a huge renovation project.
7. **Taking care of one's Physical self**: Working in the caring professions can be emotionally tiring. The Professionals require strategies for coping with the depression, anxiety, and suffering that a they experience while working with a distressed client, or patient. This is why Psychology professionals should seriously consider including severe physical activity as part of their self-care strategy for "supporting the personal self." There is significant evidence that rigorous physical exercise is good in regulating mood (Penedo & Dahn, 2005). It's a straightforward leap to the conclusion that vigorous physical activity is a cure to the mental toxins that plague the professionals' workplace.

Given the benefits of exercise, it's simple to imagine that if it were available in pill form, it would be the most popular daily medication. **Sleep**, like exercise, is an important component of overall health. According to studies published by the National Sleep Foundation (2006), a lack of sleep is associated to decreased cognitive performance as well as mood issues like anger, anxiety, and sorrow. The quantity of sleep required by each individual varies, but it is believed that people require between seven and nine hours per night. The members of the helping or caring professions are probably familiar with "sleep hygiene" practises that encourage healthy sleep. If not, they can try the following basic steps to help develop a more consistent sleeping schedule: (1) Develop an evening routine that encourages the body to relax and prepare for sleep; (2) save the bedroom for sleeping and intimacy and refrain from utilizing it for other activities such as working.

8. **Nurturing the Fun self:** Professionals are people who are attempting to do good job under difficult circumstances. There is a seemingly contradictory prescription for these folks to enjoy a long and happy career. There are numerous ways to relax, including taking bubble baths and eating chocolates, golfing or watching a fantastic basketball game, roaming aimlessly in the woods, lunching with girlfriends, and so on. The options are limitless. The most important things are to find something that nurtures oneself and to do it.
9. **Developing a Self-disciplined approach to Prioritization**: Setting priorities is an irreplaceable and valuable commodity – is critical for all Psychology professionals. If they can establish priorities, they have a better chance of getting to the priority,their own hot centre of importance, and never having time for the flotsam of life. This could be a positive outcome.
10. **Nurturing the Recreational self**: Hobbies can be a way for professionals to take care because they contain so many components of regeneration. The key to collecting or other hobbies is to divert attention away from one's own professional obligations. As a result, professionals may have a more positive outlook on work, the world, and oneself. Gardening, photography, movies, performing music, and making birdhouses are just a few of the numerous conceivable hobbies and enjoyable pastimes. High blood pressure, heart disease, depression, cancer, arthritis, and gastrointestinal system disorders are some of the current ailments that have a stress component. According to Benson (1999), religions' religious prayers, rituals, and practises can help in reducing burnout and compassion fatigue. Progressive relaxation is an old method of body relaxation introduced by Jacobson in 1929. For many years, it has been an important aspect of therapist-directed anxiety management. It entails tightening and then relaxing various muscle groups across the body.
11. **Mindfulness**: "Paying attention on purpose, in the present moment, and non-judgmentally to the unfolding of experience moment by minute" is how mindfulness is defined (Kabat-Zinn, 2003, p. 145). In therapeutic settings, mindfulness can be taught as a crucial component of therapy in programmes including dialectical behaviour therapy, mindfulness-based stress reduction (MBSR), and acceptance and commitment therapy. Mindfulness activities also help professionals take care of themselves and avoid burnout.
12. **Yoga:** Professionals can observe the state of their own body when sitting with clients which can offer clues as to when they were becoming tense, working too hard in session, or being tied to a specific outcome.
13. **Nurturing the Solitary self**: Solitude has the ability to nourish professionals profoundly. For professionals, learning to appreciate isolation can be a difficult task. There is so much media in daily lives, and more and more of professionals are living in densely populated cities around the world. Most professionals' lives have grown heavily reliant on their ability to watch a lot of television. There is a lot about television technology that people find quite enticing. Television, on the other hand, is so overstimulating that stillness feels even more foreign and unsettling. Solitude

entails switching from a well-known life channel (e.g., being plugged into the electronic world, being in close proximity to persons in need) to an often-unknown channel (silence, no human voices, aloneness). Those in the caring professions frequently have to battle the unsettling aspects of the quiet — loneliness, self-focus, and a sense of estrangement from nature. They must learn to transform their loneliness into solitude. The noises of the natural world, the outdoors, can, with time, fill up the self in a way that is refreshing. Quiet can also be a good thing. Noise pollution is a harmful by-product of technology; noise is ubiquitous. The cell phone, as well as texting, Skype, Facebook, and other forms of communication, are fantastic. The phone rings, cars pass by, and people converse all around. Noise is produced by life-enhancing machinery around us, such as loud lawn mowers, which eventually becomes the new normal. Silence is the gold of loneliness. Spiritual and religious pursuits provide a safe haven for isolation as well. Professionals can meditate and pray alone, with the focus usually being on the self-universe connection. They should emphasize the need of escaping to solitude and quiet, both from the noise of technology-filled existence and from extensive people contact in relationship-intensive jobs.

14. **Nurturing the Relaxation/ Stress-reduction self**: There are numerous sources of stress at work that contribute to excessive arousal. Professionals must maintain a continual attention on the other's demands and acute suffering. Internal sources of stress include the professional's own thoughts and self-evaluation in a range of situations. High blood pressure, heart disease, depression, cancer, arthritis, and gastrointestinal system disorders are some of the current ailments that have a stress component thereby escalating the process of burnout and compassion fatigue.
15. **Taking care of Spiritual or Religious self:** Taking care of spiritual or religious self can be an important aspect of maintaining personal self. Being spiritually or religiously active is vital as it confronts the reality of Death directly through a spiritual or religious life in a more profound way. The essential riddles of existence are addressed by an active spiritual or religious quest: What exactly is the purpose of life? Is there a heavenly presence that is active? What is the purpose of God in my life? Are people inherently good or bad? What is the best way to find forgiveness, atonement, and peace? What moral principles should I follow in my daily life? Is there such a thing as eternal life? Therefore, professionals engaged in the caring professions are directly involved in the drama of human tragedy, disappointment, and grief.
16. Professionals can analyse occupational stress levels using self-reported surveys that represent client-care versus self-care, with the goal of determining demands vs. control.
17. Professionals can examine their own self-care strengths and limitations in order to assertively foster their professional and personal well-being.
18. Professionals can use positive tactics such as spending quality time with close friends, significant others, or family members as a source of support. Maintaining a healthy balance between work and personal life, using humour to cope, Engage in quiet leisure activities outside of work environments, participate in physical activities, and take regular vacations to find delightful diversions. If they are stuck, seek supervision from other specialists in the same sector or from colleagues so that they can perceive clients' problems as intriguing. On a professional level, they can attend seminars and workshops to learn fresh approaches to handling issues that are stuck in a rut.

[a] Source: "Vicarious Traumatization: An Empirical Study of the Effects of Trauma Work on Trauma Therapists," by L. A. Pearlman and P. J. MacIan, 1995, Professional Psychology: Research and Practice, 26, pp. 558–565.

[b] In alphabetical order. Data from workshops by T. M. Skovholt in 1996.

CONCLUSION

This chapter focused on a number of important topics related to management of Burnout and Compassion fatigue. Stressors linked to numerous therapeutic concerns and client behaviours, as well as the impact of their own personal crises and life transitions escalate the process of Burnout and Compassion fatigue among Professionals. The challenges that the professional might encounter highlight the demanding nature of the assisting position and emphasise the importance of protective methods and self-care strategies for maintaining practitioner wellness and professional vitality. Professionals are more likely to recognize crucial protective factors, ranging from internal coping mechanisms to external environmental variables. Professionals need to share a dedication to self-care and a high level of proficiency in accessing useful resources by maintaining an acute awareness of the internal terrain while keeping a watchful attention on their emotional selves.

Studies conducted in the past have proved that interventions such as guided imagery, mindfulness training, educational programs, and resiliency programs are effective on combating stress occurring due to burnout and compassion fatigue. A holistic program is vital in managing the problem of burnout and compassion fatigue and in bringing out the optimal personal and professional potentials of the Psychology professionals.

Nurturance from a variety of sources, such as peers, family, and close friends, is critical during the professional development period, as well as at times of unexpected crisis, burnout, and compassion fatigue. Furthermore, activities outside of their work contexts can help to mitigate burnout and compassion fatigue, allowing them to keep a healthy sense of balance. Professionals in caring industries like counselling and therapy must be self-assured about their own health by focusing on physical, spiritual, emotional, and social well-being. As a result, the measures outlined in this chapter can assist professionals in maintaining a sense of personal congruence and energy, both of which are important components in professional wellbeing, burnout prevention, and compassion fatigue prevention.

REFERENCES

Ackerley, G. D., Burnell, J., Holder, D. C., & Kurdek, L. A. (1988). Burnout among licensed psychologists. *Professional Psychology, Research and Practice*, *19*(6), 624–631. doi:10.1037/0735-7028.19.6.624

Ackerman, D. (1999). *Deep play*. Random House.

American Psychiatric Association. (1980). *Diagnostic and statistical manual of mental disorders* (3rd ed.). Author.

American Psychiatric Association. (1994). *Diagnostic and statistical manual of mental disorders* (4th ed.). Author.

Baker, E. (2003). *Caring for ourselves: A therapist's guide to personal and professional well-being*. American Psychological Association. doi:10.1037/10482-000

Balch, J. F., & Balch, P. A. (1997). *Prescription for nutritional healing*. Avery Publishing Group.

Batson, C. D., Fultz, J., & Schoenrade, P. A. (1987). Distress and empathy: Two qualitatively distinct vicarious emotions with different motivational consequences. *Journal of Personality*, *55*(1), 19–39. doi:10.1111/j.1467-6494.1987.tb00426.x PMID:3572705

Benson, H. (1999). Power and biology of belief. Presented at the *annual convention of the American Psychological Association*, Boston, MA.

Benson-Henry Institute for Mind Body Medicine. (2010). *Eliciting the relaxation response*. Academic Press.

Boscarino, J. A. (1997). Diseases among men 20 years after exposure to severe stress: Implications for clinical research and medical care. *Psychosomatic Medicine*, *59*(6), 605–614. doi:10.1097/00006842-199711000-00008 PMID:9407579

Boscarino, J. A., Adams, R. E., & Figley, C. R. (2004). Mental health service use 1-year after the World Trade Center disaster: Implications for medical care. *General Hospital Psychiatry*, *26*(5), 346–358. doi:10.1016/j.genhosppsych.2004.05.001 PMID:15474634

Bride, B. E. (2007). Prevalence of secondary traumatic stress among social workers. *Social Work*, *52*(1), 63–70. doi:10.1093w/52.1.63 PMID:17388084

Bride, B. E., Radey, M., & Figley, C. R. (2007). Measuring compassion fatigue. *Clinical Social Work Journal*, *35*(3), 155–163. doi:10.100710615-007-0091-7

Coetzee, S. K., & Klopper, H. C. (2010). Compassion Fatigue within Nursing Practice: A Concept Analysis. *Nursing & Health Sciences*, *12*(2), 235–243. doi:10.1111/j.1442-2018.2010.00526.x PMID:20602697

Craig, C. D., & Sprang, G. (2010). Compassion satisfaction, compassion fatigue, and burnout in a national sample of trauma treatment therapists. *Anxiety, Stress, and Coping*, *23*(3), 319–339. doi:10.1080/10615800903085818 PMID:19590994

Davis, M., Eshelman, E. R., & McKay, M. (2008). *The relaxation and stress reduction workbook* (6th ed.). New Harbinger Publications.

Davis, M. H. (1983). Measuring individual differences in empathy: Evidence for a multidimensional approach. *Journal of Personality and Social Psychology*, *44*(1), 113–126. doi:10.1037/0022-3514.44.1.113

Deighton, R. M., Gurris, N., & Traue, H. (2007). Factors affecting burnout and compassion fatigue in psychotherapists treating torture survivors: Is the therapist's attitude to working through trauma relevant? *Journal of Traumatic Stress*, *20*(1), 63–75. doi:10.1002/jts.20180 PMID:17345651

Duarte, J., & Pinto-Gouveia, J. (2017b). The role of psychological factors in oncology nurses' burnout and compassion fatigue symptoms. *European Journal of Oncology Nursing*, *28*, 114–121. doi:10.1016/j.ejon.2017.04.002 PMID:28478848

Dupree, P. I., & Day, H. D. (1995). Psychotherapists' job satisfaction and job burnout as a function of work setting and percentage of managed care clients. *Psychotherapy in Private Practice*, *14*(2), 77–93.

Farber, B. (1983). The effects of psychotherapeutic practice upon the psychotherapists. *Psychotherapy (Chicago, Ill.)*, *20*(2), 174–182. doi:10.1037/h0088488

Farber, B. (1990). Burnout in psychotherapists: Incidence, types, and trends. *Psychology in Private Practice*, *8*(1), 35–44. doi:10.1300/J294v08n01_07

Figley, C. (2002). Compassion fatigue: Psychotherapists' chronic lack of self-care. *Journal of Clinical Psychology*, *58*(11), 1433–1441. doi:10.1002/jclp.10090 PMID:12412153

Figley, C. R. (1995). Compassion fatigue: Toward a new understanding of the costs of caring. In B. H. Stamm (Ed.), *Secondary traumatic stress: Self-care issues for clinicians, researchers and educators* (pp. 3–28). Sidran Press.

Figley, C. R. (1995). *Compassion fatigue as secondary traumatic stress disorder: An overview. In Compassion fatigue: Coping with secondary traumatic stress disorder*. Brunner.

Figley, C. R. (1995). Compassion fatigue as secondary traumatic stress disorder: An overview. In C. R. Figley (Ed.), *Compassion fatigue: Coping with secondary traumatic stress disorder in those who treat the traumatized* (pp. 1–20). Brunner Routledge.

Figley, C. R. (1995a). *Compassion fatigue: Coping with secondary traumatic stress disorder in those who treat the traumatized*. Brunner/Maze.

Figley, C. R. (2002a). Compassion fatigue: Psychotherapists' chronic lack of self-care. *Journal of Clinical Psychology*, *58*(11), 1433–1441. doi:10.1002/jclp.10090 PMID:12412153

Francis, L. E. (1997). Ideology and interpersonal emotion management: Redefining identity in two support groups. *Social Psychology Quarterly*, *60*(2), 153–171. doi:10.2307/2787102

Freudenberger, H. J. (1990). Hazards of psychotherapeutic practice. *Psychotherapy in Private Practice*, *8*(1), 31–34. doi:10.1300/J294v08n01_06

Geller, J. D., Norcross, J. C., & Orlinsky, D. E. (Eds.). (2005). *The psychotherapist's own psychotherapy: Patient and clinician perspectives*. Oxford University Press.

Gentry, E., Baranowsky, A. B., & Dunning, K. (1999). *Accelerated recovery program for compassion fatigue: Treatment and training protocols. Green Cross Projects*. Florida State University.

Gleichgerrcht, E., & Decety, J. (2014). The relationship between different facets of empathy, pain perception and compassion fatigue among physicians. *Frontiers in Behavioral Neuroscience*, *8*, 243. doi:10.3389/fnbeh.2014.00243 PMID:25071495

Goetz, J. L., Keltner, D., & Simon-Thomas, E. (2010). Compassion: An evolutionary analysis and empirical review. *Psychological Bulletin*, *136*(3), 351–374. doi:10.1037/a0018807 PMID:20438142

Hall, C. W., Row, K. A., Wuensch, K. L., & Godley, K. R. (2013). The Role of Self-Compassion in Physical and Psychological Well-Being. *The Journal of Psychology*, *147*(4), 311–323. doi:10.1080/00223980.2012.693138 PMID:23885635

Hamilton, S., Tran, V., & Jamieson, J. (2016). Compassion fatigue in emergency medicine: The cost of caring. *Emergen. Med. Aus.*, *28*(1), 100–103. doi:10.1111/1742-6723.12533 PMID:26777437

Harr, C., & Moore, B. (2011). Compassion fatigue among Social Work students in field placements. *Journal of Teaching in Social Work*, *31*(3), 350–363.

Hou, J. M. (2015). *Characteristics of highly resilient counselors* (Unpublished doctoral dissertation). University of Minnesota, Minneapolis, MN.

Hunt, P., Denieffe, S., & Gooney, M. (2019). Running on empathy: Relationship of empathy to compassion satisfaction and compassion fatigue in cancer healthcare professionals. *European Journal of Cancer Care, 28*(5), 13124. doi:10.1111/ecc.13124 PMID:31222849

Jacobson, E. (1929). *Progressive relaxation.* University of Chicago Press.

Jenkins, S. R., & Baird, S. (2002). Secondary traumatic stress and vicarious trauma: A validational study. *Journal of Traumatic Stress, 15*(5), 423–432. doi:10.1023/A:1020193526843 PMID:12392231

Kabat-Zinn, J. (2003). Mindfulness-based interventions in context: Past, present, and future. *Clinical Psychology: Science and Practice, 10*(2), 144–156. doi:10.1093/clipsy.bpg016

Kassam-Adams, N. (1995). The risks of treating sexual trauma: Stress and secondary trauma in psychotherapists. In B. H. Stamm (Ed.), *Secondary traumatic stress: Self-care issues for clinicians, researchers, and educators* (pp. 37–48). Sidran Press.

Linley, A., & Joseph, S. (2007). Therapy work and therapists' positive and negative well-being. *Journal of Social and Clinical Psychology, 26*(3), 385–403. doi:10.1521/jscp.2007.26.3.385

Maslach, C., & Leiter, M. P. (1997). The truth about burnout. San Francisco, CA: Jossey-Bass. Maslach, C. & Leiter, M. P. (2008). Early predictors of job burnout and engagement. *The Journal of Applied Psychology, 93*(3), 498–512. doi:10.1037/0021-9010.93.3.498 PMID:18457483

Maslach, C., Schaufeli, W. B., & Leiter, M. P. (2001). Job burnout. *Annual Review of Psychology, 52*(1), 397–422. doi:10.1146/annurev.psych.52.1.397 PMID:11148311

McCann, I. L., & Pearlman, L. A. (1990). Vicarious traumatization: A framework for understanding the psychological effects of working with victims. *Journal of Traumatic Stress, 3*(1), 131–149. doi:10.1007/BF00975140

McCarthy, W. C., & Frieze, I. H. (1999). Negative aspects of therapy: Client perceptions of therapists' social influence, burnout, and quality of care. *The Journal of Social Issues, 55*(1), 33–50. doi:10.1111/0022-4537.00103

Munroe, J. F. (1999). Ethical Issues associated with secondary trauma in therapists. In H. Stamm (Ed.), *Secondary Traumatic Stress: Self-care issues for clinicians, researchers and educators*. Sidran Press.

Nagamine, M., Shigemura, J., Fujiwara, T., Waki, F., Tanichi, M., Saito, T., Toda, H., Yoshino, A., & Shimizu, K. (2018). The relationship between dispositional empathy, psychological distress, and posttraumatic stress responses among Japanese uniformed disaster workers: A cross-sectional study. *BMC Psychiatry, 18*(1), 328. doi:10.118612888-018-1915-4 PMID:30309334

National Sleep Foundation. (2006). *Sleep-wake cycle: Its physiology and impact on health.* Author.

Neff, K. D. (2003). Development and validation of a scale to measure self-compassion. *Self and Identity, 2*(3), 223–250. doi:10.1080/15298860309027

Neff, K. D., Kirkpatrick, K. L., & Rude, S. S. (2007). Self-compassion and adaptive psychological functioning. *Journal of Research in Personality*, *41*(1), 139–154. doi:10.1016/j.jrp.2006.03.004

Negash, S., & Sahin, S. (2011). Compassion fatigue in marriage and family therapy: Implications for therapists and clients. *Journal of Marital and Family Therapy*, *37*(1), 1–13. doi:10.1111/j.1752-0606.2009.00147.x PMID:21198684

Nelson-Gardell, D., & Harris, D. (2003). Childhood abuse history, secondary traumatic stress, and child welfare workers. *Child Welfare*, *82*, 5–26. PMID:12641376

Nissen-Lie, H. A., Rønnestad, M. H., Høglend, P. A., Havik, O. E., Solbakken, O. A., Stiles, T. C., & Monsen, J. T. (2015). Love yourself as a person, doubt yourself as a therapist? *Clinical Psychology & Psychotherapy*.

Norcross, J. C., & Guy, J. D. (2007). *Leaving it at the office: A guide to psychotherapist self-care*.

Ohaeri, J. U. (2003). The burden of caregiving in families with a mental illness: A review of 2002. *Current Opinion in Psychiatry*, *16*(4), 457–465. doi:10.1097/01.yco.0000079212.36371.c0

Pearlin, L. I. (1989). The sociological study of stress. *Journal of Health and Social Behavior*, *30*(3), 241–256. doi:10.2307/2136956 PMID:2674272

Pearlman, L. A. (1995). Self-care for trauma therapists: Ameliorating vicarious traumatization. In B. H. Stamm (Ed.), *Secondary traumatic stress: Selfcare issues for clinicians, researchers, and educators* (pp. 51–64). Sidran Press.

Pearlman, L. A. (1995). Self-care for trauma therapists: Ameliorating vicarious traumatization. In B. H. Stamm (Ed.), *Secondary traumatic stress: Selfcare issues for clinicians, researchers, and educators* (pp. 51–64). Sidran Press.

Pearlman, L. A., & MacIan, P. J. (1995). Vicarious traumatization: An empirical study of the effects of trauma work on trauma therapists. *Professional Psychology, Research and Practice*, *26*(6), 558–565. doi:10.1037/0735-7028.26.6.558

Pearlman, L. A., & MacIan, P. S. (1995). Vicarious traumatization: An empirical study of the effects of trauma work on trauma therapists. *Professional Psychology, Research and Practice*, *26*(6), 558–565. doi:10.1037/0735-7028.26.6.558

Pearlman, L. A., & Saakvitne, K. W. (1995). Treating therapists with vicarious traumatization and secondary traumatic stress disorders. In C. R. Figley (Ed.), *Compassion fatigue: Coping with secondary traumatic stress disorder in those who treat the traumatized* (pp. 150–177). Brunner/Maze.

Penedo, F. J., & Dahn, J. R. (2005). Exercise and well-being: A review of mental and physical health benefits associated with physical activity. *Current Opinion in Psychiatry*, *18*(2), 189–193. doi:10.1097/00001504-200503000-00013 PMID:16639173

Radey, M., & Figley, C. R. (2007). The social psychology of compassion. *Clinical Social Work Journal*, *35*(3), 207–214. doi:10.100710615-007-0087-3

Rudolph, J. M., Stamm, B. H., & Stamm, H. E. (1997). *Compassion fatigue: A concern for mental health policy, providers, & administration.* In Poster presentation at the Annual Meeting of the International Society for Traumatic Stress Studies, Montreal, Canada.

Sabin-Farrell, R., & Turpin, G. (2003). Vicarious traumatization: Implications for the mental health of health workers? *Clinical Psychology Review, 23*(3), 449–480. doi:10.1016/S0272-7358(03)00030-8 PMID:12729680

Salston, M., & Figley, C. R. (2003). Secondary traumatic stress effects of working with survivors of criminal victimization. *Journal of Traumatic Stress, 16*(2), 167–174. doi:10.1023/A:1022899207206 PMID:12699204

Schafer, W. (1996). *Stress management for wellness.* Harcourt Brace.

Schauben, L. J., & Frazier, P. A. (1995). Vicarious trauma: The effects on female counselors of working with sexual violence survivors. *Psychology of Women Quarterly, 19*(1), 49–64. doi:10.1111/j.1471-6402.1995.tb00278.x

Showalter, S. E. (2010). Compassion Fatigue: What Is It? Why Does It Matter? Recognizing the Symptoms, Acknowledging the Impact, Developing the Tools to Prevent Compassion Fatigue, and Strengthen the Professional Already Suffering From the Effects. *The American Journal of Hospice & Palliative Care, 27*(4), 239–242. doi:10.1177/1049909109354096 PMID:20075423

Sinclair, S., Raffin-Bouchal, S., Venturato, L., Mijovic-Kondejewski, J., & Smith-MacDonald, L. (2017). Compassion fatigue: A meta-narrative review of the healthcare literature. *International Journal of Nursing Studies, 69*, 9–24. doi:10.1016/j.ijnurstu.2017.01.003 PMID:28119163

Skorupa, J., & Agresti, A. A. (1993). Ethical beliefs about burnout and continued professional practice. *Professional Psychology, Research and Practice, 24*(3), 281–285. doi:10.1037/0735-7028.24.3.281

Skovholt, T. M., Morgan, J., & Cunningham, H. N. (1989). Mental imagery in career counseling and life planning: A review of research and intervention methods. *Journal of Counseling and Development, 67*(5), 287–291. doi:10.1002/j.1556-6676.1989.tb02604.x

Skovholt, T. M., Rønnestad, M. H., & Jennings, L. (1997). Searching for Expertise in Counseling, Psychotherapy, and Professional Psychology. *Educational Psychology Review, 9*(4), 361–369. doi:10.1023/A:1024798723295

Sorenson, C., Bolick, B., Wright, K., & Hamilton, R. (2016). Understanding compassion fatigue in healthcare providers: A review of current literature. *Journal of Nursing Scholarship, 48*(5), 456–465. doi:10.1111/jnu.12229 PMID:27351469

Stamm, B. H. (1995). Preface. In B. H. Stamm (Ed.), *Secondary traumatic stress: Self-care issues for clinicians, researchers, and educators* (pp. ix–xii). Sidran Press.

Stamm, B. H. (1997). Work-related secondary traumatic stress. *PTSD Research Quarterly, 8*(2).

Stevanovic, P., & Rupert, P. A. (2004). Career-sustaining behaviors, satisfactions, and stresses of professional psychologists. *Psychotherapy (Chicago, Ill.), 41*(3), 301–309. doi:10.1037/0033-3204.41.3.301

Strauss, J. L., Hayes, A. M., Johnson, S. L., Newman, C. F., Brown, G. K., Barber, J. P., Laurenceau, J.-P., & Beck, A. T. (2006). Early alliance, alliance ruptures, and symptom change in a nonrandomized trial of cognitive therapy for avoidant and obsessive-compulsive personality disorders. *Journal of Consulting and Clinical Psychology*, *74*(2), 337–345. doi:10.1037/0022-006X.74.2.337 PMID:16649878

Stress and the Family. (2016). *Coping with Catastrophe* (C. R. Figley, Ed.). Academic Press.

Takamatsu, R. (2018). Turning off the empathy switch: Lower empathic concern for the victim leads to utilitarian choices of action. *PLoS One*, *13*(9), e0203826. doi:10.1371/journal.pone.0203826 PMID:30212541

Thoits, P. A. (1986). Social support as coping assistance. *Journal of Consulting and Clinical Psychology*, *54*(4), 416–423. doi:10.1037/0022-006X.54.4.416 PMID:3745593

Thoits, P. A. (1995). Stress, coping, and social support processes: Where are we? What next? *Journal of Health and Social Behavior*, *35*, 53–79. doi:10.2307/2626957 PMID:7560850

Thoits, P. A. (2011). Mechanisms linking social ties and support to physical and mental health. *Journal of Health and Social Behavior*, *52*(2), 145–161. doi:10.1177/0022146510395592 PMID:21673143

Thomas, J. (2013). Association of personal distress with burnout, compassion fatigue, and compassion satisfaction among clinical social workers. *Journal of Social Service Research*, *39*(3), 365–379. doi:10.1080/01488376.2013.771596

Udipi, S., Veach, P. M., Kao, J., & LeRoy, B. S. (2008). The psychic costs of empathic engagement: Personal and demographic predictors of genetic counselor compassion fatigue. *Journal of Genetic Counseling*, *17*(5), 459–471. doi:10.100710897-008-9162-3 PMID:18704664

Yu, H., Jiang, A., & Shen, J. (2016). Prevalence and predictors of compassion fatigue, burnout and compassion satisfaction among oncology nurses: A cross-sectional survey. *International Journal of Nursing Studies*, *57*, 28–38. doi:10.1016/j.ijnurstu.2016.01.012 PMID:27045562

Zhao, C., Shi, C., Zhang, L., Zhai, Z., Ren, Z., Lin, X., & Jiang, G. (2020). Establishment of online platform for psychological assistance during a public health emergency. *International Journal of Mental Health Promotion*, *22*(3), 123–132. doi:10.32604/IJMHP.2020.011077

Chapter 13
Ecological Approach to Higher Educator Wellness and Self-Care

Cara L. Metz
https://orcid.org/0000-0002-2447-2665
University of Arizona Global Campus, USA

Sarah H. Jarvie
https://orcid.org/0000-0001-9401-4275
Colorado Christian University, USA

ABSTRACT

Self-care is an important and necessary part of a teaching career. Without appropriate self-care, our wellness can suffer and develop into burnout. Educators with burnout can have more absences, be more apathetic to our work, or create an unhealthy learning environment for students. To be well, our self-care cannot happen only at a micro-level. This chapter will examine educator wellness from the perspective of the ecological model. It is important to examine all of the impacts on our wellness and understand the control we can have over our systems. This chapter will look at the impacts of wellness and how to implement self-care strategies both at a personal and a university levels to reduce the impact of burnout.

INTRODUCTION

As counselor educators, the authors focus class time on preventing burnout and encouraging self-care with their student population. Burnout is very prevalent in the helping professions. In the field of education, though, burnout can be just as prevalent as we juggle not only teaching, research, and service, but other factors like interactions with students, work-life balance, and politics, to name a few.

DOI: 10.4018/978-1-6684-2334-9.ch013

Herbert Freudenberger first defined the concept of burnout in 1975. He described it as having three components: emotional exhaustion, depersonalization, and a decreased sense of accomplishment, all of which are brought on by prolonged stress. Not only can burnout have an impact on us personally, but it can also have rippling effects on the work we do, and it can come at a cost to the university. It can result in anxiety and depression, more physical illnesses, and sick days. Burnout can cause faculty to become indifferent, make us less empathetic to the needs of students, and impact our quality of work. Further, burnout in faculty can lead to attrition and good educators leaving the field.

Sometimes as educators we do not participate in self-care nor feel supported in our efforts. Preventing burnout is one of the best ways we can maintain wellness in faculty (Shah et al., 2018). Faculty well-being not only impacts personal well-being, but it also is an asset to academic institutions (Larson et al., 2019). To prevent symptoms of burnout and work on maintaining our wellness through healthy self-care practices, we need to know where our wellness might slip, and how higher education institutions can help to maintain the wellness of their faculty and staff.

What is wellness? Wellness goes beyond just physical and mental health. Sweeny and Witmer (1991) introduced a model that expanded the idea of wellness into a wheel.They believed that wellness needed to encompass work, love, friendship, spirituality, and self-regulation. To be well, we must maintain a balance of all of these ideas, which can impact our physical and mental well-being. Because work plays an important role in our wellness, it is important to explore how our work and career can support our self-care, which will influence our wellness. In addition, a change in one area can have a profound impact or change in other areas, either for better or for worse (Myers et al., 2000). Self-care is another important aspect of maintaining wellness. Self-care is "the ability of individuals, families, and communities to promote health, prevent disease, maintain health, and to cope with illness and disability with or without the support of healthcare providers" (World Health Organization, 2021, para. 1).

This chapter will zoom out to look at wellness and the need for self-care using Conyne and Cook's (2004) ecological model, which combines Lewin's (1936) thoughts that our behavior is a product of how we interact with our environment and Bronfenbrenner's (1977) idea that we exist in environmental systems that are proximal to and distal from us (see Figure 1). Bronfenbrenner's systems included micro-, meso-, exo-, macro-, and chronosystems. When we look at what impacts our wellness, we tend to look at ourselves on a micro-level. To make a system change that supports and promotes wellness, we have to understand who the stakeholders are within the systems (Williams et al., 2018) and how they impact how we perform self-care activities and prevent burnout. Creating an environment where self-care and wellness are prioritized and even promoted through policies can enhance how we teach and our ability to meet the needs of our students. Wellness is not only the responsibility of the faculty, but also requires the commitment and support of the university.

MICROSYSTEM

After the individual, the microsystem is the innermost tier of Bronfenbrenner's (1977) ecological systems theory. In exploring the role of wellness in creating an environment conducive to implementing self-care strategies, one is probably most familiar with microsystems, which are direct interactions with the environment.

Figure 1. The ecological model

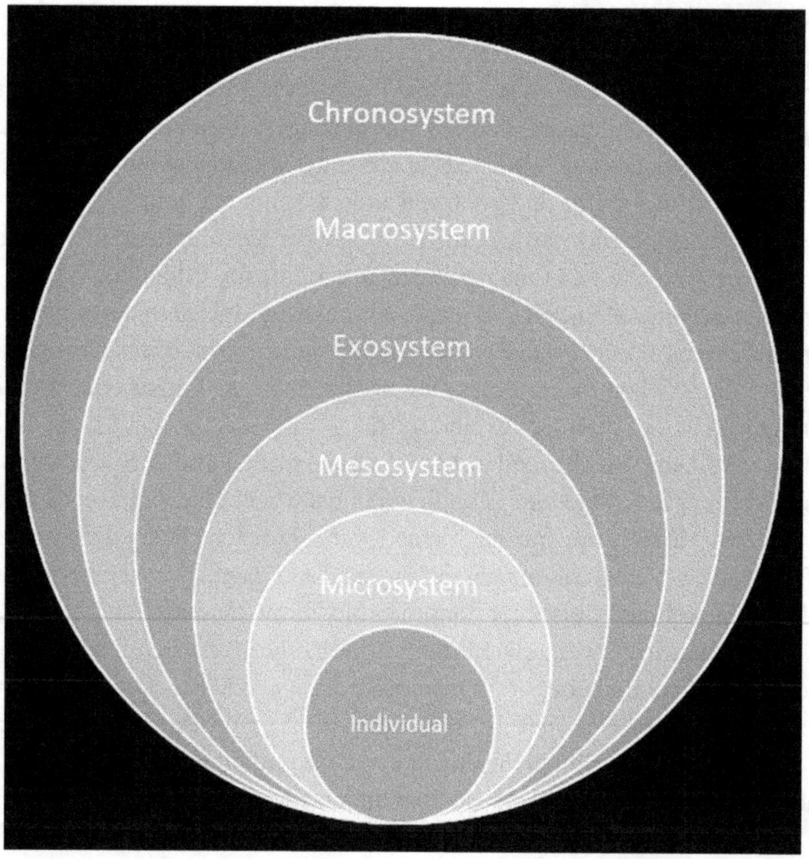

A microsystem is the smallest and most immediate environment impacting one's life. Bronfenbrenner (1977) refers to it as "the complex of relations between the developing person and environment in an immediate setting containing that person" (p. 514). The world of higher education produces unique facets of microsystems that influence one's life and can set the tone for the other systems. The multiple demands and work responsibilities can include (but are not limited to) teaching, research and writing, committee involvement, participating in university service activities, mentoring, and advising students. Thus, faculty workload is an important microsystem that can either positively or negatively influence one's self-care and wellness strategies (Johnson et al., 2018; Lease, 1999; Lackritz, 2004; Magnuson et al., 2009). For faculty on a tenure-track, there is even more pressure to maintain a strong record of teaching, research, and service (Niles et al., 2001). The stress of such a high workload can create a poorer work-life balance which directly impacts one's well-being (Johnson et al., 2018). Being able to self-examine the impact of one's workload and identify the areas that create the most stress can help one recognize what may contribute to burnout.

In terms of work-life balance, it's important to address the role of women. Women in academia seem to have more stress related to work-life balance because historically they have more child and home responsibilities than men (Cassidy-Vu et al., 2017; Stinchfield & Trepal, 2010). Stinchfield and Trepal (2010) found in their study of counselor educator female faculty members that some women delayed starting their academic careers in order to start a family and even had fewer children to obtain tenure.

The American Association of University Professors (AAUP) (2001) developed the "Statement of Principles on Family Responsibilities and Academic Work." These principles give universities guidance on developing appropriate policies and procedures that support such things as family leave, teaching schedule modifications, and policies like stopping the tenure clock for new parents. The AAUP (2001) recognizes "the conflict between work and family obligations that many faculty members experience is more acute for women faculty than for men" (pp. 339-340). The report also states that while academic culture is unique in aspects such as a flexible schedule and a potential ability to achieve a healthy work-life balance, it also poses unique challenges. The "lack of a clear boundary in academic lives between work and family has, at least historically, meant that work has been all persistent, often to the detriment of family" (AAUP, 2001, p.340). Focusing specifically on the experiences of women faculty, Ward and Wolf-Wendel (2004) found despite the challenges and frustrations of balancing raising children and academia, many found joy in their professional and personal lives. The joy was related to such things as teaching, helping students learn and grow, and being recognized for their scholarly works (Ward & Wolf-Wendel, 2004). On the flip side, while many noted the flexibility that academia can give, there are drawbacks such as "a workload that never ends, never having enough time in the day, the ambiguities of tenure expectations, and the expectations for working a 'second shift' at home" (Ward & Wolf-Wendel, 2004, p. 243). These negatives further support the importance of maintaining a work-life balance that can support one's wellness. Another theme from Ward & Wolf-Wendel's (2004) study that is significant to the area of wellness is that having a child helped give perspective on the importance of work, and for some helped change their priorities while also making them more efficient.

Additional areas of the microsystem are impacted as educators include supportive interaction from colleagues (Gasser & Shaffer, 2014; Niles et al., 2001; Stinchfield & Trepal, 2010) and leadership (Mews, 2019). Having positive interactions and support from these microsystems play an important role in maintaining wellness as a faculty member (Gonzalez & Sutton, 2013; Mews, 2019). In terms of leadership, preferred supportive interactions from leadership may depend on leadership style (Mews, 2019). Mews (2019) found that multiple leadership styles were preferred and a "situational approach may be necessary to effectively lead in a college or university setting." Taking the individual into account and not using a one-size-fits-all approach (p.65) supports the systems perspective of this chapter because it is important to view each faculty member as a unique individual.

The self-care one implements regularly is another important factor in maintaining wellness at the microsystem level (Magnuson et al., 2009; Niles et al., 2001). A longitudinal study following new assistant professors found one main theme of participant recommendations was focused on the importance of self-care (Magnuson et al., 2009). At this level, the self-care one may implement can include work-related tasks such as creating better boundaries with evening and weekend email responses and limiting how much one works on the weekend. It also may include such strategies as taking time for real breaks during the workday by getting outside for a walk or taking a lunch break that is not at one's desk or in one's office. These breaks are even more important when a person is working from home. Additionally, smaller acts of self-care like enjoying a moment with a favorite cup of tea or coffee can provide a moment of intentionality. Other small moments of self-care could include listening to a favorite song or taking a few minutes to do some breathing exercises. Self-care can be part of an individual's everyday routine, but it might take some practice to implement regularly. If faculty only focus on the microsystem, they are missing many other influences of wellness in the academic environment, and the self-care they do at this level might not be enough.

MESOSYSTEM

One's mesosystem is the relationships and connections among their microsystems. Another way of viewing it is "a mesosystem is a system of microsystems" (Bronfenbrenner, 1977, p. 515). Bronfenbrenner (1977) also stated that "a mesosystem comprises the interrelations among major settings containing the developing person at a particular point in his or her life." (p. 515). To connect this level to educator wellness, it is important to further examine work-life balance (Alexander-Albritton & Hill, 2015; Johnson et al., 2018; Leinbaugh et al., 2003; Stinchfield & Trepal, 2010) and the career support one receives from family and friends (Ropers-Huilman, 2000). If environments are not supportive of one another, it can be difficult to maintain wellness and practice self-care.

Work is viewed as one of the major life tasks of wellness (Myers, Sweeney, & Witmer, 2000). Thus, work and ultimately career satisfaction have a significant impact on wellness and one's overall well-being (Alexander-Albritton & Hill, 2015; Myers et al., 2000). "People who view their career as a calling tend to experience the highest work satisfaction" (Wrzesniewski, et al., 1997, as cited in Myers et al., 2000). When work is examined through the lens of a job, career, or calling, each can have a different impact on one's well-being. For example, according to Wrzesniewski et al. (1997), "most people see their work as either a Job (focus on financial rewards and necessity rather than pleasure or fulfillment; not a major positive part of life), a Career (focus on advancement), or a Calling (focus on enjoyment of fulfilling, socially useful work)" (p.21). Thus, it could be helpful for faculty to examine primary motivation behind work to help further assess this area of wellness.

Creating healthy boundaries is another important aspect of maintaining wellness that can be viewed as part of the mesosystem. In higher education, it can be easy to push oneself to create unhealthy boundaries such as taking on a new project, being too available to students, and pressure to publish, in addition to teaching and grading responsibilities (Yakaboski, 2019). According to Yakaboski (2019), "the relentless expansion of expectations can push work hours and stress levels higher and higher, especially for adjunct, term and untenured faculty members" (paragraph 2). There is a danger for a "do it all" mentality to become a reality for many faculty members and possibly jeopardize one's well-being with potential further risk to the department or institution (Yakaboski, 2019, paragraph 4). Hill (2004; 2009) notes that junior faculty are more likely to experience burnout because they have even more work-related stress and demands compared to more seasoned faculty. Junior faculty are tasked with learning the job in addition to performing work responsibilities; thus, it is even more important for junior faculty to prioritize their wellness.

As one continues to explore the impact of mesosystems on wellness, they must also look at how to create healthy boundaries and how to develop respect from families and employers for their boundaries and needs. Healthy work boundaries include learning to use one's time to be productive and not procrastinate despite the numerous demands (Ackerman & Gross, 2007). In their study looking at procrastination in faculty members, Ackerman & Gross (2007) found "the procrastination of some tasks leads to undue stress and anxiety and ultimately to lesser quality work because the work is completed in a hurried manner and afforded less than optimal time and attention" (p. 99). In viewing procrastination as a barrier to wellness, it is important to evaluate one's time management skills because procrastination can eventually have a negative effect on one's mental health and career success. Since there can be many future deadlines for a faculty member (i.e., publications or research for promotion or tenure), successful time management is a key (Ackerman & Gross, 2007).

Evaluating one's family commitments can be another area of importance in this level of examining one's wellness. Achieving a work-life balance is becoming increasingly difficult, especially for women in academia (Neale-McFall et al., 2020). Scholars have used a pipeline metaphor to describe the progression of one's career in academia. It's been found that typically women leak from the academic pipeline more often than men, which is referred to as the leaky pipeline (Mason et al., 2013; Neale-McFall et al., 2020; Ysseldyk et al., 2019). Neale-McFall et al. (2020) found that men in their study also alluded to work-life balance issues, and their findings include a lack of support from peers and administration as another prominent theme in work satisfaction. This further supports the idea that a supportive work environment (peers, administration, and the university in general) do have a significant impact on one's occupational satisfaction and wellness.

Looking at how leadership can create a workplace that improves cohesiveness, not only among faculty but also throughout the leadership chain, is another aspect of wellness to examine at the mesosystem level. Leadership can help generate a workplace that improves connection among faculty. A successful mentorship program in the department is one way to improve connection. In fact, Daly & Dee (2006) found mentoring to be a stronger predictor of faculty turnover than job satisfaction (as cited in Woo et al., 2019). Successful mentorship can help one navigate the university system and can even enhance their productivity, which is crucial as a faculty member (Woo et al., 2019). Additionally, creating a more collegial work environment where faculty members feel supported and share their experiences may help mitigate burnout (Woo et al., 2019). Faculty burnout should be an area of concern in the university system as it was found to be a significant predictor of high turnover intentions, which further supports the idea of organizational and institutional support (Woo et al., 2019). "When faculty are more committed to their organization, they are less likely to seek alternative employment or to leave" (p. 87, O'Meara, 2015, as cited in Woo et al., 2019).

To summarize, some examples of self-care at the mesosystem level that were explored in this section include making time for oneself in addition to one's family and finding and utilizing support for one's career from family and friends. Other ideas include creating and maintaining a work schedule and calendar that helps keep track of one's commitments; exploring one's position on whether work is a job, career, or calling; and finding ways to collaborate with colleagues for additional support. A university and its administration that can understand the idea of mesosystems can greatly influence how faculty practices self-care.

EXOSYSTEM

As one pushes out a bit further, they can examine wellness and self-care from the exosystems, the systems with which one does not directly participate, but that influence their actions and decisions. These would include the tenure system (Alexander-Albritton & Hill, 2015; Hill, 2009; Jacobs & Winslow, 2004; Lackritz, 2004; Leinbaugh et al., 2003; Magnuson et al., 2009; Stinchfield & Trepal, 2010; Wester et al., 2009) and organizational politics (Hill, et al., 2005; Magnuson et al., 2009). When it comes to self-care with respect to the exosystem, how can one create an environment that helps meet career goals while also setting appropriate boundaries personally and with colleagues?

Expectations of faculty have increased and even changed as noted by Schimanski & Alperin (2018), who mention that the review, promotion, and tenure (RPT) "processes have generally increased the value placed on research, at the expense of teaching and service, which often results in an incongruity between how faculty actually spend their time versus what is considered in their evaluation" (p. 1). This incongruence can create more stress. This shift over time in the requirements of the RPT process can also produce faculty role conflicts with tension between one's role as a teacher and researcher (Gordon, 2008, as cited in Schimanski & Alperin, 2018). These role conflicts can decrease one's job satisfaction, which can have a direct impact on professional burnout. However, it's important to note that in a review of literature, Hagedorn (1996) found faculty satisfaction is multifaceted and can be "categorized as (1) salary levels, (2) tenure and rank, (3) perceived support and interactions with superiors or facilitators, (4) job stress, (5) interaction with students, (6) social aspects and collegial relations, and (7) the 'person-environment' fit, or satisfaction with the institution" (pp. 571–572, as cited in Ropers-Hullman, 2000). These are significant characteristics that can all have an impact on the overall wellness of an individual faculty member.

In many colleges and universities, there has been an increase in Non-Tenure Track faculty (NTT). In fact, according to Curtis and Thornton (2013) (as cited in Reevy & Deason, 2014), 70 percent of faculty members are employed off the tenure track. At the ecosystem level, this is an important factor as many NTT faculty positions are dependent on institutional factors outside the faculty member's control, such as budget approvals and student enrollment, and typically are not provided benefits like health insurance or retirement (Reevy & Deason, 2014). There can also be an inequality in terms of access to resources and power for NTT versus full-time faculty. In a study examining NTT faculty and specifically looking at "perceptions related to workplace stressors and harm, organizational commitment, common coping mechanisms, and depression, anxiety and stress," Reevy and Deason (2014) found that NTT have more sources of stress than those who have full-time faculty positions (p.1). These sources of stress and perceived stressors are mostly related to their contingent positions and instability of their temporary employment. Additional stressors such as heavy workload, lack of institutional support, and lower or unequal pay were also reported as sources of stress (Reevy & Deason, 2014). Examining personal wellness of NTT, Reevy & Deason (2014) found that often unhealthy coping mechanisms are used which in turn lead to increased depression, anxiety, and stress.

Organizational politics at a university can be a barrier to wellness because negative workplace politics can be detrimental to one's health and well-being. According to Atta & Khan (2016, as cited in Ahmed et al., 2020), organizational politics are vital to a workplace as they can directly or indirectly affect behavior and attitudes. Factors such as power, conflict, and blame can all hinder work performance (Ahmed et al., 2020). They also cite factors related to the person (age, gender, and job title) and dispositional factors (autonomy and competence) as potential barriers.

In academia, like any workplace, there are spoken and unspoken rules that guide normative practices and expectations and provide policy within the institution, including a workplace hierarchy (Bisaillon & Eakin, 2014). Bisaillon and Eakin note:

While this dissension between policy and practice might be confusing or even produce anxiety for academic newcomers, such discrepancy or tension also offers opportunities to explore the informal and understated norms and contingent rules that colour and fashion academic lives. (2014, para. 4)

At the exosystem level, self-care can look at how one can best use their abilities to understand their position within their university. This may include such things as asking questions to recognize the guidelines about one's role and work expectations. Another idea is working to gain an understanding of the university's systems, including policies and procedures, to decrease ambiguity which can further contribute to work-related stress as a faculty member.

MACROSYSTEM

As one continues to expand the ecological systems, the research focuses less on the bigger systems, but when one looks at self-care and individual needs, these systems become important to understanding individual faculty differences, especially from a leadership level. To understand the faculty's needs for wellness and appropriately support those needs, one must examine the macrosystem and chronosystem. Considering these systems allows one to not only adopt ways a system can support their faculty, but also understand the issues and needs of the faculty and work on solutions that promote effective manners of self-care to maintain wellness among them.

With the macrosystem one is looking at values related to culture and social systems. The culture and values one has placed in their life will impact wellness and ripple down to affect the other systems, including how one practices self-care at a micro- and meso-level. The macrosystem influences how much self-care time one might need, what constitutes an individual's needed work-life balance, or where one places importance and value. Feeling like one's personal work-life balance is off can create stress and unhappiness (Matheson & Rosen, 2012), which can lead to burnout. Society places value on hard work and capitalism, which can mean that one spends long hours to get work done, sacrificing their health and well-being (Bone, 2015), which can create pressure to not maintain one's ideal balance. Individuals might be fed images of what health and well-being look like that might be unattainable to most. The emphasis on consumer culture with respect to health tends to send a message that one is not fit enough yet provides quick access to processed foods, and long work hours in academia can lead to a sedentary lifestyle (Bone 2005). Creating a one-size-fits-all idea of wellness both personally and within a work environment might not be an acceptable solution and could possibly do harm. Communicating the value the university places on work-life balance can help inspire change among faculty and staff (Shanafelt et al., 2021).

At the macrosystem level, policy or work culture is one important area of focus. What are the institutional policies that exist or need to be created to support faculty wellness and self-care? One should not only focus on what each faculty can do, but what is needed at an institutional level. At the macro-level, one should take the information from the other systems and begin to understand the programs that could be created and the things that can be put in place at the university to promote wellness among the faculty and staff and reduce workplace stressors (Kelloway & Day, 2005). In addition, university systems can begin to align their mission with one that encompasses self-care and overall wellness of their faculty and employees.

The macrosystem can influence what an individual chooses to do for self-care. Understanding wellness and self-care at a cultural level allows faculty to incorporate what meets their needs best and helps universities and leadership meet the needs of their diverse faculty. Understanding a person at a macrosystem level will allow for the implementation of activities that will enhance wellness at lower levels (Mabry et al., 2013) at both a personal and university level. To address the need for self-care, one has to examine from where the needs come. This does not mean knowing each faculty member's values and culture, but it can include providing the opportunity for groups to form based on interests, values, and culture to help create safe spaces where people feel supported. In addition, universities should provide the space to hear and possibly adapt to the needs of the faculty and what the university can do to improve wellness.

Another way a faculty member might demonstrate self-care at this level is to set up groups that focus on interests, values, and culture. Finding people within the university community with commonalities can help faculty members feel like they have a community and social support. Social support plays an important role in feeling satisfied within one's job (Larson et al., 2019), and social health impacts one's performance and ability to foster productive relationships and take on new opportunities (Ross & Squires, 2015; Seipel & Larson, 2018). Providing space for these types of groups can also allow people to discuss issues they might face and bring about strength to propose and make positive changes within the academic system, which can result in wellness.

As an individual faculty member, self-care at this level might include making time for spiritual activities that are valued and setting a boundary (Matheson & Rosen, 2012) for those rituals and activities that are important. Faculty feel more balanced when spirituality or religion is a part of their lives (Matheson & Rosen, 2012). At a university level, this might mean having groups that promote self-expression and healing, offering floating holidays that work around the beliefs of the faculty, or providing some flexibility in office hours. Having a workplace that respects and gives space for spirituality and its practices has been shown to improve overall wellness and offers a source of resilience. This can in turn help to relieve some of the stress experienced at work (Csiernik & Adams, 2007) and improve performance (Ross & Squires, 2015).

Creating a university culture where mental health is valued, struggles can be communicated, and work can be adapted to meet the needs of the individual is important for a workplace that values the emotional well-being of its faculty. Being able to sustain mental health is so important because those with mental health disorders are more likely to feel stress (Gunawan et al., 2018), which can impact wellness and increase the chances of burnout.

Faculty wellness can also be influenced by the culture of the university. Having a sense of community, feeling valued and appreciated, and being recognized (Shah et al., 2018) for excellence in teaching, publications, and other activities are opportunities for universities to build a culture that promotes wellness and vitality. Creating a university mission that embraces these ideas (Shah et al., 2018) is a way to reinforce with faculty a culture of wellness.

Finally, to help support the needs of the faculty and where they place value, so that faculty can create boundaries and balance, universities should work to enhance the ability of faculty to maintain a manageable workload. To do this, universities can fill positions that are open (Matheson & Rosen, 2012), hire enough support staff, and allow faculty to hire teaching and research assistants. By supporting the needs of the faculty, universities respect the faculty's work-life balance.

The macrosystem presents an opportunity to not only consider the values and culture of the faculty, but to reflect the values and the culture of the university. Through finding ways to be supportive of faculty's culture and values, a university can create a safe and supportive atmosphere where faculty can give attention to what is important to them. At the mesosystem level, faculty works to meet the needs of their wellness wheel, which can enhance their satisfaction and dedication to their work environment.

CHRONOSYSTEM

Finally, at the chronosystem level, one looks at how personal history and major life situations have happened both individually and historically. When thinking about wellness and self-care, and all of the areas that impact them, at the chronosystem one is integrating all of the other systems to understand personal wellness and its contributors. What one has experienced in their past will influence what balance looks like and what self-care strategies they use. It is important for leadership to understand how differences in age, lived experiences, and historical context will impact how an individual takes care of themselves and remains healthy. Well-being could be impacted by normative and non-normative transitions (Bronfenbrenner, 1986), such as being diagnosed with a major health condition, having someone in the family be injured or fall ill, divorces and weddings, pandemics, financial crises, and war. These transitions all impact how a person practices self-care and gets needed support (Price & McCallum, 2015). These life stressors can alter emotional well-being and induce stress and burnout (Gunawan et al., 2018).

Wellness and self-care needs change over time. For example, when people reach the age of retirement, those who report having higher mental well-being are more likely to retire later. In fact, those who feel discriminated against at their job based on their age are more likely to report being ill and stressed, which leads to more instances of burnout (McFadden et al., 2020). Understanding how to support these ever-changing needs as faculty members enter different stages of life is important. In addition, creating a healthy workplace environment is much more effective than offering occasional well-being interventions (Kelloway & Day, 2005).

Faculty and universities need to understand that when it comes to self-care, changing with the times is necessary, especially when the change is non-normative. The COVID-19 pandemic is one major example of a non-normative chronosystem change. People's lives changed dramatically, most never dealing with a situation like it before. Universities put an emphasis on meeting the needs of the students, both academically and also sometimes the students increased emotional needs, which also left many faculty drained, especially as they were simultaneously learning how to move their teaching to a mode that best suited online learning. This adaptation happened quickly, too, which made it even more difficult (Kirk-Jenkins & Hughey, 2021). There was a sense of feeling a lack of control as the universities made decisions impacting a lot of people very swiftly. Faculty had to adapt to new teaching pedagogies, learn systems they had never used before, and gain new knowledge and skills (Berdahl & Nouri, 2020) almost overnight. The pandemic not only impacted teaching load but also impacted faculty at the research level, as research funds were not as readily available, and the aspect of scholarship became even more stressful. The workload and pace required of faculty during COVID-19 was not sustainable (Roos & Borkoski, 2021).

On top of that, stressors occurred from dealing with the pandemic itself, a decrease in socialization, and limited resources. Faculty faced new challenges with childcare and supporting children at school, some of whom were learning at home online (Kirk-Jenkins & Hugey, 2021). What one did for wellness prior to the pandemic might not have been possible or looked very different. The ability for faculty to adapt, find new ways to participate in self-care activities, feel supported by the university, and have their needs met to feel safe was very important to maintain all areas of wellness. Looking at what the university level, changes could include increased flexibility (Matheson & Rosen, 2012); training opportunities to learn new systems; and providing groups to enhance socialization, share ideas, decrease isolation, and find others who were dealing with the same stressors.

The self-care needs for each faculty will be different, so the balance someone requires will also be different. For example, faculty who have children or grandchildren might need opportunities for flexible work hours to accommodate the needs of their children and the needs of their occupation or have reliable childcare that would meet the demands of their job. A system that supports these needs also supports the well-being of these faculty who no longer must choose one over the other. A university system can provide flexibility (Matheson & Rosen, 2012) with respect to when grading is done, office hours, office modality, the use of virtual options, research directions and schedules, and career paths. When given the time by the university, whether through a flexible schedule or paid time off to participate in wellness activities, faculty are more likely to participate in self-care activities (Marby et al., 2013; Terrell, 2015). Because people who feel supported in meeting their needs outside of the office will be happier and more productive while at work, this system is one that cannot be ignored. In addition, universities can have their faculty create their own self-care goals for the year, as a part of their annual goal setting. This can include a section of goal setting that asks what the university can do to help them achieve their goals.

At the chronosystem level, one looks at how lived experiences throughout their lives impact well-being and what to do to practice healthy self-care. The COVID-19 pandemic was a non-normative life situation that reflects how universities and individuals address self-care needs to be flexible and adaptable. It has shown that when big changes are made, the impact of faculty wellness cannot be overlooked.

FUTURE RESEARCH RECOMMENDATIONS

It is important to gain a complete understanding of wellness and self-care. Most research has focused on the micro- and meso-levels of maintaining wellness but ignore or just begin to scratch the surface of the larger levels, such as the exosystem, macrosystem, and chronosystem. At the upper levels, wellness and self-care are not mere personal choices, but they depend on university policy. If universities can understand the needs and issues that exist at these levels, they can begin to address the core needs of the faculty instead of implementing programs and policies that put a Band-Aid over burnout to address wellness. Future research should examine these three levels to identify how universities can help faculty as a whole, support the self-care and wellness needs at the individual level, and gain perspective of what policies and programs can be implemented that will contribute to overall wellness.

In addition, future research can examine the policies and procedures that various universities already have in place by taking a deep dive into the opportunities that have been developed. Program evaluations should be considered to find the opportunities that are working so that more universities can implement them with their own faculty as a new layer of university-supported self-care. Research should also focus on what is not working and why some programs are not accomplishing the wellness goals they set. A comprehensive look at various programs can also identify the holes that still need to be addressed.

CONCLUSION

Wellness is important to have as faculty. Being able to maintain work wellness can help faculty prevent burnout, which can lead to turnover, health issues, and not serving students to the best of their abilities. Faculty can maintain wellness by practicing appropriate self-care strategies. Self-care, though, happens at not only a personal level, but must be supported in many ways by universities. When thinking about self-care in the education profession, it is important to understand each faculty member as a whole and how the environmental systems impact wellness and self-care strategies. Having leadership who understand the unique needs of the faculty can help create an environment that not only promotes self-care but develops a system that is conducive to wellness. Wellness and self-care cannot happen in a vacuum and, when working, they cannot happen without the support of leadership and the university. To create a productive environment that values wellness, one must understand wellness as a whole and how it relates to everyone who works within the system.

REFERENCES

Ackerman, D., & Gross, B. (2007). I can start that JME manuscript next week, can't I? The task characteristics behind why faculty procrastinate. *Journal of Marketing Education, 29*(2), 97–110. doi:10.1177/0273475307302012

Ahmed, S., Farooqi, M. T. K., & Iqbal, A. (2020). Influence of organizational politics on university teachers' performance. *Global Social Sciences Review, 5*(2), 341–355. doi:10.31703/gssr.2020(V-II).33

Alexander-Albritton, C., & Hill, N. R. (2015). Familial and institutional factors: Job satisfaction for female counselor educators. *Counselor Education and Supervision, 54*(2), 109–121. doi:10.1002/ceas.12008

American Association of University Professors. (2001). *Statement of principles on family responsibilities and academic work.* https://www.aaup.org/file/Family_and_Academic_Work.pdf

Bergdahl, N., & Nouri, J. (2021). Covid-19 and crisis-prompted distance education in Sweden. *Tech Know Learn, 26*(3), 443–459. doi:10.100710758-020-09470-6

Bisaillon, L., & Eakin, J. (2014, November 12). *Strategies for understanding and navigating the "academic underlife."* University Affairs. https://www.universityaffairs.ca/career-advice/career-advice-article/strategies-understanding-navigating-academic-underlife/

Bone, K. D. (2015). The bioecological model: Applications in holistic workplace well-being management. *International Journal of Workplace Health Management, 8*(4), 256–271. doi:10.1108/IJWHM-04-2014-0010

Borders, L. D., Young, J. S., Wester, K. L., Murray, C. E., Villalba, J. A., Lewis, T. F., & Mobley, A. K. (2011). Mentoring promotion/tenure-seeking faculty: Principles of good practice within a counselor education program. *Counselor Education and Supervision, 50*(3), 171–188. doi:10.1002/j.1556-6978.2011.tb00118.x

Bronfenbrenner, U. (1977). Toward an experimental ecology of the human development. *The American Psychologist, 32*(7), 513–531. doi:10.1037/0003-066X.32.7.513

Bronfenbrenner, U. (1986). Ecology of the family as a context for human development: Research perspectives. *Developmental Psychology, 22*(6), 723–742. doi:10.1037/0012-1649.22.6.723

Cassidy-Vu, L., Beck, K., & Moore, J. B. (2017). Burnout in female faculty members. *Journal of Primary Care & Community Health, 8*(2), 97–99. doi:10.1177/2150131916669191 PMID:27650035

Conyne, R. K., & Cook, E. P. (2004). *Ecological counseling: An innovative approach to conceptualizing person-environment interaction*. American Counseling Association.

Csiernik, R., & Adams, D. W. (2007). Spirituality, stress, and work. In J. Coates, J. R. Graham, & B. Swarzentruber (Eds.), *Spirituality and social work: Selected Canadian readings* (pp. 243–251). Canadian Scholars' Press, Inc.

Freudenberger, H. J. (1975). The staff burn-out syndrome in alternative institutions. *Psychotherapy (Chicago, Ill.)*, *12*(1), 73–82. doi:10.1037/h0086411

Gasser, C. E., & Shaffer, K. S. (2014). Career development of women in academia: Traversing the leaky pipeline. *The Professional Counselor*, *4*(4), 332–352. doi:10.15241/ceg.4.4.332

Gonzalez, G. M., & Sutton, M. (2013). The role of supportive leaders at top performing universities: Best practice lessons from American institutions for Indonesian higher education. *International Journal of Leadership and Change*, *1*(1), 5–13.

Guawan, E., Deo, P., Hidayat, T., Pandia, V., Iskandar, S., Yuni, P. S., Sylviana, N., Akbar, I., Farenia, R., Wahyu, K., Purba, A., & Hatta, S. I. D. I. (2018). Factors correlated with occupational stress among university lecturers. *Medicine & Health*, *13*(2), 95–102. doi:10.17576/MH.2018.1302.9

Hill, N. R., Leinbaugh, T., Bradley, C., & Hazler, R. (2005). Female counselor educators: Encouraging and discouraging factors in academia. *Journal of Counseling and Development*, *83*(3), 374–380. doi:10.1002/j.1556-6678.2005.tb00358.x

Jacobs, J. A., & Winslow, S. E. (2004). Overworked faculty: Job stresses and family demands. *The Annals of the American Academy of Political and Social Science*, *596*(1), 104–129. doi:10.1177/0002716204268185

Johnson, S. J., Willis, S. M., & Evans, J. (2019). An examination of stressors, strain, and resilience in academic and non-academic U.K. university job roles. *International Journal of Stress Management*, *26*(2), 162–172. doi:10.1037tr0000096

Kelloway, E. K., & Day, A. (2005). Building healthy workplaces: Where we need to be. *Canadian Journal of Behavioural Science / Revue Canadienne Des Sciences Du Comportement*, *37*(4), 309–312. https://doi-org.proxy-library.ashford.edu/10.1037/h0087265

Kirk-Jenkins, A. J., & Hughey, A. W. (2021). Abrupt adaption: A review of the impact of the COVID-19 pandemic on faculty in higher education. *Journal of the Professoriate*, *12*(1), 104–121.

Lackritz, J. R. (2004). Exploring burnout among university faculty: Incidence, performance, and demographic issues. *Teaching and Teacher Education*, *20*(7), 713–729. doi:10.1016/j.tate.2004.07.002

Larson, L. M., Seipel, M. T., Shelley, M. C., Gahn, S. W., Ko, S. Y., Schenkenfelder, M., Rover, D. T., Schmittmann, B., & Heitmann, M. M. (2019). The academic environment and faculty well-being: The role of psychological needs. *Journal of Career Assessment*, *27*(1), 167–182. doi:10.1177/1069072717748667

Lease, S. H. (1999). Occupational role stressors, coping, support, and hardiness as predictors of strain in academic faculty: An emphasis on female faculty. *Research in Higher Education*, *40*(3), 285–307. doi:10.1023/A:1018747000082

Leinbaugh, T., Hazler, R. J., Bradley, C., & Hill, N. R. (2003). Factors influencing counselor educators' subjective sense of well-being. *Counselor Education and Supervision*, *43*(1), 52–64. doi:10.1002/j.1556-6978.2003.tb01829.x

Lewin, K. (1936). *Principles of topological psychology*. McGraw-Hill. doi:10.1037/10019-000

Mabry, L., Elliot, D. L., MacKinnon, D. P., Thoemmes, F., & Kuehl, K. S. (2013). Understanding the durability of a fire department wellness program. *American Journal of Health Behavior*, *37*(5), 693–702. doi:10.5993/AJHB.37.5.13 PMID:23985292

Magnuson, S., Norem, K., & Lonneman-Doroff, T. (2009). The 2000 cohort of new assistant professors of counselor education: Reflecting at the culmination of six years. *Counselor Education and Supervision*, *49*(1), 54–71. doi:10.1002/j.1556-6978.2009.tb00086.x

Mason, M. A., Wolfinger, N. H., & Goulden, M. (2013). *Do babies matter: Gender and family in the ivory tower*. Rutgers University Press. doi:10.36019/9780813560823

Matheson, J. L., & Rosen, K. H. (2012). Marriage and family therapy faculty members' balance of work and personal life. *Journal of Marital and Family Therapy*, *38*(2), 394–416. doi:10.1111/j.1752-0606.2009.00137.x PMID:22512300

McFadden, P., Moriarty, J., Schröder, H., Gillen, P., Manthorpe, G., & Mallett, J. (2020). Growing older in social work: Perspective on systems of support to extend working lives -Findings from a UK survey. *British Journal of Social Work*, *50*(2), 405–426. doi:10.1093/bjsw/bcz165

Mews, J. G. (2019). Effective leadership in higher education: A review of leadership style preferences among faculty and staff within the United States. *Open Journal of Leadership*, *8*(02), 58–74. doi:10.4236/ojl.2019.82004

Myers, J. E., Sweeney, T. J., & Witmer, J. M. (2000). The Wheel of Wellness counseling for wellness: A holistic model for treatment planning. *Journal of Counseling and Development*, *78*(3), 251–266. doi:10.1002/j.1556-6676.2000.tb01906.x

Neale-McFall, C., Hermann, M. A., & Eckart, E. (2020). Predictive variables of faculty retention in the counselor education field: A gender perspective. *Journal of Education and Training Studies*, *8*(10), 1–9. doi:10.11114/jets.v8i10.4989

Niles, S. G., Akos, P., & Cutler, H. (2001). Counselor educators' strategies for success. *Counselor Education and Supervision*, *40*(4), 276–291. doi:10.1002/j.1556-6978.2001.tb01260.x

Price, D., & McCallum, F. (2015). Ecological influences on teachers' well-being and "fitness.". *Asia-Pacific Journal of Teacher Education*, *43*(3), 195–209. doi:10.1080/1359866X.2014.932329

Reevy, G., & Deason, G. (2014). Predictors of depression, stress, and anxiety among non-tenure track faculty. *Frontiers in Psychology*, *5*(701), 1–17. doi:10.3389/fpsyg.2014.00701 PMID:25071667

Roos, B. H., & Borkoski, C. C. (2021). Attending to the teacher in teaching: Prioritizing faculty well-being. *Perspectives of the ASHA Special Interest Groups*, *6*(4), 831–840. doi:10.1044/2021_PERSP-21-00006

Ropers-Huilman, B. (2000). Are you satisfied yet? Women faculty members' interpretations of their academic work. *New Directions for Institutional Research, 2000*(105), 21–32. doi:10.1002/ir.10502

Ross, K. T., & Squires, P. (2015). Tone at the top: Leadership as the foundation of organizational health and wellness. *People & Strategy, 38*(1), 36–41.

Schimanski, L. A., & Alperin, J. P. (2018). The evaluation of scholarship in academic promotion and tenure processes: Past, present, and future. *F1000 Research, 7*(1605), 1–20. doi:10.12688/f1000research.16493.1 PMID:30647909

Seipel, M. T., & Larson, L. M. (2018). Supporting non-tenure-track faculty well-being. *Journal of Career Assessment, 26*(1), 154–171. doi:10.1177/1069072716680046

Shah, D. T., Williams, V. N., Thorndyke, L. E., Marsh, E. E., Sonnino, R. E., Block, S. M., & Viggiano, T. R. (2018). Restoring faculty vitality in academic medicine when burnout threatens. *Academic Medicine, 93*(7), 979–984. doi:10.1097/ACM.0000000000002013 PMID:29166355

Shanafelt, T., Trockel, M., Rodriguez, A., & Logan, D. (2021). Wellness-centered leadership: Equipping health care leaders to cultivate physician well-being and professional fulfillment. *Academic Medicine, 96*(5), 641–651. doi:10.1097/ACM.0000000000003907 PMID:33394666

Stinchfield, T. A., & Trepal, H. (2010). Academic motherhood for counselor educators: Navigating through the academic pipeline. *International Journal for the Advancement of Counseling, 32*(2), 91–100. doi:10.100710447-009-9086-0

Sweeney, T. J., & Witmer, J. M. (1991). Beyond social interest: Striving toward optimum health and wellness. *Individual Psychology: The Journal of Adlerian Theory. Research & Practice, 47*(4), 527–540.

Ward, K., & Wolf-Wendel, L. (2004). Academic motherhood: Managing complex roles in research universities. *Review of Higher Education, 27*(2), 233–257. doi:10.1353/rhe.2003.0079

Wester, K. L., Trepal, H. C., & Myers, J. E. (2009). Wellness of counselor educators: An initial look. *Journal of Humanistic Counseling, Education, and Supervision, 48*(1), 91–109. doi:10.1002/j.2161-1939.2009.tb00070.x

Williams, S. A. S., Conyers, A., & Garcia, F. (2018). Practical applications of ecological consultation in higher education: Diversity and inclusion initiatives. *Public Administration Quarterly, 42*(2), 183–212.

Woo, H., Kim, H., & Park, S. (2019). Burnout and turnover intentions among junior counseling faculty: Moderating role of mentoring. *Journal of Employment Counseling, 58*(2), 85–94. doi:10.1002/joec.12114

World Health Organization. (2021). *What do we mean by self-care?* https://www.who.int/reproductive-health/self-care-interventions/definitions/en/

Wrzesniewski, A., McCauley, C., Rozin, P., & Schwartz, B. (1997). Jobs, careers, and callings: People's relations to their work. *Journal of Research in Personality, 31*(1), 21–33. doi:10.1006/jrpe.1997.2162

Yakaboski, T. (2019, November 13). *Making space under the weight of growing expectations.* Inside Higher Ed. https://www.insidehighered.com/advice/2019/11/13/how-set-boundaries-support-your-personal-life-and-career-opinion

Ysseldyk, R., Greenaway, K. H., Hassinger, E., Zutrauen, S., Lintz, J., Bhatia, M. P., Frye, M., Starkenburg, E., & Tai, V. (2019). A leak in the academic pipeline: Identity and health among postdoctoral women. *Frontiers in Psychology*, *10*(1297), 1–17. doi:10.3389/fpsyg.2019.01297 PMID:31231285

ADDITIONAL READING

Bronfenbrenner, U. (1979). *The ecology of human development: Experiments by nature and design*. Harvard University Press.

Conyne, R. K., & Cook, E. P. (2004). *Ecological counseling: An innovative approach to conceptualizing person-environment interaction*. American Counseling Association.

Lewin, K. (1936). *Principles of topological psychology*. McGraw-Hill. doi:10.1037/10019-000

Nagoski, E., & Nagoski, A. (2020). *Burnout: The secret to unlocking the stress cycle*. Ballantine Books.

Sweeney, T. J., & Witmer, J. M. (1991). Beyond social interest: Striving toward optimum health and wellness. *Individual Psychology: The Journal of Adlerian Theory, Research & Practice*, *47*(4), 527–540.

KEY TERMS AND DEFINITIONS

Burnout: Emotional exhaustion, depersonalization, and a decreased sense of accomplishment that is caused by a prolonged period of stress.

Chronosystem: This system consists of all of our personal history and major life situations have happened both personally and historically, both normative and non-normative.

Exosystem: Systems we do not have direct participation with but they do influence our actions and decisions that impact us.

Macrosystem: Our values related to our cultural and social systems.

Mesosystem: A system of the relationships and connections among our microsystems.

Microsystem: the smallest and most immediate environment impacting one's life.

Self-Care: The practice of taking care of oneself to maintain health and well-being.

Wellness: Physical and mental well-being that is influenced by our personal balance between work, love, friendship, spirituality, and our ability to self-regulate.

Chapter 14
My Black Is TOO Precious to Crack!
The Importance of Self-Care

Antione D. Tomlin
Anne Arundel Community College, USA

ABSTRACT

This chapter will explore the experiences of a Black, male, full-time, tenure-track faculty member at a community college. The chapter will delve into his experiences as a Black faculty in part-time (adjunct positions) and his current full-time tenure-track faculty position. There is no doubt that as a Black man in America, he is fighting two pandemics right now, that is, COVID-19 and racism, and this is top of mind for him as he frames this chapter. With a focus on race and gender, this chapter examines his challenges and successes as a Black man who teaches. Additionally, it shares the importance of protecting space and time as a Black academic to prevent burnout. Lastly, this chapter will provide strategies that would be helpful to Black academics and administration that can help one to cope with challenges before situations occur.

INTRODUCTION

Historically, higher education has been an environment built for the benefit and success of non-Black folks (Wagoner & Star, 2021). As a Black male, tenure-track faculty, I have come to know that this notion of higher education being built for the success of non-Blacks does not only apply to students. As a Black Man, I come to Academia with a very different perspective on what it takes to excel in higher education (Tomlin & Hoey, 2021). Being a Black male in America is exhausting. Coupling my Black maleness with my profession is a genuine struggle, as I have to work twice as hard to demonstrate my expertise (Nyunt et al., 2022). While reflecting on my experiences, I note, "as a Black male educator, I find myself constantly fighting for equity and inclusion" (Tomlin, 2022c).

DOI: 10.4018/978-1-6684-2334-9.ch014

My name is Dr. Antione D. Tomlin, and I am a native of Baltimore. I was born and raised in Baltimore City, Maryland. I come from a low-income neighborhood, and growing up, my family did not have much. However, I learned how to be grateful for all I had and make do with what I earned. My adult life is no different; sure, my finances have changed. However, I still believe that a massive part of my resourcefulness comes from being grateful for what I have and honoring my past while continuing to make do with what I have. Early on, as a young adjunct faculty member, this mindset may have in some ways been a detriment to my career trajectory. However, I do not regret any of the experiences I share in this chapter, as each lived experience contributes to the shaping and molding of the professional and academic I am today. This chapter will explore those experiences and share how said experiences create opportunities for me to learn more about taking care of my Blackness as a faculty member in academia.

WHAT IT MEANS TO BE BLACK FACULTY

Black faculty, be it full-time or part-time, have unique experiences that create challenges and obstacles to excelling and create barriers to recruitment and retention of Black faculty due to racism and whiteness that deters cultural change (Bhopal, 2022). While I am a full-time tenure track faculty member now, I did not start my career this way. I was adjunct teaching in multiple departments across multiple institutions. Additionally, I held many jobs in student affairs, as I needed to pay the bills. My passion was in teaching; however, it felt like I had no opportunities to move into a full-time faculty position. One experience was in my early twenties; I taught every level of English from developmental to African American literature II at this community college. When it came time to apply for the one full-time position in the English department, not only did they hire a white colleague, representative of what the majority of the department already looked like, I did not even get an interview. I had been teaching in this department for three years at that point. At that moment, I realized full-time employment was not going to be in my future there. I stopped trying and started applying to other institutions. The following year I was offered a full-time assistant professor position, and I accepted. The institution that had crushed my hopes and dreams of being full-time came to me and said we have a full-time temp position posted, and the person who gets this position has the potential to apply for the next full-time position that comes around; you should apply. I was shocked, appalled, and offended all in the same breath. Not only did the English department know I was leaving, they knew where I was going and the amazing opportunity I had to continue developing as a faculty, but also to have stable and secure full–time employment. It was then that this institution showed me they only cared about my Blackness and expertise when it was helpful to them. They had gotten an order from senior administration to, in other words, sprinkle some brown into the all-white English department. I respectfully declined and have never looked back. This was just one experience I faced that I would absolutely classify as a challenge of mine as a Blackacdemic. The following section will provide additional personal examples of challenges I face as a Black faculty person related to dealing with stereotype threat, being the token Black person, being hired for diversity and managed for assimilation, and feeling that I was not allowed to be tired or say no.

Challenges Black Faculty [I] Face

There is no doubt that COVID-19 has been challenging for all faculty (Manturuk & Reavis, 2022). Moreover, Black faculty have dealt with the challenges of the global pandemic and the challenges of the racial pandemic in the United States. This section will share some of the challenges that Black faculty face in academia while sharing some of my narratives and experiences for observation and learning. This section of the chapter will review how my personal experiences have been impacted by stereotype threat, feeling like the token Black person, being hired for diversity and managed for assimilation, and feeling like I am not allowed to be tired or say no. While this section illustrations some of the challenges Black faculty may face, it does not outline possible solutions or strategies, as I will outline these approaches in a later section.

Stereotype Threat

I started teaching in higher education when I was 21 years old. While finishing up my master's degree, I had an opportunity to teach. I fell in love with teaching and have been in the profession since I stepped foot into my first classroom many years ago. However, at 21, you can imagine that most of my colleagues were older than me. While now I live by the philosophy that age does not equate to wisdom and knowledge when I was 21, I felt intimidated by my older colleagues, many of whom did not look like me. I was young and Black, and being in a majority white space with colleagues much older than me made me less confident in my abilities and the way I showed up. I felt I did not have support, and that further isolated me. I became anxious to navigate that space; as I was afraid, I would confirm a negative stereotype about people who looked like me or belonged to another intersecting identity of mine. In short, stereotype threat was real for me being Black in white space (Anderson, 2022).

Token Black Person

Black faculty working in especially non-Black spaces could be found in positions that classify them as tokens (see Kanter, 1977 for more on tokenism). I will admit, I know that I am valued in many spaces and places in higher education. I also know that there are not many Black males in general with PhDs, and my education and experiences allow me access to many places I would have been denied had I not obtained a doctorate. However, I am a Black PhD, and I still have to fight! (Tomlin, 2022c). I have to fight against stereotypes, racism, tokenism, and more. There are many times I feel I am asked to do something because of the color of my skin. I am asked to "diversify" or add some brown perspective to a committee, I am asked to mentor others who look like me because I am the only Black faculty, I am asked about how to manage and support students of color because I am assumed to be the expert, all things that my non-Black colleagues are not asked to do (Griffin & Harris, 2011). While all of these things are important, and I help when I can, these things are not written into my contract as responsibilities of my full-time job. In fact, as a faculty member, teaching excellence is the most significant determining factor on if one is awarded promotion and tenure. In this way, all things that create an atmosphere that pushes me to a box or to feel tokenized do not support my growth and development, as the things mentioned above are not scored in the promotion and tenure application process. Therefore, when asked to do some of the things above, it feels like my long-term success is being jeopardized and sabotaged by the folks who make these requests of me, my white colleagues.

Hired for Diversity Managed for Assimilation

The idea of hiring for diversity has always been fascinating to me. Partly my interest comes from how organizations and institutions define diversity, equity, inclusion, and anti-racism (DEIA). While DEIA may be at the forefront of many organizations and institutions missions, visions, and goals, I am not sure as a society, and especially as a profession [higher education] we have a good grasp on how to talk the talk and walk the walk (Tomlin, 2022b; Grier-Reed & Quinones, 2021). This uncertainty or lack of clarity of what DEIA means to institutions creates situations I like to refer to as Black faculty being hired for diversity and managed for assimilation. That is, Black faculty hired to bring their expertise, perspectives, and different approaches to the institution but micromanaged and met with hyper resistance and lack of support with every idea posed that does not align with current or traditional institutional thinking, frameworks and culture. In other words, the Black faculty member was actually hired to be a number or Black body, not for their expertise.

Not Allowed to Be Tired/Say No

When I was younger, especially when I first started teaching, I felt honored and grateful for the opportunity and space to be a young, Black academic. I did not feel I could say no because I thought I would be reprimanded or retaliated against. Therefore, I always said yes, and I became the yes man. However, I quickly learned that the yes approach was not sustainable and made me miserable. While there are strategies to help Black faculty cope, I had to start saying no because I was getting burnt out (Tomlin, 2022c; Zambrana et al., 2021). In my experiences, I am sent special requests to speak at events, review materials, sit on committees in addition to my full-time teaching responsibilities. These requests come from peers as well as senior leadership and administration. I always want to do the work to support students and colleagues. However, I realized long ago, I cannot save the world or even attempt to save the world if I am not practicing self-care and declining opportunities that I do not have the mental capacity to handle in the moment or opportunities that do not illuminate my passions and core values.

THE SHIFT: I STAND IN MY BLACKNESS

As a Black faculty, the workload, expectations, and standards are inequitably set, measured, and rewarded from my perspective. When higher education sees my Black skin, all expectations and standards double for me to be considered decent. In my faculty positions over my tenure in academic affairs, I have seen non-Black colleagues get by and be promoted and rewarded based on doing next to nothing. They are not only subpar and mediocre, but they would also perform below the bare minimum, and it was more than okay (Haynes, et al., 2020).

However, I have learned that if I do not support myself and learn to speak up in ways that benefit me, I will not excel within the profession the way that my non-Black colleagues are. Here I share two examples where I felt I was not treated equitable compared to my non-Black, and in this case, specifically my white colleagues.

I started as a full-time faculty at one institution and was assigned release time to run and coordinate the developmental reading and writing tutoring center. This was an excellent opportunity for me, as it allowed me to use my tutoring expertise and leadership to provide a new mission and vision for the center. I was awarded 3 load hours or credits per semester to supervise the lab. While my position included hiring, training, and staffing all tutors year-round, I was not given release time during the summer or winter. I thought it was expected that the job needed to be done, so it was on me to get it done, even during the winters and summers. So, for three years, I essentially worked for free during the winters and summers to ensure the developmental reading and writing tutoring center ran smoothly. My name and reputation was attached to the center, so I went above and beyond to put my all into seeing the lab become a resource and support for all students on campus. As I was rotating out of my position during the spring semester of my third year, a white colleague was rotating into the position. In a department meeting, the faculty member taking over asked me how many hours/credits of release time I got for my leadership in the lab over the summers. Quickly, I responded and said none. My white colleague looked very confused and surprised. Immediately, my white female department chair at the time said, "Oh, maybe it slipped my mind to say something. You should have gotten something" She then directed her conversation to my white colleague and said, "lets talk to so and so, we have to get you release time for the summer!" Not only at that point was I shocked, but angry. I could not believe I had been working for FREE every winter and summer when I could have been compensated for my time and expertise. This was the moment that taught me that when additional obligations are expected, I can expect or request additional compensation as faculty. This also taught me to stand up and ask for what I want or need. Even though I worked to create the tutoring center, I wanted to because my name and reputation were attached, that doesn't mean that I should work for free or stress myself out about every small thing.

The second example I will share here is when I was applying for tenure-track. At this particular institution, only a certain percentage of faculty could be awarded tenure or tenure-track at any given time. The year that tenure-track slots became available, I was able to apply; however, only three spots were available. When I had to apply, the process had moved to a remote process because of the COVID-19 global pandemic. Before this time, the process was entirely in person, with all documents being submitted as hard copies. Since this was my first time applying for tenure-track, naturally, I had many questions about the process and the detail of content that needed to be submitted with my application and electronic binder that needed to be reviewed. To my surprise, none of my logistical questions could be answered, not even about how the process was implemented previously. I was floored. As the only Black full-time faculty member in the English and developmental English department, I thought to myself, either there is a secret society that no one wants me to be apart of, or we have some work to do with aiding faculty in preparing for success during the promotion and tenure process. I went to my department chair, the same person mentioned in the previous example above [white woman], and inquired more about the process, supports in place to help me navigate, and other colleagues who might be willing to help me understand and navigate the process. She knew nothing, and there was very little help in providing guidance in that moment. Months go by, and I start to figure some things out on my own. Then, at a department meeting, one of my white male colleagues is overwhelmed and wants to know more about what he needs to do to get his materials and application together to apply for one of the tenure-track positions. With excitement, our department chair jumps at the opportunity to help and go out of her way to not only ask around but reach out to some of her close friends who were granted tenure and since retired from the college to come back and answer any questions that [we] might have. Again, I was surprised, and at this point, I should not have been. Over and over, I have been shown that my professional growth, questions, and expertise is less than or valued beneath my white colleagues. Here again, is another example that opened my eyes to some of the persistent inequitable practices. Intentionally or unintentionally, my career as a Black faculty is impacted by how I am not supported in majority-white spaces.

BLACK FACULTY CANNOT DO IT ALONE: WHAT NON-BLACK COLLEAGUES AND ADMINISTRATORS NEED TO KNOW

Here I offer advice to non-Black colleagues and administrators on supporting Black faculty. I have read many pieces that claim to support faculty of color. Still, the recommendations and tips lean more to what Black faculty should do to navigate a space and be okay, as if we are not already exhausted from being Black in higher education. So, this section will be directly addressed to non-Black colleagues and administrators and what they can do to support Black faculty. Below, I provide four tips for non-Black faculty to support Black faculty.

Ask Us [Black Faculty] What We Need

As a Black faculty member, I can honestly say I am not sure I am asked what I need. I am not saying that this doesn't happen. However, I am saying that often non-Black colleagues see that I am doing the job or jobs that need to be done, and they assume that all is well. While most times all is well, there are times when I am not okay (Tomlin, 2022c). So, non-Black colleagues, take the time to genuinely check on Black colleagues and see what is happening in our worlds and how you might collaborate on current or future projects. Showing that you care and are willing to support goes a long way.

Go the Extra Mile, it Matters

I appreciate when my non-Black colleagues show consistency and commitment to supporting me as a colleague. Showing up, authentically, being willing to be an ally, and learning from past events and mistakes allows me to build bonds with non-Black colleagues that foster trust and security. As a Black male faculty member, I always have to "watch my back" and always think that I am the only one who has my best interests at heart, noted from some of the previous examples in this chapter. To this point, when non-Black colleagues show up in ways that show they want to listen, learn, and help, it allows me, as a Black faculty to feel that I have some support in carrying my load in navigating what it means for me to work in academia, which is exhausting. So, non-Black colleagues, please take a moment to go the extra mile to support Black colleagues; it can be the difference between that colleague staying and leaving.

Set Clear Standards for ALL Faculty

Clear expectations, guidelines, policies, and standards should be implemented across and institution an apply to all faculty. However, it is not uncommon to hear from many Black faculty and their experiences of feeling that they have to work a great deal harder than non-Black colleagues to get ahead and be treated equitably (Tomlin, 2022c). When setting clear standards, we must think about work tasks/obligations, requirements for promotion and tenure, and what resources and supports are available to all. Just as I noted for K-12 teachers, structure and detailed manuals and descriptions need to be created to communicate clear expectations (Tomlin, 2021), I argue the same is true for all faculty as well. Additionally, this goes by the handbook or faculty manual. More clear and outlined documents should be created for the different aspects of faculty responsibilities (e.g., community service, college service, department service, teaching excellence, etc.) and how these obligations are directly related to promotion and tenure.

CONCLUSION

Just as the point was made for student affairs and student support staff, the same is true for academic affairs and faculty: working while Black is hard! (Tomlin, 2022a). As Black faculty, we take great pride in our work, profession, and reputation. However, we must also take great pride in our physical and mental health. We must give ourselves permission to say no, lean into enjoying the breaks and time off, and lastly, commit to being more in the moment and present when possible. As faculty in general, we live for the future. We are constantly planning, reviewing, and editing things that will allow our future classes, semesters, and years to improve while also preparing and planning to apply for promotion and tenure cycles. Black faculty have to do all of the mentioned and navigate an environment not set up for their success or pay professional taxes for promotion and tenure (Arnold et. al, 2021). We [Black faculty] must intentionally put ourselves, our mental, and our physical health first. If we don't, then who will? So, protect your space, time, energy, and effort. Lastly, not everything will be black and white. In fact, there is much gray space and area to be explored in higher education. Additionally, the black and white that we oftentimes want so bad, when those colors meet and blend it creates the color gray. So, we must learn not to stress about the gray area or things outside of our control. However, we can learn to plan and find our way through the gray space. Let's stop letting the unknown future stress us out and learn to hold situations more lightly and take it easy.

REFERENCES

Anderson, E. (2022). *Black in White Space: The Enduring Impact of Color in Everyday Life*. University of Chicago Press.

Arnold, N., Osanloo, A. F., & Sherman Newcomb, W. (2021). Paying Professional Taxes for Promotion and Tenure: The Costs of Justice Work for Black Faculty. *Journal of Research on Leadership Education*.

Bhopal, K. (2022). Academics of colour in elite universities in the UK and the USA: The 'unspoken system of exclusion'. *Studies in Higher Education*, 1–11. doi:10.1080/03075079.2021.2020746

Grier-Reed, T., Said, R., & Quiñones, M. (2021). From Antiblackness to Cultural Health in Higher Education. *Education Sciences*, *11*(2), 11. doi:10.3390/educsci11020057

Griffin, K. A., Bennett, J. C., & Harris, J. (2011). Analyzing Gender Differences in Black Faculty Marginalization through a Sequential Mixed-Methods Design. *New Directions for Institutional Research*, *151*(151), 45–61. doi:10.1002/ir.398

Haynes, C., Taylor, L., Mobley, S. D. Jr, & Haywood, J. (2020). Existing and Resisting: The Pedagogical Realities of Black, Critical Men and Women Faculty. *The Journal of Higher Education*, *91*(5), 698–721. doi:10.1080/00221546.2020.1731263

Kanter, R. (1977). Some effects of proportions on group life: Skewed sex ratios and responses to token women. *American Journal of Sociology*, *82*(5), 965–990. doi:10.1086/226425

Manturuk, K., & Reavis, G. (2022). Pedagogical implications of COVID-19: A case study of what faculty learned about teaching well by teaching remotely during the COVID-19 pandemic. In J. S. McKeown, K. Bista, & R. Y. Chan (Eds.), *Global higher education during COVID-19: Policy, society, and technology* (pp. 154–166). STAR Scholars. https://starscholars.org/product/global-education/

Nyunt, G., O'Meara, K., Bach, L., & LaFave, A. (2022). Tenure Undone: Faculty Experiences of Organizational Justice When Tenure Seems or Becomes Unattainable. *Equity & Excellence in Education*, 1–15. doi:10.1080/10665684.2021.2010013

Tomlin, A. D. (2021). *When they see us: Narratives of black male teachers*. Dissertation. University of Maryland.

Tomlin, A. D. (Ed.). (2022a). *Working while black: The untold stories of student affairs practitioners*. Information Age Publishing.

Tomlin, A. D. (2022b, January 12). 4 Strategies to Foster Equity and Inclusion in the Classroom. *Interfolio*. https://www.interfolio.com/resources/blog/four-strategies-to-foster-equity-and-inclusion-in-the-classroom/

Tomlin, A. D. (2022c). I'm a black PhD, and I still have to fight! In A. Allen & J. Stewart (Eds.), *We are not okay: Black faculty experiences & higher education strategies*. Cambridge University Press. doi:10.1017/9781009064668.005

Tomlin, A. D., & Hoey, D. M. (2021). *4 Tips for gaining/progressing in an administrative appointment*. Available online: https://www.interfolio.com/resources/blog/four-tips-for-progressing-in-an-administrative-appointment/

Wagoner, R. L., & Star, H. (2021). Confronting Ourselves: An Autoethnographic Approach to Whiteness in Higher Education. In K. R. Roth & Z. S. Ritter (Eds.), *Whiteness, Power, and Resisting Change in US Higher Education*. Palgrave Studies in Race, Inequality and Social Justice in Education. Palgrave Macmillan. doi:10.1007/978-3-030-57292-1_3

Zambrana, R. E., Valdez, R. B., Pittman, C. T., Bartko, T., Weber, L., & Parra-Medina, D. (2021). Workplace stress and discrimination effects on the physical and depressive symptoms of underrepresented minority faculty. *Stress and Health*, *37*(1), 175–185. doi:10.1002mi.2983 PMID:32926523

Chapter 15
Educare Is Loving Care

Karis LeToi Clarke
https://orcid.org/0000-0002-1014-8338
Clark Atlanta University, USA

Noran L. Moffett
https://orcid.org/0000-0002-3007-9309
Fayetteville State University, USA

Nurah-Talibah N. Moffett
Georgia State University, USA

ABSTRACT

Educators have the best job in the world. They have the responsibility of helping others find their purpose in life. Every profession there is depends on them. Why is it that people with the greatest responsibility tend to not make time to care for themselves? We have often heard you cannot pour from an empty cup. In order for you to be effective and make a difference in the lives of others, you must be certain you are up for the task. The responsibility of helping others achieve their goals sometimes means putting yours on the back burner. This can lead to burnout. Educators must be better to themselves so they can be good to their students.

EDUCARE IS LOVING CARE

Educators have the best job in the world. We have the responsibility of helping others find their purpose in life. Every profession there is depends on us. Why is it that people with the greatest responsibility tend to not make time to care for themselves? I have often heard you cannot pour from an empty cup. In order for you to be effective and make a difference in the lives of others, you must be certain you are up for the task. It is my goal to be the person God created me to me. I wholeheartedly know it is my purpose to support educators. Alas, I will admit there are times when I do not practice what I preach. The

DOI: 10.4018/978-1-6684-2334-9.ch015

responsibility of helping others achieve their goals sometimes means putting yours on the back burner. This can lead to burnout. To not burnout on the work I am so passionate about I am seeking ways to help others like me be better. We must be better to ourselves so we can be good to our students.

Let us get underway by acknowledging the trials of faculty in higher education. One of these challenges is high student to faculty ratios (Blix, Cruise, Mitchell, and Blix, 2016). Research shows that 20% of 265 university faculty members reported exhaustion, with more female faculty members experiencing emotional exhaustion, and men showing higher mean depersonalization (Lackritz, 2015). In another study, faculty members often complained about the many demands placed on their time and the effect and impact on the condition of their teaching, they still stove for excellence (Birkhead, 2020). Furthermore, students have proclaimed that their academic performance is better when they have increased access to faculty (Bryan, Weaver, Anderson-Johnson, & Lindo, 2013), and positive exchanges with their academic and administrative teams (Graunke & Woosley, 2015). Therefore, when faculty try to provide excellent service, in addition to multiple work demands, they increase their risk for burnout. The perception of minimal resources for too many people leads to increased competition and stress (Doughty, 2016). Universities might have traditionally been regarded as low stress academics has indicated that stress is alarmingly widespread and, on the rise, (Levecque, Anseel, De, Van & Gisle, 2017). Stress can be worsened when individuals have to put personal goals on hold to meet higher education goals. While higher education seeks to foster knowledge advancement and human development through research communities, staff often must sacrifice pursuing a family, or achieving other personal goals outside of academia (Mason, Wolfinger, & Goulden, 2013). It is for these reasons self-care must be a priority.

Self-care is a matter of survival as it sustains and fosters good health (Taylor & Renpenning, 2011). It is also an ethic, to ensure that one can function responsibly, especially in relation to others. Ethics is the study of "oughts" and relationships, including how we ought to relate to ourselves, to others, and to the earth (Marino, 2020). It is useful to think of these "oughts" as a code of values to guide an individual's choices and actions, which determine the "purpose and the course" of one's life (Rand, 1964, pp. 188-190). Values are wide-ranging even in a singular context. They project into actions and prompt debate as to what is acceptable conduct, and what is right or wrong. Values in ethics can veer into complex directions when individual confront uncomfortable scenarios, and they have to make tough choices. In higher education teaching and research, ethics mater when individual has to negotiate between their core values and principles, requiring compromise with commonly held beliefs, and the peculiarities of individual situations (Healey et al, 2013). That is a potential cause for personal tension between beliefs and actions. Thattension increases when individuals have to prioritize community values, and academic or professional goals over self-care needs. However, the ethics of care respects the claims of the particular which happens in relationship with others and calls into question, the universalistic and abstract rules of the dominant (Held, 2016). By extension, the ethics of self-care respects the particular, even the personal, sometimes over the universal and dominant. Contrary to popular belief, the personal aspect of self-care is not an indulgent, escapist time to engage in mindless pleasure-seeking (White, 2014).

Self-care is an ethic because it is a social responsibility. It is a duty to care for the self because it allows one to be a responsible citizen (Foucault, 2007). It requires knowing the "self" and knowing rules of acceptable conduct or principles (Foucault, Martin, Gutman, & Hutton, 1998). These principles are not preset values, but an interior life which must be worked out by an individual, to be able to act responsibly. Responsible, ethical self-care begins with facing the inner life and knowing the self. That is the basis for turning to authentic leadership, to frame how individuals in higher education may practice self-care. Authentic leadership emphasizes self-knowledge as essential to ethical leadership of self and others. It can help to foster resilience and balance in higher education.

Some occupations embed self-care within the work ethic. Conscious and purposeful self-care in some human service occupations is an "ethical duty" if professionals are expected to provide good treatment to clients (Willams et al., 2020, p. 322). In that sense, self-care is a way of acting responsibly to others. After all, Irvine (2019, p. 127) asked, "how can we hope to care for others if we, ourselves are crippled by ill health, burnout, or resentment?" Norcross and Barnett (2017) argued that self-care goes beyond the management of such problems and encompasses action to present difficulties from even occurring. Likewise, for professionals and students in higher education, self-care can be seen as a means to preempt stress and challenges. Self-care is a continuous, proactive process for sustaining well-being throughout student life or career development. It requires self-knowledge and strength of effort (Braime, 2016). Authentic leadership offers individuals an ethical way of organizing self-care practices, which can sustain well-being.

As an educator of 16 years, self-care resonates with me because I see it as a way of life. Educators provide service to others. One cannot help someone else unless he or she helps oneself. In my profession, I have found that compassion fatigue and stress can challenge self-care efforts. Further, I recognize that self-care is just as relevant for educators as it is for higher education students. Students' work, assignments, and school demands pose similar stress risks to the professionals in higher education. Self-care is not simply taking a break to treat the self, relax, or grab a moment from busy routines. Self-care is proactive and planned. It requires tremendous discipline for success (Braime, 2016). I would like to share my self-care plan, which I must admit is a work-in-progress that others can adjust to their own situations in higher education. My plan has resulted from reflecting and analyzing that self-care is not reactionary, but intentional.

I fully understand that my self-care plan will not meet the needs of every demographic in higher education. Self-care practices are not generalizable (Braime, 2016). They are personalized actions which are shaped by one's values. Self-care has an experiential component in that it includes reflection and action in conjunction with real world encounters. It requires a kind of "self-critical, self-reflective, self-transformative" attitude to the self, and relationships with others, in a deliberate "way of thinking that is itself a practice, an exercise, or an activity that serves also to guide subsequent action" (Hroch, 2013, p. 5). From that lens, this chapter suggests that self-care is value-driven and action-directed. The dilemma of self-care may be the tension between values and actions which are in conflict, or values which contradict each other. It can also be the tension in meeting higher education professional or academic goals, through actions which may clash with attending to all of one's basic needs. It is my assertion that authentic leadership can help with that tension.

Self-care is the performance or practice of activities that individuals initiate and perform on their own behalf to maintain life, health, and well-being (Denyes, Orem, & Bekel, 2001, p. 249). It requires planning, because it explicitly includes the complex processing of self-awareness and self-regulation, balancing connections between the self and others, balancing connections with the larger community through civic and professional involvement (Baker, 2003). This complex process facilitates holistic wellness. Authentic leadership is a useful theoretical framework for fostering well-being and self-development in higher education, because it attends to self-awareness and self-regulation as a means of promoting and maintaining resilience (Avolio, Gardner, Walumbwa, Luthans, & May, 2014).

Authentic leadership draws upon positive ethical climates and psychological capital such as hope, resilience, self-efficacy, and self-confidence to promote leadership and self-development (Dimovski,

Ferjan, Maric, Uhan, Jovanovic, & Janezic, 2012). Authentic leadership can facilitate self-leadership which is necessary for effective self-care (Clapp-Smith, Vogelgesang, & Avey, 2019). When one adopts an Authentic Leadership framework in one's life, it helps to create balance and avoid burnout (Laschinger, Wong, & Grau, 2013). Research shows the benefits of authentic leadership: a professional reported that authentic leadership helped her to manage guilt about her inability to work longer hours, she ceased comparing herself to co-workers who could work longer, and she prevented burnout by attaining balance between her work and family life (Vitello-Cicciu et al., 2014). A similar study reported that Authentic Leadership assists people through its positive effects on "occupational coping self-efficacy" with job demands, and the development of resilience and practices to protect against burnout and poor mental health (Laschinger, Borgogni, Consiglio, & Read, 2015). Authentic Leadership has also been shown to improve individuals' well-being, job satisfaction, and learning (Bamford, Wong, & Laschinger, 2013).

The Authentic Leadership construct has four dimensions: self-awareness, balanced processing, internalized moral perspective, and relational transparency. Self-awareness in Authentic Leadership refers to the extent to which individuals understand their sense-making of the world, their personal strengths and limitations, and their impact on others (Illies, Morgeson, & Nahrgang, 2015). The individual addresses questions such as: who am I, what are my values, what is my purpose, what drives me, are my actions consistent with what I value, how do others see me, and is this consistent with how I wish to be seen (Shirey, 2015, para. 15).

Self-awareness can inform balanced processing, which is the ability for individuals to analyze data before coming to a decision, with the willingness and openness to seek out views which challenge one's fundamental position (Walumbwa, Avolio, Gardner, Wernsing, & Peterson, 2018). Balanced processing harnesses an internalized moral perspective. An internalized moral perspective refers to an individual's ability to set a high standard for moral and ethical conduct (Avolio et al., 2014). This standard manifests in ethical decisions, behaviors, and interactions with others (Waite, Mckinney, Smith-Glasgow, & Meloy, 2014). Also, this standard comes from the individual's virtues, where intentionality about developing a particular attitude is purposefully strengthened and developed through all interactions (Ciulla & Forsyth, 2021).

An internalized moral perspective helps individuals remain true to their core values. The "authentic" individual acts on personal values and convictions, and by doing what they say they are going to do, they earn respect, trust, and credibility for adhering to their beliefs (Wilson, 2014). When actions are aligned with an internalized moral perspective, then one minimizes the tensions which may exist between actions and values (Gardner, Avolio, & Walumbwa, 2015). These AL principles strengthen relational transparency. Relational transparency is a concept which describes the extent to which an individual can present the true self to others, and by doing so, is open to others being true to themselves (Rego, Sousa, Marques, & Cunha, 2012). Therefore, although authentic leadership addresses individual self-management and wellness, their self-management is in relation to strong connections with other people.

For individuals in Higher Education, these authentic leadership principles can offer ways of managing or aligning higher education duties and responsibilities with one's needs, values, and principles. Authentic leadership can be a strategic approach to ethical self-care in higher education, as authentic leadership places emphasis on knowing and developing the self. This is not an individualistic course of action, but part of ethical relations with others. An authentic leadership outlook encourages individuals to prioritize and schedule necessary activities to care for the self and enhance self-development, so they can be their "best selves" possible and function at an optimal state.

Kutafakari from Swahili means meditation and connotes a care for the self that suggests a practice requiring work, repetition, attention, and effort of body and mind (Hroch, 2013, p. 3). I examined a range of examples of self-care practices and resources for higher education, then engaged in a self-study process (Lassonde, Galman, & Kosnik, 2019) in which the following questions were asked: what is self-care in higher education for me, and how can I practice self-care ethically? My analysis of self-care practices from a range of sources led me to frame these authentic leadership questions:

1. Self-awareness: What is optimum emotional, mental, social, and physical wellness for me?
2. Balanced processing: What are the resources to help me foster and sustain this wellness by incorporating sensible self-care practices into my agenda?
3. Internalized moral perspective: How do these self-car practices harness my core values to help me achieve balance with myself and others?
4. Relational transparency: How can I hold myself accountable to my colleagues, peers, mentees, and mentors in HE; family and friends in my domestic life; wider community?

These questions can be the start of a template for a self-care plan. Such a plan can be part of an orientation package for students or a routine professional development activity for employees in higher education.

The authentic leadership dimensions are aligned to strategic emotional, mental, social, and physical self-care practices (Table 1). The table is a practical application of AL. It highlights some self-care practices which have been helpful my experiences in higher education. Some sections of the plan include practices which are already mastered habits. Good habits should not be omitted from a self-care plan. As part of self-awareness, they can be strengthened, or recognized for their roles in sustaining well-being. Then there are practices which are goals. I recommend filling out a few sections which need the most attention. Guise (2014) is a self-help resource with strategies to transform goals into mini-habits. Mini-habits can eventually become long-lasting, healthy habits. This plan does not specify timelines for executing goals. However, a SMART goal strategy (Lawlor, 2012) can support the inclusion of a time-frame for accomplishing these goals.

Self-awareness is important in all categories of self-care, as individuals need to understand where they stand in order to develop and adhere to an effective self-care plan. Balanced processing is evident in all self-care categories in terms of being mindful of the necessary resources to achieve self-care goals. An internalized moral perspective helps individuals protect the time carved out to practice self-care, in order to achieve maximum results. When individuals hold themselves to ethical standards, they can be true to themselves in their efforts to achieve personal and professional goals for self-care. Relational transparency serves to harness support for these goals. Individuals can identify someone, or a small, trusted team to whom they will be accountable. This fourth dimension of authentic leadership solidifies commitment to self-care goals through the support and trust of others. The following section presents examples of self-care practices which can be part of a comprehensive self-care plan. Just as students plan out their course schedules for the semesters ahead, or instructors and staff plan ways to implement occupational goals for the year, this sampling can help to shape a self-care plan, instead of leaving self-care to chance.

Table 1. Exemplar of an authentic leadership self-care plan for professionals in higher education

Authentic Leadership Elements	Emotional	Mental	Social	Physical
Self-awareness What is optimum wellness for me?	*Reflection*	*Meditation*	*Decluttering calendar events*	*Basic needs: exercise, sleep, medical checkups, sensible nutrition*
Goal **Habit** **Mastery**	*Yes*	*Yes*	*Yes*	*Needs improvement*
Balanced processing What are the resources to help me foster and sustain wellness?	*Spiritual practices*	*Mindfulness family-time*	*Consult a financial planner*	*Sanitation and safe dwelling spaces*
Goal		*Yes*	*Yes*	
Habit				
Mastery	*Yes*			*Yes*
Internalized moral perspective: How do these practices harness by core values to have balance with myself and others?	*Self-empathy*	*Purposeful-allocate a set time for play*	*Resume planning*	*Sports*
Goal		*Needs improvement*	*Yes*	
Habit	*Yes*			*Needs improvement*
Mastery				
Relational transparency How can I hold myself accountable to my others in my life?	*Emotional regulation*	*Generosity-volunteer*	*Network*	*Eco-practices-recycling*
Goal	*Yes*			
Habit		*Needs improvement*		*Needs improvement*
Mastery			*Yes*	

POSSIBLE PATHWAYS TO HOLISTIC SELF-CARE

Emotional Self-Care

Emotional self-care is an approach to wellness which fosters, reinforces, and sustains healthy emotional states for those studying and working in higher education. Higher Education is a center of intellectual work that sometimes excludes emotion and adding emotion to public academic talk can be perceived as a threat to academic enterprise (Neumann, 2016). Furthermore, there are ongoing challenges to emotional composure in terms of stressful interpersonal encounters, and urgent program requirements, in research or evaluations, for instructors and students (Bloch, 2012). Reflection (Miller & McGowen, 2020; Valente & Marotta, 2015; Irvine, 2019), spiritual practices (Baker, 2003; Flarity, Gentry, & Mesnikoff, 2013; Yoder, 2010), emotional regulation (Christou-Champi, Farrow, & Webb, 2015; Koole & Rothermund,

2011), and self-empathy (Robinson et al., 2016; Neff & Pommier, 2013), are some of the ways to manage risks to emotional wellness. Awareness of the emotional states which could sabotage higher education goals and practicing our management of these states, is sound higher education resilience (Woods, 2019). Emotional wellness is about showing kindness to oneself just as one might show care and concern to a friend (Robinson et al., 2016).

Mental Self-Care

Mental self-care practices are vital to combatting stress and burnout that may be associated with higher education (University at Buffalo, 2017). Deficiencies in practicing mental self-care may result in stress, negative self-talk, anxiety, worry, and withdrawal (The Crisis Intervention and Suicide Prevention Centre of BC, 2013). This can occur because higher education has several "important" activities that are competing for time. The decision to make carefully scheduled time to care for the self and put other matters on hold, can also create some mental tension (Tan & Castillo, 2014). Managing this tension requires mental fortitude. It may be a constant inner battle and individuals may feel so overwhelmed that they decide to put more time into completing tasks or meeting the needs of others, rather than being involved in self-care (Fowler, 2015). However, some sensible mental self-care includes practices such as meditation (Pembrook, 2016), mindfulness (Kabat-Zinn, 2015), generosity (Fowler, 2015; Maloney, 2014), and purposeful decision making (Tan & Castillo, 2014; University of Michigan, 2016).

Social Self-Care

Social self-care in higher education is strategic decision-making to ensure that social encounters are meeting one's higher education goals while fostering wellness and managing stress risks. Academic work can be lonely and isolating (Wilshire, 1990). Conversely, the pressure to participate in a range of social activities can be overwhelming, time-consuming, and financially demanding. Time is critical to higher education success (Grove, 2017). Social supports can strengthen the higher education experience (Wilcox, Winn, & Fyvie-Gauld, 2015). Social wellness can include planning one's resume or a professional dossier, much like the teaching dossier (Kenny and Berenson, 2014), legal and financial planning using SMART goals (Lawlor, 2012), or accessing financial supports, time management in terms of networking or social budgeting (Davenport & Scott, 2016), and critical friends (Braun, 2017; Costa & Kallick, 2003). These are just a few of the ways one can work towards academic and professional goals, while maintaining balance and resilience. Volunteering is one of the networking strategies that can strengthen a dossier while providing social engagement. These selected examples of social self-care, or epimeleia heatou, sometimes requires attending to the lessons of a master in terms of support from a trusted guide, counselor, or friend (Foucault, 1997, p. 287).

Physical Self-Care

Higher education poses several risks to physical well-being. Higher education can contribute to sedentary lifestyles, as well as poor nutrition and sleeping habits, for both students and professionals (Buckworth & Nigg 2010; Yang, An, & Zhu, 2016). Physical self-care includes practices such as exercise, sleep, medical checkups, sensible nutrition, responsible sexual habits and substance use, maintenance of sanitary, comfortable dwelling spaces, and protective measures from criminality. These practices tend to lend themselves to primary physiological needs so individuals can find a wealth of traditional, well documented, scientifically supported resources for physical wellness, in most higher education wellness departments. Yet physical wellness can go beyond these traditional principles of wellness. Physical self-care can also include practices which ensure a balanced relationship with the physical, natural environment whether it is in terms of exercising in the outdoors, or seeking outdoor nature spaces for peace and restoration, or even relationships with pets. For others, it can be activism in eco-conscious aspects of their lives. Although more research is needed to better describe relationships between the body in the natural environment and how environmental awareness becomes embodied (Humberstone, 2013), individuals who make environmentally friendly choices in various aspects of their daily lives, often articulate their decisions (eating, travelling, etc.), in terms of how these decisions impact their lives and the environment (Hroch, 2013). This aspect of physical wellness is increasingly making its way in traditional guidelines for meeting physiological needs for wellness, however, ordinary practices which are considered "environmentally-friendly" ways of eating, managing waste, using energy, or traveling are complex (Hroch, 2013). They raise the intersections of ethical self-care and eco-ethics (Gasper, 2014). This is an area of research, which the academic literature does not represent fully, but it is worth exploring beyond this article, as a facet of physical wellness.

CONCLUSION

This chapter was guided by a critical-reflective approach to the literature. The author sought to address self-care in higher education, and the ways in which faculty can practice self-care ethically. I was drawn to the tension between self-care and higher education goals for academics. I came to realize that a self-care plan is not a self-indulgent course of activities; an excuse to avoid responsibilities and miss deadlines; a justification for inappropriate workplace behaviors; a self-isolating activity; or a dabble with fashionable self-help trends without a commitment to one's needs. A self-care plan is hard work. Considering the level of discipline required to make self-care work, some individuals may find it difficult to practice care of the self while pursuing academic or career goals in higher education. Through a review of authentic leadership to practice self-care, I realized that higher education goals and self-care goals do not need to stand in opposition. They can and should co-exist, to strengthen and support each other.

It is my recommendation to view authentic leadership as a series of principles to guide imperative self-care. Authentic leadership reiterates the ethics of self-care. Authentic leadership shows that responsible, ethical self-care begins with knowing the self, practicing the self, and becoming the self. Self-care is an ethic. It is a duty, a necessity, and a responsibility to well-being. Higher education has a range of risks, which can lead to attrition or illness. Proactively practicing self-care can manage and preempt these risks. The ethics of self-care, inherently means that the sense of duty to self, is a way of being dutiful to others. Self-care occurs in relation to others, and so do the implications of ill health, poor finances, and emotional suffering, especially to our loved ones.

Emotional, mental, social, and physical self-care can help individuals maintain wellness. Considering a spectrum of wellness, reacting, injury, and illness, higher education students and professionals need to practice self-care so as not to descend into attrition or illness. Self-care, as an ethic, "ought" to be a priority for basic survival and resilience while students and professionals pursue their higher education goals. Self-care allows individuals to align their inner core values to be their best selves, thriving in balance and harmony, peace, and joy.

SUMMARY RECOMMENDATIONS

The revolutionary need for educators to embrace the foundations of self-care should be promoted for those who seek doctoral degrees at the state of admission to the program of study to avoid the dissertation syndrome (Moffett et al., 2018). Furthermore, the recommendations cited by Johnson-Arnold for self-car of doctoral professionals should be considered by programs of study from admissions to completion of the program of study. Additionally, the research study on doctoral candidates seeking leadership degrees on the suggested eight dimensions of self-care should be institutionalized in P-12 and Higher Education to support the preparation of educational leaders at the master's and the doctoral levels. For example, the movement into leadership roles should include some inventory of the HELP Model developed by Moffett and Johnson-Arnold in the award-winning dissertation (Johnson-Arnold, 2020). For example, this study used a mixed-methods research design inclusive of the following findings:

Findings suggested that students have experienced a decline in health since beginning coursework due to challenges associated with the additional demands of graduate studies, and participants believe institutions are not demonstrating a commitment to the health and wellness of graduate students.

Consequently, it is highly improbable to suggest the self-care or educare in educational settings can emphatically occur with n unhealthy leader and unhealthy administration. Most emphatically, it is unlikely that the care of educators and others in the environment can be systematically and fundamentally assured without an inventory of the type of personality characteristics and internal and external self-care inventory of the leadership in the organization.

REFERENCES

Avolio, B. J., Gardner, W. L., Walumbwa, F. O., Luthans, F., & May, D. R. (2014). Unlocking the mask: A look at the process by which authentic leaders impact follower attitudes and behaviors. *The Leadership Quarterly*, *15*(6), 801–823. doi:10.1016/j.leaqua.2004.09.003

Baker, E. K. (2003). *Taking care of ourselves: A therapist's guide to personal and professional well-being*. American Psychological Association. doi:10.1037/10482-000

Bamford, M., Wong, C. A., & Laschinger, H. (2013). The influence of authentic leadership and areas of work life on work engagement of registered nurses. *Journal of Nursing Management*, *21*(3), 529–540. doi:10.1111/j.1365-2834.2012.01399.x PMID:23406200

Birkhead, T. (2020). *I feel like a marked man*. Retrieved from https://www.caut.ca/bulletin/articles/2020/04/i-feel-like-a-marked-man

Blix, A. G., Cruise, R. J., Mitchell, B. N., & Blix, G. G. (2016). Occupational stress among university teachers. *Educational Research*, *36*(2), 157–169. doi:10.1080/0013188940360205

Bloch, C. (2016). *Passion and paranoia: Emotions and the culture of emotion in academia*. Routledge. doi:10.4324/9781315599618

Braime, H. (2016). *From coping to thriving: How to turn self-care into a way of life*. Create Space Independent Publishing Platform.

Braun, R. (2017). *Critical friends in self-studies* [Blog post]. The Research Associate (RA) Notebooks. Retrieved from http://tirap.ucal-garyblogs.ca/2017/01/28/critical-friends-in-self-studies

Bryan, V., Weaver, S., Anderson-Johnson, P., & Lindo, J. (2013). The effect of interpersonal relationships between nursing students and lecturers on learning outcomes at a Jamaican nursing school. *Caribbean Journal of Nursing, 1*(1), 41-48. Retrieved from http://ojs.mona.uwi.edu/index.php/cjn/article/view/3690/3218

Buckworth, J. P. D., & Nigg, C. P. D. (2004). Physical activity, exercise, and sedentary behavior in college students. *Journal of American College Health, 53*(1), 28–34. doi:10.3200/JACH.53.1.28-34 PMID:15266727

Christou-Champi, S., Farrow, T. F., & Webb, T. L. (2015). Automatic control of negative emotions: Evidence that structured practice increases the efficiency of emotion regulation. *Cognition and Emotion, 29*(2), 319–331. doi:10.1080/02699931.2014.901213 PMID:24678930

Ciulla, J. B., & Forsyth, D. R. (2021). Leadership ethics. In A. Bryman, D. Collinson, K. Grint, B. Jackson, & M. Uhl-Bien (Eds.), *The Sage Handbook of Leadership* (pp. 352–364). Sage.

Clapp-Smith, R., Vogelgesang, G. R., & Avey, J. B. (2019). Authentic leadership and positive psychological capital: The mediating role of trust at the group level of analysis. *Journal of Leadership & Organizational Studies, 15*(3), 227–240. doi:10.1177/1548051808326596

Costa, A. L., & Kallick, B. (2003). Through the lens of a critical friend. *Educational Leadership, 51*(2), 49–51.

Davenport, B., & Scott, S. J. (2016). *Declutter your mind: How to stop worrying, relieve anxiety, and eliminate negative thinking*. Oldtown Publishing LLC.

Denyes, M. J., Orem, D. E., & Bekel, G. (2001). Self-Care: A Foundational Science. *Nursing Science Quarterly, 14*(1), 48–54. doi:10.1177/089431840101400113 PMID:11873354

Dimovski, V., Ferjan, M., Maric, M., Uhan, M., Jovanovic, M., & Janezic, M. (2012). Authentic leadership to the future. *Skola Biznisa, 1*(1), 1–14. doi:10.5937kolbiz1201001D

Doughty, H. A. (2016). *Book review/The slow professor.* Retrieved from https://www.caut.cabulletin/articles/2016/09/the-slow-professor.

Flarity, K., Gentry, J. E., & Mesnikoff, N. (2013). The effectiveness of an educational program on preventing and treating compassion fatigue in emergency nurses. *Advanced Emergency Nursing Journal, 35*(3), 247–258. doi:10.1097/TME.0b013e31829b726f PMID:23899949

Foucault, M., Martin, L. H., Gutman, H., & Hutton, P. H. (1997). *Technologies of the self: A seminar with Michel Foucault*. University of Massachusetts Press.

Foucault, M., & Rabinow, P. (2007). *Ethics: Subjectivity and truth.* New Press.

Fowler, M. (2015). Dealing with compassion fatigue. When children hurt, we hurt too. And this can wear us out. *NJEA Review, 88*, 32–35.

Gardner, W. L., Avolio, B. J., & Walumbwa, F. O. (2005). *Authentic leadership theory and practice: Origins, effects and development*. Elsevier.

Gasper, D. (2014). Future global ethics: Environmental change, embedded ethics, evolving human identity. *Journal of Global Ethics*, *10*(2), 135–145. doi:10.1080/17449626.2014.933442

Graunke, S. S., & Woosley, S. A. (2005). An exploration of the factors that affect the academic success of college sophomores. *College Student Journal*, *39*(2), 367–376.

Grove, J. (2017). The teaching survey 2017: results and analysis. *Times Higher Education*. Retrieved from https://www.timeshighereducation.com/features/the-teaching-survey-2017-results-and-analysis

Guise, S. (2014). *Mini habits: Smaller habits, bigger results*. Kindle E. Book.

Healey, R. L., Bass, T., Caulfield, J., Hoffman, A., McGinn, M. K., Miller-Young, J., & Haigh, M. (2013). Being ethically minded: Practicing the scholarship of teaching and learning in an ethical manner. *Teaching & Learning Inquiry: The Issotl Journal*, *1*(2), 23–32. doi:10.20343/teachlearninqu.1.2.23

Held, V. (2016). *The ethics of care: Personal, political, and global*. Oxford University Press.

Hroch, P. (2013). Encountering the "ecopolis" Foucault's epimeleia heautou and environmental relations. *ETopia online initiative of TOPIA: Canadian Journal of Cultural Studies*. Retrieved from https://etopia.journals.yorku.ca/index.php/etopia/article/view/36563/33222

Humberstone, B. (2013). Adventurous activities, embodiment and nature: Spiritual, sensual and Sustainable? Embodying environmental justice. *Motriz*, *19*(3), 565–571. doi:10.1590/S1980-65742013000300006

Ilies, R., Morgeson, F. P., & Nahrgang, J. D. (2015). Authentic leadership and eudaemonic well-being: Understanding leader-follower outcomes. *The Leadership Quarterly*, *16*(3), 373–394. doi:10.1016/j.leaqua.2005.03.002

Irvine, C. (2019). The ethics of self-care. In T. R. Cole, T. J. Goodrich, & E. R. Gritz (Eds.), *Faculty health in academic medicine: physicians, scientists, and the pressures of success* (pp. 127–146). Humana Press.

Johnson-Arnold, L. P. (2020). Practicing Holistic Health and Self-Care Throughout the Dissertation Journey: Practical Applications and Self-Reflections for Doctoral Students. In *Creating a Framework for Dissertation Preparation: Emerging Research and Opportunities* (pp. 1-22). IGI Global. doi:10.4018/978-1-5225-9707-0.ch001

Johnson-Arnold, L.P. (2020). *Self-Care Practices and Perceptions of Holistic Health Among Selected Educational Leadership Graduate Students Attending Historically Black Colleges and Universities of Minority Serving Institutions*. Academic Press.

Kabat-Zinn, J. (2015). *Wherever you go, there you are: mindfulness meditation in everyday life*. Hachette Books.

Kenny, N., & Berenson, K. (2014). *Creating a teaching dossier*. Taylor Institute for Teaching and Learning Educational Development Unit. Retrieved from http://ucalgary.ca/taylorinstitute/edu/sites/default/files/Teaching%20Dossier%20Handout_0.pdf

Koole, S. L., & Rothermund, K. (2011). "I feel better but I don't know why" The psychology of implicit emotion regulation. *Cognition and Emotion, 25*(3), 389–399. doi:10.1080/02699931.2010.550505 PMID:21432681

Lackritz, J. R. (2015). Exploring burnout among university faculty: Incidence, performance, and demographic issues. *Teaching and Teacher Education, 20*(7), 713–729. doi:10.1016/j.tate.2004.07.002

Laschinger, H. K., Borgogni, L., Consiglio, C., & Read, E. (2015). The effects of authentic leadership, six areas of worklife, and occupational coping self-efficacy on new graduate nurses' burnout and mental health: A cross-sectional study. *International Journal of Nursing Studies, 52*(6), 1080–1089. doi:10.1016/j.ijnurstu.2015.03.002 PMID:25801311

Laschinger, H. K., Wong, C. A., & Grau, A. L. (2013). Authentic leadership, empowerment and burnout: A comparison in new graduates and experienced nurses. *Journal of Nursing Management, 21*(3), 541–552. doi:10.1111/j.1365-2834.2012.01375.x PMID:23405976

Lassonde, C. A., Galman, S., & Kosnik, C. M. (2019). *Self-study research methodologies for teacher educators*. Sense Publishers.

Lawlor, K. B. (2012). Smart goals: How the application of smart goals can contribute to achievement of student learning outcomes. *Developments in Business Simulation and Experiential Learning, 39*, 259–267.

Levecque, K., Anseel, F., De, B. A., Van, H. J., & Gisle, L. (2017). Work organization and mental health problems in PhD students. *Research Policy, 46*(4), 868–879. doi:10.1016/j.respol.2017.02.008

Maloney, J. V. (2014). Nursing and philanthropy. *Nursing Administration Quarterly, 38*(4), 280–282. doi:10.1097/NAQ.0000000000000052 PMID:25208143

Marino, G. D. (2020). *Ethics: The essential writings*. Modern Library.

Mason, M. A., Wolfinger, N. H., & Goulden, M. (2013). *Do babies matter? Gender and family in the ivory tower*. Rutgers University Press.

Miller, M. N., & McGowen, R. (2020). Strategies to avoid burnout in professional practice: Some practical suggestions. *The Psychiatric Times, 27*(2), 25–25.

Neff, K. D., & Pommier, E. (2013). The relationship between self-compassion and other-focused concern among college undergraduates, community adults, and practicing meditators. *Self and Identity, 12*(2), 160–176. doi:10.1080/15298868.2011.649546

Neumann, A. (2016). Professing passion: Emotion in the scholarship of professors at research universities. *American Educational Research Journal, 43*(3), 381-421. Retrieved January from https://www.jstor.org/stable/4121764

Norcross, J. C., & Barnett, J. E. (2017). *Self-care as ethical imperative. The Register Report: Spring 2008*. The Guilford Press.

Pembroke, N. (2016). Contributions from Christian ethics and Buddhist philosophy to the management of compassion fatigue in nurses. *Nursing & Health Sciences, 18*(1), 120–124. doi:10.1111/nhs.12252 PMID:26694199

Rand, A., & Branden, N. (1970). *The virtue of selfishness: A new concept of egoism.* Signet/New American Library.

Rego, A., Sousa, F., Marques, C., & Cunha, M. (2012). Authentic leadership promoting employees' psychological capital and creativity. *Journal of Business Research, 65*(3), 429–437. doi:10.1016/j.jbusres.2011.10.003

Robinson, K. J., Mayer, S., Allen, A. B., Terry, M., Chilton, A., & Leary, M. R. (2016). Resisting self-compassion: Why are some people opposed to being kind to themselves? *Self and Identity, 15*(5), 505–524. doi:10.1080/15298868.2016.1160952

Shirey, M. R. (2015). Enhance your self-awareness to be an authentic leader. *American Nurse Today, 10*(8). http://www.americannursetoday.com/enhance-self-awareness-authentic-leader/

Tan, S. Y., & Castillo, M. (2014). Self-care and beyond: A brief literature review from a Christian perspective. *Journal of Psychology and Christianity, 33*(1), 90–95.

Taylor, S. G., & Renpenning, K. M. (2021). *Self-care science, nursing theory, and evidence-based practice.* Retrieved from http://lghttp.48653.nexcesscdn.net/80223CF/springer-

The Crisis Intervention and Suicide Prevention Centre of BC. (2013). *Coping & self-care.* Retrieved from https://crisiscentre.bc.ca/coping-and-self-care/

University at Buffalo. (2017). *Introduction to self-care.* Retrieved from https://socialwork.buffalo.edu/resources/self-care-starter-kit/introduction-to-self-care.htm

University of Michigan. (2017). *Ten things you can do for your mental health* Retrieved from https://www.uhs.umich.edu/tenthings

Valente, V., & Marotta, A. (2015). The impact of yoga on the professional and personal life of the psychotherapist. *Contemporary Family Therapy, 27*(1), 65–80. doi:10.100710591- 004-1971-4

Vitello-Cicciu, J. M., Weatherford, B., Gemme, D., Glass, B., & Seymour-Route, P. (2014). The effectiveness of a leadership development program on self-awareness in practice. *The Journal of Nursing Administration, 44*(3), 170–174. doi:10.1097/nna.0000000000000046

Waite, R., Mckinney, N., Smith-Glasgow, M., & Meloy, F. (2014). The embodiment of authentic leadership. *Journal of Professional Nursing, 30*(4), 282–291. doi:10.1016/j.profnurs.2013.11.004

Walumbwa, F. O., Avolio, B. J., Gardner, W. L., Wernsing, T. S., & Peterson, S. J. (2018). Authentic leadership: Development and validation of a theory-based measure. *Journal of Management, 34*(1), 89–126. doi:10.1177/0149206307308913

White, R. (2014). Foucault on the care of the self as an ethical project and a spiritual goal. *Human Studies: A Journal for Philosophy and the Social Sciences, 37*(4), 489-504. doi:10.1007/s10746-014-9331-3

Wilcox, P., Winn, S., & Fyvie-Gauld, M. (2015). 'It was noting to do with the university, it was just the people': The role of social support in the first-year experience of higher education. *Studies in Higher Education, 30*(6), 707–722.

Williams, I. D., Richardson, T. A., Moore, D. D., Gambrel, L. E., & Keeling, M. L. (2020). Perspectives on self-care. *Journal of Creativity in Mental Health*, *5*(3), 320–338. doi:10.1080/15401383.2010.507700

Wilshire, B. W. (1990). *The moral collapse of the university: Professionalism, purity, and alienation.* State University of New York Press.

Wilson, M. (2014). Critical reflection on authentic leadership and school leader development from a virtue ethical perspective. *Educational Review*, *66*(4), 482–496. doi:10.1080/00131911.2013.812062

Woods, C. (2019). Employee wellbeing in the higher education workplace: A role for emotion scholarship. *Higher Education*, *60*(2), 171–185. doi:10.100710734-009-9293-y

Yoder, E. A. (2010). Compassion fatigue in nurses. *Applied Nursing Research*, *23*(4), 191–197. doi:10.1016/j.apnr.2008.09.003

Compilation of References

Abbas, A., Dian, E., & Suhariadi, F. (2022). Social Perspective: Leadership in Changing Society. In M. I. Hassan, S. S. Roy, U. Chatterjee, S. Chakraborty, & U. Singh (Eds.), *Social Morphology, Human Welfare and Sustainability*. Springer.

Abbas, A., Ekowati, D., & Suhariadi, F. (2021a). Individual psychological distance: A leadership task to assess and cope with invisible change. *Journal of Management Development*, *40*(3), 168–189. doi:10.1108/JMD-09-2020-0304

Abbas, A., Ekowati, D., & Suhariadi, F. (2021b). Managing Individuals, Organizations Through Leadership: Diversity Consciousness Roadmap. In B. Christiansen & H. Chandan (Eds.), *Handbook of Research on Applied Social Psychology in Multiculturalism* (Vol. 1, pp. 47–71). IGI Global. doi:10.4018/978-1-7998-6960-3.ch003

Abbas, A., Ekowati, D., Usman, I., Saud, M., & Setia, S. (2020). Technology and stress: A proposed framework for coping stress in Indonesia higher education: Technology in Education. *International Journal of Innovation. Creativity and Change*, *13*(4), 373–390.

Abbas, A., Eliyana, A., Ekowati, D., Saud, M., Raza, A., & Wardani, R. (2020). Data set on coping strategies in the digital age: The role of psychological well-being and social capital among university students in Java Timor, Surabaya, Indonesia. *Data in Brief*, *30*, 10558. doi:10.1016/j.dib.2020.105583 PMID:32368599

Abbas, A., Saud, M., Ekowati, D., & Suhariadi, F. (2021). Social Psychology and Fabrication: A Synthesis of Individuals, Society, and Organization. In B. Christiansen & H. Chandan (Eds.), *Handbook of Research on Applied Social Psychology in Multiculturalism* (Vol. 1, pp. 89–109). IGI Global. doi:10.4018/978-1-7998-6960-3.ch005

Abbas, A., Saud, M., Ekowati, D., Usman, I., & Suhariadi, F. (2021). Servant leadership: A strategic choice for organisational performance. An empirical discussion from Pakistan. *International Journal of Productivity and Quality Management*, *34*(4), 468–485. doi:10.1504/IJPQM.2021.120599

Abbas, A., Saud, M., Suhariadi, F., Usman, I., & Ekowati, D. (2020). Positive leadership psychology: Authentic and servant leadership in higher education in Pakistan. *Current Psychology (New Brunswick, N.J.)*, •••, 1–11. doi:10.100712144-020-01051-1

Abdel Latif, M. M. (2022). Coping with COVID-19-related online English teaching challenges: Teacher educators' suggestions. *ELT Journal*, *76*(1), 20–33. doi:10.1093/elt/ccab074

Abdullah, N. H., Ismail, N., & Ismail, N. (2021). A Study of the Work-Life Balance among the Female Academics at Polytechnics. *BITARA International Journal of Civilizational Studies and Human Sciences*, *4*(1), 130–145.

Abrahams, Z. (2019). *The future of remote work: When it's done right, telework can improve employee productivity, creativity and morale, psychologists' research finds*. American Psychological Association. https://www.apa.org/monitor/2019/10/cover-remote-work

Abrell, T. (2020, September 12). A year-round guide to self-advocacy. *Forbes.* https://www.forbes.com/sites/ellevate/2020/10/01/a-year-round-guide-to-self-advocacy/

Abu Bakar, M. R., Norazmi, N. A., & Ahmad, M. M. (2020). Level of Job Stress, Job Satisfaction and Organizational Commitment amongst Polytechnic Tuanku Syed Sirajuddin Lecturers. *Jurnal Dunia Pengurusan, 2*(3), 94–100.

Ackerley, G. D., Burnell, J., Holder, D. C., & Kurdek, L. A. (1988). Burnout among licensed psychologists. *Professional Psychology, Research and Practice, 19*(6), 624–631. doi:10.1037/0735-7028.19.6.624

Ackerman, D. (1999). *Deep play.* Random House.

Ackerman, D., & Gross, B. (2007). I can start that JME manuscript next week, can't I? The task characteristics behind why faculty procrastinate. *Journal of Marketing Education, 29*(2), 97–110. doi:10.1177/0273475307302012

Administration for Children & Families. (n.d.). *Secondary traumatic stress.* https://www.acf.hhs.gov/trauma-toolkit/secondary-traumatic-stress

Ahmed, S., Farooqi, M. T. K., & Iqbal, A. (2020). Influence of organizational politics on university teachers' performance. *Global Social Sciences Review, 5*(2), 341–355. doi:10.31703/gssr.2020(V-II).33

Albulescu, I., & Albulescu, M.University's Contribution to Local and Regional Development by Providing Educational Services for Adults. (2014). The University in the Community. The University's Contribution to Local and Regional Development by Providing Educational Services for Adults. *Procedia: Social and Behavioral Sciences, 142*, 5–11. doi:10.1016/j.sbspro.2014.07.578

Alderton, M. (2021, July 31). *Teachers are feeling burned out. artificial intelligence can help.* Retrieved from https://www.usatoday.com/story/life/2021/07/31/education-can-enhanced-through-technology-like-ai/7939422002/

Alexander-Albritton, C., & Hill, N. R. (2015). Familial and institutional factors: Job satisfaction for female counselor educators. *Counselor Education and Supervision, 54*(2), 109–121. doi:10.1002/ceas.12008

Alli, B. (2008). *Fundamental Principles of Occupational Health and Safety.* International Labour Organziation.

Allies, S. (2020). *Supporting Teacher Wellbeing: A Practical Guide for Primary Teachers and School Leaders.* Routledge. doi:10.4324/9780429330698

American Association of University Professors. (2001). *Statement of principles on family responsibilities and academic work.* https://www.aaup.org/file/Family_and_Academic_Work.pdf

American Psychiatric Association. (1980). *Diagnostic and statistical manual of mental disorders* (3rd ed.). Author.

Amitai, A., Vervaet, R., & Houtte, M. V. (2020). When teachers experience burnout: Does a multi-ethnic student population put out or spark teachers' fire? *Pedagogische Studiën*, (97), 125–145.

Anderson, D., Cameron-Standerford, A., Bergh, B., & Bohjanen, S. (2019). Teacher evaluation and its impact on wellbeing: Perceptions of Michigan teachers and administrators. *Education, 139*(3), 139–150.

Anderson, E. (2022). *Black in White Space: The Enduring Impact of Color in Everyday Life.* University of Chicago Press.

Apple, M. W. (2012). Rethinking Education, Rethinking Culture, Rethinking Media: Rethinking Popular Culture and Media, edited by Elizabeth Marshall & Ozlem Sensoy (Milwaukee: Rethinking Schools, 2011). Educational Policy, 26(2), 339–346. doi:10.1177/0895904811417593

Ardalan, G. (2017). Spreading happiness: A preschool classroom in Washington, DC, investigates citizenship and makes a statement—"Be Happy! *YC Young Children, 72*(2), 64–71.

Arnett, J. J. (2000). Emerging adulthood: A theory of development from the late teens through the twenties. *The American Psychologist, 55*(5), 469–480. doi:10.1037/0003-066X.55.5.469 PMID:10842426

Arnold, N., Osanloo, A. F., & Sherman Newcomb, W. (2021). Paying Professional Taxes for Promotion and Tenure: The Costs of Justice Work for Black Faculty. *Journal of Research on Leadership Education.*

Arnold, M. B. (1960). *Emotion and personality*. Columbia University Press.

Asociación de Fabricantes de Medicamentos de Libre Acceso AFAMELA. (2017). *The economics of self-care in Mexico*. https://www.selfcarefederation.org/resources/value-otc-self-care-mexico

Aust, B., & Ducki, A. (2004). Comprehensive health promotion interventions at the workplace: Experiences with health circles in Germany. *Journal of Occupational Health Psychology, 9*(3), 258–270. doi:10.1037/1076-8998.9.3.258 PMID:15279520

Avolio, B.J., & Gardner, W.L. (2005). Authentic leadership development: getting to the root of positive forms of leadership. *The Leadership Quarterly, 16*(3), 315-338.

Avolio, B. J., Gardner, W. L., Walumbwa, F. O., Luthans, F., & May, D. R. (2014). Unlocking the mask: A look at the process by which authentic leaders impact follower attitudes and behaviors. *The Leadership Quarterly, 15*(6), 801–823. doi:10.1016/j.leaqua.2004.09.003

Aziz, A. R. A. (2014). *Happiness Sustainable among Lecturers at the Malaysian Research University. Universiti Teknologi Malaysia*. Skudai. doi:10.1016/j.sbspro.2014.01.918

Azman & Kutty. (2016). Imposing global university rankings on local academic culture. In The global academic rankings game. New York: Routledge Taylor & Francis Group.

Azreen, H.A., Norudin, M., & Zuraida, M. (2016). Impak Beban Kerja Terhadap Prestasi Kerja Pensyarah: Kes Kajian Di Politeknik Sultan Mizan Zainal Abidin (Psmza). *e-Academia Journal UiTMT, 5*(1), 1-12.

Bachman, J. G., & Schulenberg, J. (1993). How part-time work intensity relates to drug use, problem behavior, time use, and satisfaction among high school seniors: Are these consequences or merely correlates? *Developmental Psychology, 29*(2), 220–235. doi:10.1037/0012-1649.29.2.220

Badakar, C. M., Thakkar, P. J., Hugar, S. M., Kukreja, P., Assudani, H. G., & Gokhale, N. (2017). Evaluation of the relevance of Piaget's cognitive principles among parented and orphan children in Belagavi City, Karnataka, India: A comparative study. *International Journal of Clinical Pediatric Dentistry, 10*(4), 346–350. doi:10.5005/jp-journals-10005-1463 PMID:29403227

Baker, R., & Ibrahim, H. I. (2014). Work Stress in Police Organizations: A Review in the perspective of emotional intelligence. *Journal of the Humanities*, (23), 1–24.

Baker, E. (2003). *Caring for ourselves: A therapist's guide to personal and professional well-being*. American Psychological Association. doi:10.1037/10482-000

Bakker, A. B., Schaufeli, W. B., Leiter, M. P., & Taris, T. W. (2008). Work engagement: An emerging concept in occupational health psychology. *Work and Stress, 22*(3), 187–200. doi:10.1080/02678370802393649

Balch, J. F., & Balch, P. A. (1997). *Prescription for nutritional healing*. Avery Publishing Group.

Bamford, M., Wong, C. A., & Laschinger, H. (2013). The influence of authentic leadership and areas of work life on work engagement of registered nurses. *Journal of Nursing Management, 21*(3), 529–540. doi:10.1111/j.1365-2834.2012.01399.x PMID:23406200

Bamonti, P. M., Keelan, C. M., Larson, N., Mentrikoski, J. M., Randall, C. L., Sly, S. K., Travers, R. M., & McNeil, D. W. (2014). Promoting ethical behavior by cultivating a culture of self-care during graduate training: A call to action. *Training and Education in Professional Psychology*, *8*(4), 253 - 260. doi:10.1037/tep0000056

Bani Hidayat Mohd Shafie. (2020). Pelaksanaan PdPc Dalam Talian (OLL) Semasa Perintah Kawalan Pergerakan (PKP) Fasa 1 Dan 2 Covid-19. *Jurnal Dunia Pendidikan*, *2*(2), 213-221. doi:10.1287/orsc.2018.1235

Barile, N. (n.d.). Beyond the classroom. *Exercise and the brain: How fitness impacts learning*. https://www.wgu.edu/heyteach/article/exercise-and-brain-how-fitness-impacts-learning1801.html

Barnett, J., & N. Cooper. (2009). Creating a culture of selfcare. *Clinical Psychology: Science and Practice*, *16*(1), 16 – 20. . doi:10.1111/j.1468-2850.2009.01138.x

Barni, D., Danioni, F., & Benevene, P. (2019). Teachers' self-efficacy: The role of personal values and motivations for teaching. *Frontiers in Psychology*, *10*, 1645. Advance online publication. doi:10.3389/fpsyg.2019.01645 PMID:31354604

Batson, C. D., Fultz, J., & Schoenrade, P. A. (1987). Distress and empathy: Two qualitatively distinct vicarious emotions with different motivational consequences. *Journal of Personality*, *55*(1), 19–39. doi:10.1111/j.1467-6494.1987.tb00426.x PMID:3572705

Bayer Consumer Health. (2018). *Self-care. Better daily health for individuals and societies. A global policy blueprint*. https://www.bayer.com/sites/default/files/2020-04/self-care-policy-paper-2018-08-16.pdf

Becker, G. S. (1993). *Human capital: A theoretical and empirical analysis, with special reference to education* (3rd ed.). University of Chicago press. doi:10.7208/chicago/9780226041223.001.0001

Beddow, K. (2019, July 21). *Spilling coffee*. Calmer Classrooms. https://www.calmerclassrooms.co.uk/coffee/

Beltman, S., Mansfield, C., & Price, A. (2011). Thriving not just surviving: A review of research on teacher resilience. *Educational Research Review*, *6*(3), 185 – 207. doi:10.1016/j.edurev.2011.09.001

Benson, H. (1999). Power and biology of belief. Presented at the *annual convention of the American Psychological Association*, Boston, MA.

Benson-Henry Institute for Mind Body Medicine. (2010). *Eliciting the relaxation response*. Academic Press.

Berbiglia, V. A., & Banfield, B. (2013). Self-care deficit theory of nursing. *Nursing Theorists and Their Work-E-Book*, *30*(1), 240.

Bergdahl, N., & Nouri, J. (2021). Covid-19 and crisis-prompted distance education in Sweden. *Tech Know Learn*, *26*(3), 443–459. doi:10.100710758-020-09470-6

Berson, Y. & Oreg, S. (2016). The role of school principals in shaping children's values. *Psychological Science*, *27*(12), 1539 – 1549.

Bhaskaran, R. P. (2017). Language complexity and Multilingual education in India – a Policy Perspective1. *Issues and Ideas in Education*, *5*(2), 199–214. doi:10.15415/iie.2017.52013

Bhopal, K. (2022). Academics of colour in elite universities in the UK and the USA: The 'unspoken system of exclusion'. *Studies in Higher Education*, 1–11. doi:10.1080/03075079.2021.2020746

Birkhead, T. (2020). *I feel like a marked man*. Retrieved from https://www.caut.ca/bulletin/articles/2020/04/i-feel-like-a-marked-man

Birren, J. E., & Cunningham, W. R. (1985). Research on the psychology of aging: Principles, concepts and theory. In The handbooks of aging. Handbook of the psychology of aging. Van Nostrand Reinhold Co.

Bisaillon, L., & Eakin, J. (2014, November 12). *Strategies for understanding and navigating the "academic underlife."* University Affairs. https://www.universityaffairs.ca/career-advice/career-advice-article/strategies-understanding-navigating-academic-underlife/

Blaschka, A. (2020). This Is The Best Way To Avoid COVID Burnout. *Forbes*. https://www.forbes.com/sites/amyblaschka/2020/07/30/this-is-the-best-way-to-avoid-covid-burnout/?sh=35e055a0509d

Blix, A. G., Cruise, R. J., Mitchell, B. N., & Blix, G. G. (2016). Occupational stress among university teachers. *Educational Research, 36*(2), 157–169. doi:10.1080/0013188940360205

Bloch, C. (2016). *Passion and paranoia: Emotions and the culture of emotion in academia*. Routledge. doi:10.4324/9781315599618

Boice, K. L., Jackson, J. R., Alemdar, M., Rao, A. E., Grossman, S., & Usselman, M. (2021). Supporting teachers on their STEAM journey: A collaborative STEAM teacher training program. *Education Sciences, 11*(3), 105. doi:10.3390/educsci11030105

Bondanini, G., Giorgi, G., Ariza-Montes, A., Vega-Muñoz, A., & Andreucci-Annunziata, P. (2020). Technostress dark side of technology in the workplace: A scientometric analysis. *International Journal of Environmental Research and Public Health, 17*(21), 8013. doi:10.3390/ijerph17218013 PMID:33143270

Bone, K. D. (2015). The bioecological model: Applications in holistic workplace well-being management. *International Journal of Workplace Health Management, 8*(4), 256–271. doi:10.1108/IJWHM-04-2014-0010

Borders, L. D., Young, J. S., Wester, K. L., Murray, C. E., Villalba, J. A., Lewis, T. F., & Mobley, A. K. (2011). Mentoring promotion/tenure-seeking faculty: Principles of good practice within a counselor education program. *Counselor Education and Supervision, 50*(3), 171–188. doi:10.1002/j.1556-6978.2011.tb00118.x

Borror, J. (2020). Developing as a teacher. In Teacher Self-Care. Cambridge Scholars Publishing.

Borror, J. Ransdell, S., Binaco, J., & Feeser, A. (2020). The impact of transitioning to online learning and virtual conferences on students and educators during the coronavirus pandemic. *Distance Learning Journal, 18*(1).

Boscarino, J. A. (1997). Diseases among men 20 years after exposure to severe stress: Implications for clinical research and medical care. *Psychosomatic Medicine, 59*(6), 605–614. doi:10.1097/00006842-199711000-00008 PMID:9407579

Boscarino, J. A., Adams, R. E., & Figley, C. R. (2004). Mental health service use 1-year after the World Trade Center disaster: Implications for medical care. *General Hospital Psychiatry, 26*(5), 346–358. doi:10.1016/j.genhosppsych.2004.05.001 PMID:15474634

Boujut, E., Bruchon-Schweitzer, M., & Dombrowski, S. U. (2012). Coping among students: Development and validation of an exploratory measure. *Psychology (Irvine, Calif.), 3*(8), 562–568. doi:10.4236/psych.2012.38084

Boyatzis, R., & McKee, A. (2005). *Resonant leadership*. Harvard Business School Press.

Brackett, M. A., Floman, J. L., & Bradley, C. (2018). *Emotion revolution for education leaders - survey.* Unpublished data. Yale University.

Brackett, M., & Cipriano, C. (2020, April 7). *Teachers Are Anxious and Overwhelmed. They Need SEL Now More Than Ever.* EdSurge. https://www.edsurge.com/news/2020-04-07-teachers-are-anxious-and-overwhelmed-they-need-sel-now-more-than-ever

Brackett, M., Cannizarro, M., & Levy, S. (2020). *The pandemic's toll on school leadership is palpable. Here's what is needed for a successful school year.* Retrieved from: https://www.edsurge.com/news/2020-07-16-the-pandemic-s-toll-on-school-leaders-is-palpable-here-s-what-s-needed-for-a-successful-school-year

Bradberry, T. (2021, June 24). *70% of Employees Say They Are Disengaged at Work. Here's How to Motivate Them.* World Economic Forum. https://www.weforum.org/agenda/2016/11/70-of-employees-say-they-are-disengaged-at-work-heres-how-to-motivate-them/#:%7E:text=The%20scariest%20thing%20is%20how%20prevalent%20this%20lack,happen.%20When%20they%20don%E2%80%99t%2C%20the%20bottom%20line%20suffers

Braime, H. (2016). *From coping to thriving: How to turn self-care into a way of life.* Create Space Independent Publishing Platform.

Braun, R. (2017). *Critical friends in self-studies* [Blog post]. The Research Associate (RA) Notebooks. Retrieved from http://tirap.ucal-garyblogs.ca/2017/01/28/critical-friends-in-self-studies

Bressi, S. K., & Vaden, E. R. (2017). Reconsidering self care. *Clinical Social Work Journal, 45*(1), 33–38. doi:10.100710615-016-0575-4

Bride, B. E. (2007). Prevalence of secondary traumatic stress among social workers. *Social Work, 52*(1), 63–70. doi:10.1093w/52.1.63 PMID:17388084

Bride, B. E., Radey, M., & Figley, C. R. (2007). Measuring compassion fatigue. *Clinical Social Work Journal, 35*(3), 155–163. doi:10.100710615-007-0091-7

Bronfenbrenner, U. (1977). Toward an experimental ecology of the human development. *The American Psychologist, 32*(7), 513–531. doi:10.1037/0003-066X.32.7.513

Bronfenbrenner, U. (1986). Ecology of the family as a context for human development: Research perspectives. *Developmental Psychology, 22*(6), 723–742. doi:10.1037/0012-1649.22.6.723

Brown, A. M. (2017). *Emergent strategy: Shaping change, changing worlds.* AK Press.

Brown, D. (2021). *Covid-19: Five ways to avoid lockdown eye strain.* BBC News. https://www.bbc.com/news/uk-55933168

Brown, K. W., & Ryan, R. M. (2003). The benefits of being present: Mindfulness and its role in psychological wellbeing. *Journal of Personality and Social Psychology, 84*(4), 822 – 848. doi: . doi:10.1037/0022-351484.4.822

BrunetteA. (2004). https://www.wcu.edu/WebFiles/PDFs/CEAP-HS-BK_Self-CareForTeachers.pdf

Bryan, V., Weaver, S., Anderson-Johnson, P., & Lindo, J. (2013). The effect of interpersonal relationships between nursing students and lecturers on learning outcomes at a Jamaican nursing school. *Caribbean Journal of Nursing, 1*(1), 41-48. Retrieved from http://ojs.mona.uwi.edu/index.php/cjn/article/view/3690/3218

Buckworth, J. P. D., & Nigg, C. P. D. (2004). Physical activity, exercise, and sedentary behavior in college students. *Journal of American College Health, 53*(1), 28–34. doi:10.3200/JACH.53.1.28-34 PMID:15266727

Buettner, D. (2017). *The blue zones solution: Eating and living like the world's healthiest people.* National Geographic Books.

Buttner, A. (2021, April 19). *The state of the teacher shortage in 2021.* Frontline Education. https://www.frontlineeducation.com/blog/teacher-shortage-2021/

Calderon, V. J. (2020, June 1). *U.S. Parents Say COVID-19 Harming Child's Mental Health.* Gallup. https://news.gallup.com/poll/312605/parents-say-covid-harming-child-mental-health.aspx

Callaghan, D. (2006). Basic conditioning factors' influences on adolescents' healthy behaviors, self-efficacy, and self-care. *Issues in Comprehensive Pediatric Nursing*, *29*(4), 191–204. doi:10.1080/01460860601087156 PMID:17190774

Callaghan, D. M. (2005). The influence of spiritual growth on adolescents' initiative and responsibility for self-care. *Pediatric Nursing*, *31*(2), 91–97. PMID:15934561

Cameron, D. (2021). *History of Workplace Health and Safety*. Staysafe. https://staysafeapp.com/blog/2020/08/21/history-workplace-health-and-safety

Cancio, E. J., Larsen, R., Mathur, S. R., Estes, M. B., Johns, B., & Chang, M. (2018). Special education teacher stress: Coping strategies. *Education & Treatment of Children*, *41*(4), 457–482. doi:10.1353/etc.2018.0025

Caprara, G. V., Barbaranelli, C., Borgogni, L., & Steca, P. (2003). Efficacy beliefs as determinants of teachers' job satisfaction. *Journal of Educational Psychology*, *95*(4), 821–832. doi:10.1037/0022-0663.95.4.821

Cardozo-Gaibisso, L., & Harman, R. (2019). Preparing in-service teachers to work with linguistically and culturally diverse youth. Handbook of Research on Engaging Immigrant Families and Promoting Academic Success for English Language Learners, 361-377. doi:10.4018/978-1-5225-8283-0.ch018

Carpenter, D. (2020, February 14). *3 ways to build real empathy for others in your life*. Verywell Mind. Retrieved from https://www.verywellmind.com/how-to-develop-empathy-in-relationships-1717547

Carpenter, J. P., & Green, T. D. (2017). Mobile instant messaging for professional learning: Educators' perspectives on and uses of Voxer. *Teaching and Teacher Education*, *68*, 53–67. doi:10.1016/j.tate.2017.08.008

Carver-Thomas, D., & Darling-Hammond, L. (2019). The trouble with teacher turnover: How teacher attrition affects students and schools. *Education Policy Analysis Archives*, *27*(36), 1–28. doi:10.14507/epaa.27.3699

Cassidy-Vu, L., Beck, K., & Moore, J. B. (2017). Burnout in female faculty members. *Journal of Primary Care & Community Health*, *8*(2), 97–99. doi:10.1177/2150131916669191 PMID:27650035

CDC. (n.d.). *Healthy eating for a healthy weight*. https://www.cdc.gov/healthyweight/healthy_eating/index.html

Chance, M. R. (2015). *Social fabrics of the mind*. Psychology Press. doi:10.4324/9781315728186

Chandler, C. (2020). *Working from home occupational health and safety implications*. https://www.lexology.com/library/detail.aspx?g=9fbe1053-b59e-4fe9-b6c1-5e45d8489042

Chaney, S. C., & Mechael, P. (2020). *Digital Self-care: A Framework for Design, Implementation & Evaluation*. Self-Care Trailblazer Group. https://www.psi.org/wp-content/uploads/2020/09/Digital-Self-Care.pdf

Chee Keong, C., Muhammad Faizal, A. G., & Abdullah, Z. (2018). Cabaran amalan komuniti pembelajaran dalam kalangan guru sekolah rendah berprestasi tinggi Malaysia. *Jurnal Kurikulum & Pengajaran Asia Pasifik*, *6*(3), 1–14.

Cherry, K., & Susman, D. (2020, June 10). *What Are the Pros and Cons of Autocratic Leadership?* Verywell Mind. https://www.verywellmind.com/what-is-autocratic-leadership-2795314#:%7E:text=Because%20autocratic%20leaders%20make%20decisions,hurt%20the%20group%20from%20performing

Christou-Champi, S., Farrow, T. F., & Webb, T. L. (2015). Automatic control of negative emotions: Evidence that structured practice increases the efficiency of emotion regulation. *Cognition and Emotion*, *29*(2), 319–331. doi:10.1080/02699931.2014.901213 PMID:24678930

Ciulla, J. B., & Forsyth, D. R. (2021). Leadership ethics. In A. Bryman, D. Collinson, K. Grint, B. Jackson, & M. Uhl-Bien (Eds.), *The Sage Handbook of Leadership* (pp. 352–364). Sage.

Clapp-Smith, R., Vogelgesang, G. R., & Avey, J. B. (2019). Authentic leadership and positive psychological capital: The mediating role of trust at the group level of analysis. *Journal of Leadership & Organizational Studies*, *15*(3), 227–240. doi:10.1177/1548051808326596

Cleveland Clinic. (2021). *6 tips to help combat computer vision syndrome*. https://health.clevelandclinic.org/computers-and-blurry-vision-5-fixes-for-your-tech-induced-eyestrain/

Coetzee, S. K., & Klopper, H. C. (2010). Compassion Fatigue within Nursing Practice: A Concept Analysis. *Nursing & Health Sciences*, *12*(2), 235–243. doi:10.1111/j.1442-2018.2010.00526.x PMID:20602697

Cohen, P. (1997). Rethinking the youth question. In *Rethinking the youth question* (pp. 179–249). Palgrave. doi:10.1007/978-1-349-25390-6_8

Coleman, J. S. (1988). Social Capital in the Creation of Human Capital. *American Journal of Sociology*, *94*, 95–120. doi:10.1086/228943

Compassion Resilience Toolkit. (2021, May 10). https://compassionresiliencetoolkit.org/

Conyne, R. K., & Cook, E. P. (2004). *Ecological counseling: An innovative approach to conceptualizing person-environment interaction*. American Counseling Association.

Cook, C., Miller, F., Fiat, A., Renshaw, T., Frye, M., Joseph, G., & Decano, P. (2017). Promoting secondary teachers' well-being and intentions to implement evidence-based practices: Randomized evaluation of the achiever resilience curriculum. *Psychology in the Schools*, *54*(1), 13–28. doi:10.1002/pits.21980

Cooper, C. L., & Marshall, J. (1978). *Understanding executive stress*. Springer. doi:10.1007/978-1-349-03030-9

Costa, A. L., & Kallinick, B. (2020, September 12). *Describing 16 habits of mind*. https://www.habitsofmindinstitute.org

Costa, A. L. (2001). *Developing Minds: A Resource Book for Teaching Thinking*. Hawker Brownlow Education.

Costa, A. L., & Kallick, B. (2003). Through the lens of a critical friend. *Educational Leadership*, *51*(2), 49–51.

Craig, C. D., & Sprang, G. (2010). Compassion satisfaction, compassion fatigue, and burnout in a national sample of trauma treatment therapists. *Anxiety, Stress, and Coping*, *23*(3), 319–339. doi:10.1080/10615800903085818 PMID:19590994

Cronkleton, E. (2021). Yoga for osteoporosis: 5 beneficial poses. *Healthline*. https://www.healthline.com/health/osteoporosis/yoga-for-osteoporosis#12

Csiernik, R., & Adams, D. W. (2007). Spirituality, stress, and work. In J. Coates, J. R. Graham, & B. Swarzentruber (Eds.), *Spirituality and social work: Selected Canadian readings* (pp. 243–251). Canadian Scholars' Press, Inc.

Cunningham, P. M. (1998). The social dimension of transformative learning. *PAACE Journal of Lifelong Learning*, *7*, 15–28.

Czarnitzki, D., Grimpe, C., & Toole, A. A. (2014). Delay and secrecy: Does industry sponsorship jeopardize disclosure of academic research? *Industrial and Corporate Change*, *24*(1), 251–279. doi:10.1093/icc/dtu011

Czeisler, M. E., Lane, R. I., Petrosky, E., Wiley, J. F., Christensen, A., Njai, R., Weaver, M. D., Robbins, R., Facer-Childs, E. R., Barger, L. K., Czeisler, C. A., Howard, M. E., & Rajaratnam, S. M. W. (2020). Mental health, substance use, and suicidal ideation during the Covid-19 pandemic – United States, June 24-30, 2020. *MMWR. Morbidity and Mortality Weekly Report*, *69*, 1049–1057. doi:10.15585/mmwr.mm6932a1 PMID:32790653

Dada, J. O., Babatunde, S. O., & Adeleye, R. O. (2019). Assessment of academic stress and coping strategies among built environment undergraduate students in Nigerian higher education. *Journal of Applied Research in Higher Education, 11*(3), 367–378. doi:10.1108/JARHE-06-2018-0100

Dalky, H. F., & Gharaibeh, A. (2018). *Depression, anxiety, and stress among college students in Jordan and their need for mental health services*. doi:10.1111/nuf.12316

Damin, Z. A., Isa, K., Jaes, L., Kadir, Z. A., & Abdul, H. A. R. (2020). Analysis of Stress Contributing Factors in Work Organizations in Public Institutions of Higher Learning. *Journal of Social Transformation and Regional Development., 2*(3), 11–23. doi:10.30880/jstard.2020.02.03.002

Davenport, B., & Scott, S. J. (2016). *Declutter your mind: How to stop worrying, relieve anxiety, and eliminate negative thinking*. Oldtown Publishing LLC.

David, S., & Congleton, C. (2013, November). Emotional agility. *Harvard Business Review*. https://hbr.org/2013/11/emotional-agility

David, S. A. (2017). *Emotional agility: get unstuck, embrace change, and thrive in work and life*. Penguin Life Publishing.

Davidson, R.J. (2003). Alterations in Brain and Immune Function Produced by Mindfulness Meditation. *Psychosomatic Medicine, 65*(1), 564 – 570.

Davis, M. H. (1983). Measuring individual differences in empathy: Evidence for a multidimensional approach. *Journal of Personality and Social Psychology, 44*(1), 113–126. doi:10.1037/0022-3514.44.1.113

Davis, M., Eshelman, E. R., & McKay, M. (2008). *The relaxation and stress reduction workbook* (6th ed.). New Harbinger Publications.

Day, C. (2020, January 4). *Making a vision book*. https://www.calvalynday.com/

de Oliveira, M. M., Santos, M. C., & Kiker, B. F. (2000). The role of human capital and technological change in overeducation. *Economics of Education Review, 19*(2), 199–206. doi:10.1016/S0272-7757(99)00020-5

De Stasio, S., Fiorilli, C., Benevene, P., Uusitalo-Malmivaara, L., & Di Chiacchio, C. (2017). Burnout in special needs teachers at kindergarten and primary school: Investigating the role of personal resources and work wellbeing. *Psychology in the Schools, 54*(5), 472–486. doi:10.1002/pits.22013

Deb, S., Strodl, E., & Sun, H. (2015). Academic stress, parental pressure, anxiety and mental health among Indian high school students. *International Journal of Psychology and Behavioral Sciences, 5*(1), 26–34.

Deepti, B., & Hemant, T. (2018). A Study of Causes of Stress and Stress Management among Youth. *International Journal of Management and Social Sciences, 11*(3), 108–117. doi:10.21013/jmss.v11.n3.p1

Deighton, R. M., Gurris, N., & Traue, H. (2007). Factors affecting burnout and compassion fatigue in psychotherapists treating torture survivors: Is the therapist's attitude to working through trauma relevant? *Journal of Traumatic Stress, 20*(1), 63–75. doi:10.1002/jts.20180 PMID:17345651

Delgado, P. (2020, November 2). *Teacher training, the Great Challenge of Online Education - Observatory: Institute for the Future of Education*. Retrieved from https://observatory.tec.mx/edu-news/teacher-training-challenge

DeMatthews, D., Carrola, P., Reyes, P., & Knight, D. (2021). School Leadership Burnout and Job-Related Stress: Recommendations for District Administrators and Principals. *The Clearing House: A Journal of Educational Strategies, Issues and Ideas, 94*(4), 159–167. doi:10.1080/00098655.2021.1894083

DeMause, L. (1995). *The history of childhood, Master Work*. Rowman & Littlefield Published.

Demerouti, E., Bakker, A. B., Nachreiner, F., & Schaufeli, W. B. (2001). The job demands-resources model of burnout. *The Journal of Applied Psychology*, *86*(3), 499–512. doi:10.1037/0021-9010.86.3.499 PMID:11419809

Denyes, M. J., Orem, D. E., & Bekel, G. (2001). Self-Care: A Foundational Science. *Nursing Science Quarterly*, *14*(1), 48–54. doi:10.1177/089431840101400113 PMID:11873354

DePaul, K. (2019). *Remote Work Health Risks: What You Need to Know*. Remote Co. https://remote.co/remote-work-health-risks-what-need-know/#:~:text=Carpal%20Tunnel%20Syndrome,problem%20called%20Carpal%20Tunnel%20 Syndrome

Dewey, J. (1986, September). Experience and education. *The Educational Forum*, *50*(3), 241–252. doi:10.1080/00131728609335764

Di Donato, M., Iles, R., Buchbinder, R., Xia, T., & Collie, A. (2021). Prevalence, Predictors and Wage Replacement Duration Associated with Diagnostic Imaging in Australian Workers with Accepted Claims for Low Back Pain: A Retrospective Cohort Study. *Journal of Occupational Rehabilitation*, 1–9. PMID:33913056

Dickler, J. (2021, March 1). *More teachers plan to quit as Covid stress overwhelms educators*. CNBC. https://www.cnbc.com/2021/03/01/more-teachers-plan-to-quit-as-covid-stress-overwhelms-educators.html

Dimovski, V., Ferjan, M., Maric, M., Uhan, M., Jovanovic, M., & Janezic, M. (2012). Authentic leadership to the future. *Skola Biznisa*, *1*(1), 1–14. doi:10.5937kolbiz1201001D

Donesky, D., Norton, L., Fisher, E., & Bunker-Alberts, M. (2021). Health services and the Project RoomKey COVID-19 initiative for the unhoused: A university and community partnership. *Journal of Professional Nursing*, *37*(6), 1175–1179. doi:10.1016/j.profnurs.2021.10.008 PMID:34887037

Doughty, H. A. (2016). *Book review/The slow professor*. Retrieved from https://www.caut.cabulletin/articles/2016/09/the-slow-professor.

Duarte, J., & Pinto-Gouveia, J. (2017b). The role of psychological factors in oncology nurses' burnout and compassion fatigue symptoms. *European Journal of Oncology Nursing*, *28*, 114–121. doi:10.1016/j.ejon.2017.04.002 PMID:28478848

Dugas, D. (2017). The perils of feeling in-between: The experiences of emerging adult novice teachers. *Journal of Adult Development*, *24*(3), 189–198. doi:10.100710804-016-9257-2

Dupree, P. I., & Day, H. D. (1995). Psychotherapists' job satisfaction and job burnout as a function of work setting and percentage of managed care clients. *Psychotherapy in Private Practice*, *14*(2), 77–93.

Edelman, A. (2021, June 6). Biden wants to fix the nation's teacher shortage. Educators say the problem is worsening. *NBC News*.

Educator Policy Innovation Center. (2016). *Smart solutions to Minnesota's teacher shortage: Developing and sustaining a diverse and valued educator workforce*. EPIC. https://educationminnesota.org/wp-content/uploads/2021/08/EPIC-Recruitment-Retention-Report.pdf

EHS Insight Resources. (2019). *A Brief History of Occupational Health and Safety*. https://www.ehsinsight.com/blog/a-brief-history-of-occupational-health-and-safety#:~:text=In%20the%20United%20States%2C%20occupational,of%20 their%20job%20or%20industry

Elder, G. H. (1998). The life course and human development. In W. Damon & R. M. Lerner (Eds.), *Theoretical models of human development* (pp. 939–991). John Wiley & Sons Inc.

Elizabeth, S. (2020). *How to handle the stress of working from home*. Access from https://www.verywellmind.com/the-stress-of-working-fromhome-4141174

El-Osta, Webber, Gnani, Banarsee, Mummery, Mated, & Smith. (2019). The Self-care Matrix: A Unifying Framework for Self-Care. *SelfCare*, *10*(3), 38–56.

Engin, G. (2020). An examination of primary school students' academic achievements and motivation in terms of parents' attitudes, teacher motivation, teacher self-efficacy and leadership approach. *International Journal of Progressive Education*, *16*(1), 257–276. doi:10.29329/ijpe.2020.228.18

Epstein, R. M., & Krasner, M. S. (2013). Physician resilience: What it means, why it matters, and how to promote it. *Academic Medicine*, *88*, 301 – 303. doi:10.1097/ACM.0b013e31828cff0

Erskine, J. A. K., & Georgiou, G. J. (2017). *Leadership Styles: Employee Stress, Well being, Productivity, Turnover and Absenteeism*. Understanding Stress at Work.

ESFI. (2021). *Electrical Safety While Working From Home*. https://www.esfi.org/electrical-safety-while-working-from-home/

Estrada-Muñoz, C., Vega-Muñoz, A., Castillo, D., Müller-Pérez, S., & Boada-Grau, J. (2021). Technostress of Chilean teachers in the context of the COVID-19 pandemic and Teleworking. *International Journal of Environmental Research and Public Health*, *18*(10), 5458. doi:10.3390/ijerph18105458 PMID:34065219

Etel, E., & Yagmurlu, B. (2015). Social competence, theory of mind, and executive function in institution-reared Turkish children. *International Journal of Behavioral Development*, *39*(6), 519–529. doi:10.1177/0165025414556095

Etzion, D. (2003). Annual vacation: Duration of relief from job stressors and burnout. *Anxiety, Stress, and Coping*, *16*(2), 213 – 26. . doi:10.1080/10615806.2003.10382974

European Agency for Safety and Health at Work. (2009). *Heath circles, an effective and enjoyable way to conduct risk assessments*. https://osha.europa.eu/en/publications/health-circles-effective-and-enjoyable-way-conduct-risk-assessment/view

Faller, G. (2021). Future Challenges for Work-Related Health Promotion in Europe: A Data-Based Theoretical Reflection. *International Journal of Environmental Research and Public Health*, *18*(20), 10996. doi:10.3390/ijerph182010996 PMID:34682748

Fancourt, D., Opher, S., & de Oliveira, C. (2020). Fixed-effects analyses of time-varying associations between hobbies and depression in a longitudinal cohort study: Support for social prescribing? *Psychotherapy and Psychosomatics*, *89*(2), 111–113. doi:10.1159/000503571 PMID:31658464

Farber, B. (1983). The effects of psychotherapeutic practice upon the psychotherapists. *Psychotherapy (Chicago, Ill.)*, *20*(2), 174–182. doi:10.1037/h0088488

Farber, B. (1990). Burnout in psychotherapists: Incidence, types, and trends. *Psychology in Private Practice*, *8*(1), 35–44. doi:10.1300/J294v08n01_07

Farrace, B. (2020, June 3). *Principals say pandemic conditions are accelerating their plans to leave the profession*. https://blog.nassp.org/2020/08/21/principals-say-pandemic-conditions-are-accelerating-their-plans-to-leave-the-principalship/

Farzan, A. N., & Taylor, A. (2020). Students in England fell behind by average of three months during shutdown, study finds. *Washington Post*. https://www.washingtonpost.com/world/2020/09/01/studentsengland-fell-behind-three-months-coronavirus-study/

Felitti, V. J., Anda, R. F., Anda, R. F., Nordenberg, D., Williamson, D. F., Spitz, A. M., Edwards, V., Koss, M. P., & Marks, J. S. (1998, May 1). Relationship of childhood abuse and household dysfunction to many of the leading causes of death in adults. *American Journal of Preventive Medicine*, *14*(4), 245–258. https://www.ajpmonline.org/article/S0749-3797(98)00017-8/fulltext

Figley, C. (2002). Compassion fatigue: Psychotherapists' chronic lack of self-care. *Journal of Clinical Psychology*, *58*(11), 1433–1441. doi:10.1002/jclp.10090 PMID:12412153

Figley, C. R. (1995). *Compassion fatigue as secondary traumatic stress disorder: An overview. In Compassion fatigue: Coping with secondary traumatic stress disorder*. Brunner.

Figley, C. R. (1995). Compassion fatigue as secondary traumatic stress disorder: An overview. In C. R. Figley (Ed.), *Compassion fatigue: Coping with secondary traumatic stress disorder in those who treat the traumatized* (pp. 1–20). Brunner Routledge.

Figley, C. R. (1995). Compassion fatigue: Toward a new understanding of the costs of caring. In B. H. Stamm (Ed.), *Secondary traumatic stress: Self-care issues for clinicians, researchers and educators* (pp. 3–28). Sidran Press.

Figley, C. R. (1995a). *Compassion fatigue: Coping with secondary traumatic stress disorder in those who treat the traumatized*. Brunner/Maze.

Fink, D., & Brayman, C. (2006). School leadership succession and the challenges of change. *Educational Administration Quarterly*, *42*, 62 – 89. doi:10.1177/0031316

Fisher, Frey, & Lapp. (2011). Focusing on the Participation and Engagement Gap: A Case Study on Closing the Achievement Gap. *Journal of Education for Students Placed at Risk*, *16*, 56 – 64.

Fitzsimons, P. (1999). *Human capital theory and education*. Macmillan.

Fix, G. M., Rikkerink, M., Ritzen, H. T. M., Pieters, J. M., & Kuiper, W. A. J. M. (2021). Learning within sustainable educational innovation: An analysis of teachers' perceptions and leadership practices. *Journal of Educational Change*, *22*(1), 131–145. doi:10.100710833-020-09410-2

Flannery, M. E. (2020, August 14). *Safety concerns over covid-19 driving some educators out of the profession*. NEA. https://www.nea.org/advocating-for-change/new-from-nea/safety-concerns-over-covid-19-driving-some-educators-out

Flarity, K., Gentry, J. E., & Mesnikoff, N. (2013). The effectiveness of an educational program on preventing and treating compassion fatigue in emergency nurses. *Advanced Emergency Nursing Journal*, *35*(3), 247–258. doi:10.1097/TME.0b013e31829b726f PMID:23899949

Folkman, S., & Lazarus, R. S. (1988). Coping as a mediator of emotion. *Journal of Personality Social Psychology*, *54*(3), 466. doi:10.1037/0022-3514.54.3.466

Folkman, S., Lazarus, R. S., Pimley, S., & Novacek, J. (1987). Age differences in stress and coping processes. *Psychology and Aging*, *2*(2), 171–184. doi:10.1037/0882-7974.2.2.171 PMID:3268206

Forbes, H. T. (2013). *Help for Billy: A beyond consequences approach to helping children in the classroom*. BookBaby.

Forster, V. (2020). Are Your Eyes Hurting During The Coronavirus Pandemic? You May Have "Computer Vision Syndrome". *Forbes Magazine*. https://www.forbes.com/sites/victoriaforster/2020/06/01/are-your-eyes-hurting-during-the--coronavirus-pandemic-you-may-have-computer-vision-syndrome/?sh=32dcb8326cf9

Foucault, M., Martin, L. H., Gutman, H., & Hutton, P. H. (1997). *Technologies of the self: A seminar with Michel Foucault*. University of Massachusetts Press.

Foucault, M., & Rabinow, P. (2007). *Ethics: Subjectivity and truth.* New Press.

Fowler, M. (2015). Dealing with compassion fatigue. When children hurt, we hurt too. And this can wear us out. *NJEA Review, 88*, 32–35.

Francis, L. E. (1997). Ideology and interpersonal emotion management: Redefining identity in two support groups. *Social Psychology Quarterly, 60*(2), 153–171. doi:10.2307/2787102

Freire, P. (2018). *Pedagogy of the oppressed (50th anniversary edition).* Bloomsbury Academic.

Freudenberger, H. J. (1975). The staff burn-out syndrome in alternative institutions. *Psychotherapy (Chicago, Ill.), 12*(1), 73–82. doi:10.1037/h0086411

Freudenberger, H. J. (1990). Hazards of psychotherapeutic practice. *Psychotherapy in Private Practice, 8*(1), 31–34. doi:10.1300/J294v08n01_06

Freud, S. (1953). *Three essays on the theory of sexuality (1905).* Imago Publishing.

Fuglseth, A. M., & Sørebø, Ø. (2014). The effects of technostress within the context of employee use of ICT. *Computers in Human Behavior, 40*, 161–170. doi:10.1016/j.chb.2014.07.040

Furlong, A. (2013). *Youth studies: An introduction* (Vol. 1). Routledge, Taylor & Francis Group Inc.

Gahlann, V. S. (2014). The Effect of Role Overload and Role Ambiguity on Job Performance of IT Professionals in India. *The IUP Journal of Management Research, 13*(3), 37–49.

Galderisi, S., Heinz, A., Kastrup, M., Beezhold, J., & Sartorius, N. (2015). Toward a new definition of mental health. *World Psychiatry; Official Journal of the World Psychiatric Association (WPA), 14*(2), 213–233. doi:10.1002/wps.20231 PMID:26043341

Gallup. (2014). *State of America's schools report.* https://www.gallup.com/education/269648/state-america-schools-report.aspx

García, E., & Weiss, E. (2019, April 16). *U.S. schools struggle to hire and retain teachers: The second report in "The perfect storm in the teacher labor market" series.* Economic Policy Institute. https://www.epi.org/publication/u-s-schools-struggle-to-hire-and-retain-teachers-the-second-report-in-the-perfect-storm-in-the-teacher-labor-market-series/

Gardner, W. L., Avolio, B. J., & Walumbwa, F. O. (2005). *Authentic leadership theory and practice: Origins, effects and development.* Elsevier.

Garis Panduan Amalan Baik. Staf Akademik. (2014). Retrieved on 14 March 2022. https://www2.mqa.gov.my/qad/garispanduan/2017/GGP%20Academic%20Staff(BM).upload%20website%2013.10.17.pdf

Garis Panduan Beban Staf Akademik. (n.d.). Retrieved on 14 March 2022. https://www2.mqa.gov.my/qad/garispanduan/2015/Garis%20Panduan%20Beban%20Staf%20Akademik.pdf

Gasper, D. (2014). Future global ethics: Environmental change, embedded ethics, evolving human identity. *Journal of Global Ethics, 10*(2), 135–145. doi:10.1080/17449626.2014.933442

Gasser, C. E., & Shaffer, K. S. (2014). Career development of women in academia: Traversing the leaky pipeline. *The Professional Counselor, 4*(4), 332–352. doi:10.15241/ceg.4.4.332

Geller, J. D., Norcross, J. C., & Orlinsky, D. E. (Eds.). (2005). *The psychotherapist's own psychotherapy: Patient and clinician perspectives.* Oxford University Press.

Gentry, E., Baranowsky, A. B., & Dunning, K. (1999). *Accelerated recovery program for compassion fatigue: Treatment and training protocols. Green Cross Projects*. Florida State University.

Gewin, V. (2021). Pandemic burnout is rampant in academia. *Nature, 591*(7850), 489–491. doi:10.1038/d41586-021-00663-2 PMID:33723408

Ghavifekr, S., & Pillai, N. S. (2016). The relationship between school's organizational climate and teacher's job satisfaction: Malaysian experience. *Asia Pacific Education Review, 17*(1), 87–106. doi:10.100712564-015-9411-8

Ghazali, D., & Sufean, H. (2016). *Metodologi Penyelidikan Dalam Pendidikan: Amalan dan Analisis Kajian*. Penerbit Universiti Malaya.

Giardina., . . . (2021). When do elementary students need masks in school? Model-estimated risk of in-school SARS-CoV-2 transmission and related infections among household members before and after student vaccination. MedRxiv. doi:10.1101/2021.08.04.21261576

Gill, J. (2020). Long-distance leadership: Principals support teachers as they dive into remote learning. *Learning Professional, 41*(3), 26–29.

Glass, T. E., Bjork, L., & Brunner, C. C. (2000). *The study of the American school superintendency, 2000: A look at the superintendent of education in the new millennium*. American Association of School Administrators.

Gleason, A. M. (2021). *Remote Monitoring of a Work-From-Home Employee to Identify Stress: A Case Report*. Workplace Health & Safety. https://journals.sagepub.com/doi/abs/10.1177/2165079921997322

Gleichgerrcht, E., & Decety, J. (2014). The relationship between different facets of empathy, pain perception and compassion fatigue among physicians. *Frontiers in Behavioral Neuroscience, 8*, 243. doi:10.3389/fnbeh.2014.00243 PMID:25071495

Glock, S., Kleen, H., & Morgenroth, S. (2019). Stress Among Teachers: Exploring the Role of Cultural Diversity in Schools. *Journal of Experimental Education, 87*(4), 696–713. doi:10.1080/00220973.2019.1574700

Goetz, J. L., Keltner, D., & Simon-Thomas, E. (2010). Compassion: An evolutionary analysis and empirical review. *Psychological Bulletin, 136*(3), 351–374. doi:10.1037/a0018807 PMID:20438142

Gonzalez, G. M., & Sutton, M. (2013). The role of supportive leaders at top performing universities: Best practice lessons from American institutions for Indonesian higher education. *International Journal of Leadership and Change, 1*(1), 5–13.

Gordon, S. P., Oliver, J., & Solis, R. (2016). Successful innovations in educational leadership preparation. *International Journal of Educational Leadership Preparation, 11*(2), 51 – 70.

Grant, M. (1990). The effect of nursing consultation on anxiety, side effects, and self-care of patients receiving radiation therapy. *Oncology Nursing Forum, 17*(3), 31–36. PMID:2342981

Graunke, S. S., & Woosley, S. A. (2005). An exploration of the factors that affect the academic success of college sophomores. *College Student Journal, 39*(2), 367–376.

Green, R. L. (2013). A response to the call for effective leadership in today's schools: Three essentials: preparation, competency, and dispositions. *National Forum of Applied Educational Research Journal, 26*(1&2), 3 – 16.

Greenberg, L. S., Watson, J. C., Elliot, R., & Bohart, A. C. (2001). Empathy. *Psychotherapy (Chicago, Ill.), 38*(4), 380–384. doi:10.1037/0033-3204.38.4.380

Greenstein, M. (2020). *Tips for eye health while working from home*. https://www.kshb.com/news/coronavirus/tips-for-eye-health-while-working-from-home

Grier-Reed, T., Said, R., & Quiñones, M. (2021). From Antiblackness to Cultural Health in Higher Education. *Education Sciences*, *11*(2), 11. doi:10.3390/educsci11020057

Griffin, K. A., Bennett, J. C., & Harris, J. (2011). Analyzing Gender Differences in Black Faculty Marginalization through a Sequential Mixed-Methods Design. *New Directions for Institutional Research*, *151*(151), 45–61. doi:10.1002/ir.398

Grove, J. (2017). The teaching survey 2017: results and analysis. *Times Higher Education*. Retrieved from https://www.timeshighereducation.com/features/the-teaching-survey-2017-results-and-analysis

Grubb, W. N., & Flessa, J. J. (2006). A job too big for one: Multiple principals and other nontraditional approaches to school leadership. *Educational Administration Quarterly*, *42*(4), 518 – 550. doi:10.1177/0013161X06290641

Guawan, E., Deo, P., Hidayat, T., Pandia, V., Iskandar, S., Yuni, P. S., Sylviana, N., Akbar, I., Farenia, R., Wahyu, K., Purba, A., & Hatta, S. I. D. I. (2018). Factors correlated with occupational stress among university lecturers. *Medicine & Health*, *13*(2), 95–102. doi:10.17576/MH.2018.1302.9

Guise, S. (2014). *Mini habits: Smaller habits, bigger results*. Kindle E. Book.

Gutierrez, S. B., & Quispe-Orihuela, K. (2021). Weight gain and physical inactivity during the COVID-19 pandemic. *Revista Panamericana de Salud Pública*, *45*, 1. Advance online publication. doi:10.26633/RPSP.2021.136 PMID:34703462

Gyatso, T. (2021, April 26). The Monk in the Lab. *The New York Times*. https://www.nytimes.com/2003/04/26/opinion/the-monk-in-the-lab.html

Hairul Akmal Mohd Halim. (2014). *Stres sebagai moderator ke atas hubungan antara gaya kepimpinan ketua dengan tingkah laku buli* (Master Dissertation). Universiti Teknologi Malaysia, Skudai.

Hall, C. W., Row, K. A., Wuensch, K. L., & Godley, K. R. (2013). The Role of Self-Compassion in Physical and Psychological Well-Being. *The Journal of Psychology*, *147*(4), 311–323. doi:10.1080/00223980.2012.693138 PMID:23885635

Hamilton, S., Tran, V., & Jamieson, J. (2016). Compassion fatigue in emergency medicine: The cost of caring. *Emergen. Med. Aus.*, *28*(1), 100–103. doi:10.1111/1742-6723.12533 PMID:26777437

Hand & Wrist Center. (2020). *4 Hand-Wrist Stretches for Remote Workers During COVID-19*. https://northfloridahandandwrist.com/4-hand-wrist-stretches-for-remote-workers-during-covid-19/

Hansraj, K. K. (2014). Assessment of Stresses in the Cervical Spine Caused by Posture and Position of the Head. *Surgical Technology International*, *25*, 277–279. PMID:25393825

Hargreaves, A. (1998). The emotional politics of teaching and teacher development: with implications for educational leadership. *International Journal of Leadership in Education*, *1*(4), 315 – 336.

Hargreaves, A. (2001). Emotional geographies of teaching. *Teachers College Record*, *103*(6), 1056 – 1080. . doi:10.1111/0161-4681.00142

Harr, C., & Moore, B. (2011). Compassion fatigue among Social Work students in field placements. *Journal of Teaching in Social Work*, *31*(3), 350–363.

Harter, J., & Arora, R. (2008). Social time crucial to daily emotional well-being in U.S. *Gallup*. https://news.gallup.com/poll/107692/social-time-crucial-daily-emotional-wellbeing.aspx

Haryati, R., & Rahardjo, S. N. (2013). *Influence of Corporate social responsibility, Environmental Performance and Corpor*. Fakultas Ekonomika dan Bisnis.

Hascher, T., & Waber, J. (2021). Teacher well-being: A systematic review of the research literature from the year 2000–2019. *Educational Research Review, 34,* 100411. . 2021.100411 doi:10.1016/j.edurev

Haslam, S. A., & Reicher, S. (2006). Stressing the group: Social Identity and the unfolding dynamics of responses to stress. *The Journal of Applied Psychology*, *91*(5), 1037–1052. doi:10.1037/0021-9010.91.5.1037 PMID:16953766

Hasselquist, L., & Graves, N. A. (2020). CTE teacher retention: Lessons learned from mid-career teachers. *Career and Technical Education Research*, *45*(1), 3–16. doi:10.5328/cter45.1.3

Hatlevik, O. E. (2016). Examining the relationship between teachers' self-efficacy, their digital competence, strategies to evaluate information, and use of ICT at school. *Scandinavian Journal of Educational Research*, *61*(5), 555–567. doi:10.1080/00313831.2016.1172501

Hawk, N., & Martin, B. (2011). Understanding and reducing stress in the superintendency. *Educational Management Administration and Leadership*, *39*(3), 364 – 389. doi:10.1177/17411432039400

Haynes, C., Taylor, L., Mobley, S. D. Jr, & Haywood, J. (2020). Existing and Resisting: The Pedagogical Realities of Black, Critical Men and Women Faculty. *The Journal of Higher Education*, *91*(5), 698–721. doi:10.1080/00221546.2020.1731263

Haywoode, A. (2018). City Connects prompts data-driven action in community schools in the Bronx. *Phi Delta Kappan*, *99*(5), 44–46. doi:10.1177/0031721718754812

Healey, R. L., Bass, T., Caulfield, J., Hoffman, A., McGinn, M. K., Miller-Young, J., & Haigh, M. (2013). Being ethically minded: Practicing the scholarship of teaching and learning in an ethical manner. *Teaching & Learning Inquiry: The Issotl Journal*, *1*(2), 23–32. doi:10.20343/teachlearninqu.1.2.23

Healthcare. (2021). *Pandemic Weight Gain — It's a Thing.* https://www.muhealth.org/our-stories/pandemic-weight-gain-its-thing

Healthline. (2020a). *4 Simple Tips to Avoid Developing 'Tech Neck' During COVID-19.* https://www.healthline.com/health-news/4-simple-tips-to-avoid-developing-tech-neck-during-covid-19#How-to-treat-tech-neck

Healthline. (2020b). *12 Ways to Calm Your Anxiety.* https://www.healthline.com/health/how-to-calm-anxiety

Hedge, A. (2020). Getting Back Pain While Working From Home? An Ergonomics Expert Offers Advice. *Time Magazine.* https://time.com/5821252/back-pain-work-from-home-tips/

He, J. (2020). Progress and Prospect of Research on University-Industry Cooperation: From the Perspective of Researchers. *American Journal of Industrial and Business Management*, *10*(05), 920–934. doi:10.4236/ajibm.2020.105062

Held, V. (2016). *The ethics of care: Personal, political, and global.* Oxford University Press.

Helliwell, J. F., & Putnam, R. D. (2004). The social context of well–being. *Philosophical Transactions of the Royal Society of London. Series B, Biological Sciences*, *359*(1449), 1435–1446. doi:10.1098/rstb.2004.1522 PMID:15347534

Helmke, S. (2020). Address the stress: How leaders can support teachers in an extraordinary year. *Learning Professional*, *41*(5), 36–37.

Hickman, A. (2019). *How to Manage the Loneliness and Isolation of Remote Workers.* Gallup. https://www.gallup.com/workplace/268076/manage-loneliness-isolation-remote-workers.aspx

Hicks-Moore, S. (2005). Relaxing music at mealtime in nursing homes. *Journal of Gerontological Nursing*, *31*(12), 26–32. doi:10.3928/0098-9134-20051201-07 PMID:16375095

Hill, N. R., Leinbaugh, T., Bradley, C., & Hazler, R. (2005). Female counselor educators: Encouraging and discouraging factors in academia. *Journal of Counseling and Development, 83*(3), 374–380. doi:10.1002/j.1556-6678.2005.tb00358.x

Holmes, B., Parker, D., & Gibson, J. (2019). Rethinking teacher retention in hard-to-staff schools. *Contemporary Issues in Education Research, 12*(1), 27–33. doi:10.19030/cier.v12i1.10260

Hong, X., Liu, Q., & Zhang, M. (2021). Dual stressors and female pre-school teachers' job satisfaction during the covid-19: The mediation of work-family conflict. *Frontiers in Psychology, 12*, 691498. Advance online publication. doi:10.3389/fpsyg.2021.691498 PMID:34168602

Hooks, B. (1994). *Teaching to transgress: Education as the practice of freedom.* Routledge.

Horowitz, A. (2010). Do humans ape? or Do apes human? Imitation and intention in humans and other animals. *Journal of Comparative Psychology, 17*(3), 325–336. doi:10.1037/0735-7036.117.3.325 PMID:14498809

Hou, J. M. (2015). *Characteristics of highly resilient counselors* (Unpublished doctoral dissertation). University of Minnesota, Minneapolis, MN.

Houlden, S., & Veletsianos, G. (2021, October 14). *Coronavirus pushes universities to switch to online classes - but are they ready?* Retrieved from https://theconversation.com/coronavirus-pushes-universities-to-switch-to-online-classes-but-are-they-ready-132728

Houtman, I., Jettinghof, K., Cedillo, L., & the World Health Organization. Occupational and Environmental Health Team. (2007)‹ *Raising awareness of stress at work in developing countries: advice to employers and worker representatives.* World Health Organization. https://apps.who.int/iris/handle/10665/42956

Hroch, P. (2013). Encountering the "ecopolis" Foucault's epimeleia heautou and environmental relations. *ETopia online initiative of TOPIA: Canadian Journal of Cultural Studies.* Retrieved from https://etopia.journals.yorku.ca/index.php/etopia/article/view/36563/33222

Huan, V. S., See, Y. L., Ang, R. P., & Har, C. W. (2008). The impact of adolescent concerns on their academic stress. *Educational Review, 60*(2), 169–178. doi:10.1080/00131910801934045

Humberstone, B. (2013). Adventurous activities, embodiment and nature: Spiritual, sensual and Sustainable? Embodying environmental justice. *Motriz, 19*(3), 565–571. doi:10.1590/S1980-65742013000300006

Hunter, J. (2013, April). Is mindfulness good for business? *Mindful Magazine*, 52-59.

Hunt, P., Denieffe, S., & Gooney, M. (2019). Running on empathy: Relationship of empathy to compassion satisfaction and compassion fatigue in cancer healthcare professionals. *European Journal of Cancer Care, 28*(5), 13124. doi:10.1111/ecc.13124 PMID:31222849

Husky, M. M., Kovess-Masfety, V., & Swendsen, J. D. (2020). Stress and anxiety among university students in France during Covid-19 mandatory confinement. *Comprehensive Psychiatry, 102*, 152191. doi:10.1016/j.comppsych.2020.152191 PMID:32688023

Hynes, C. A., Baird, A. A., & Grafton, S. T. (2006). Differential role of the orbital frontal lobe in emotional versus cognitive perspective-taking. *Neuropsychologia, 44*(3), 374–383. doi:10.1016/j.neuropsychologia.2005.06.011 PMID:16112148

IES. (2020, February). *Infographic: HOW TO GROW Teacher Wellbeing in Your Schools.* IES—REL Regional Educational Laboratory Program. https://ies.ed.gov/ncee/edlabs/infographics/pdf/REL_PA_How_To_Grow_Teacher_Wellbeing_in_Your_Schools.pdf

Ilić-Kosanović, T. (2021). Work-life balance of teaching staff at higher education during COVID 19 pandemic. *Serbian Journal of Engineering Management*, *6*(1), 63–71. doi:10.5937/SJEM2101064I

Ilies, R., Morgeson, F. P., & Nahrgang, J. D. (2015). Authentic leadership and eudaemonic well-being: Understanding leader-follower outcomes. *The Leadership Quarterly*, *16*(3), 373–394. doi:10.1016/j.leaqua.2005.03.002

Ingusci, E., Signore, F., Giancaspro, M. L., Manuti, A., Molino, M., Russo, V., Zito, M., & Cortese, C. G. (2021). Workload, Techno Overload, and Behavioral Stress During COVID-19 Emergency: The Role of Job Crafting in Remote Workers. *Frontiers in Psychology*, *12*, 12. doi:10.3389/fpsyg.2021.655148 PMID:33912116

International Baccalaureate PD. (n.d.). *Professional development.* International Baccalaureate®. https://www.ibo.org/professional-development/

International Labor Organization. (2017). *The future of work.* International Labor Organization. https://www.ilo.org/global/topics/future-of-work/langen/index.htm

International Labor Organization. (2020). *Defining and measuring remote work, telework, work at home, and home-based work.* https://www.ilo.org/global/statistics-and- databases/publications/WCMS_747075/lang--en/index.htm

Irvine, C. (2019). The ethics of self-care. In T. R. Cole, T. J. Goodrich, & E. R. Gritz (Eds.), *Faculty health in academic medicine: physicians, scientists, and the pressures of success* (pp. 127–146). Humana Press.

Isa, Muda, Paim, Alavi, Shah, & Jamil. (2021). Kelaziman Punca Tekanan Pensyarah Di Universiti Awam Malaysia. *Journal of Social Sciences and Humanities, 18*(2), 84-97.

Ishak, A. A., & Talaat, A. Z. M. A. (2020). Online learning: A survey of readiness and motivation among logistics and supply chain management diploma students. *World Journal of Education*, *2*(4), 68–82.

Ismail, N. H., & Noor, A. (2016). Occupational stress and its associated factors among academician in a research university, Malaysia. *Malaysian Journal of Public Health Medicine*, *16*(1), 81–91.

Jacobs, J. A., & Winslow, S. E. (2004). Overworked faculty: Job stresses and family demands. *The Annals of the American Academy of Political and Social Science*, *596*(1), 104–129. doi:10.1177/0002716204268185

Jacobson, E. (1929). *Progressive relaxation.* University of Chicago Press.

James, J. (2021). *Remote work exhaustion: 13 tips to reduce fatigue.* The Enterprises Project. https://enterprisersproject.com/article/2021/1/remote-work-13-tips-reduce-fatigue

Janis, I. L. (1989). Stress inoculation in health care. In Stress reduction and prevention (pp. 67-99). Springer. doi:10.1007/978-1-4899-0408-9_3

Janssens, M., Janssens, E., Eshuis, J., Lataster, J., Simons, M., Reijnders, J., & Jacobs, N. (2021). Companion animals as buffer against the impact of stress on affect: An experience sampling study. *Animals (Basel)*, *11*(8), 2171. doi:10.3390/ani11082171 PMID:34438629

Jenkins, S. R., & Baird, S. (2002). Secondary traumatic stress and vicarious trauma: A validational study. *Journal of Traumatic Stress*, *15*(5), 423–432. doi:10.1023/A:1020193526843 PMID:12392231

Jennings, P. A., & Greenberg, M. (2009). The prosocial classroom: Teacher social and emotional competence in relation to child and classroom outcomes. *Review of Educational Research*, *79*, 491–525.

Jennings, P. A., Frank, J. L., Snowberg, K. E., Coccia, M. A., & Greenberg, M. T. (2013). Improving Classroom Learning Environments by Cultivating Awareness and Resilience in Education (CARE): Results of a Randomized Controlled Trial. *School Psychology Quarterly*, *28*(4), 374–390. . doi:10.1037/spq0000035

Jha, P. N., & Shenoy, P. V. (2016). Digitization of Indian Education process: A hope or hype. *IOSR Journal of Business and Management, 18*(10), 131–139. doi:10.9790/487X-181003131139

Johns Hopkins Medicine. (n.d.). *The science of sleep: Understanding what happens when you sleep.* https://www.hopkinsmedicine.org/health/wellness-and-prevention/the-science-of-sleep-understanding-what-happens-when-you-sleep

Johnson-Arnold, L. P. (2020). Practicing Holistic Health and Self-Care Throughout the Dissertation Journey: Practical Applications and Self-Reflections for Doctoral Students. In *Creating a Framework for Dissertation Preparation: Emerging Research and Opportunities* (pp. 1-22). IGI Global. doi:10.4018/979-1-5225-9707-0.ch001

Johnson-Arnold, L.P. (2020). *Self-Care Practices and Perceptions of Holistic Health Among Selected Educational Leadership Graduate Students Attending Historically Black Colleges and Universities of Minority Serving Institutions.* Academic Press.

Johnson, S. J., Willis, S. M., & Evans, J. (2019). An examination of stressors, strain, and resilience in academic and non-academic U.K. university job roles. *International Journal of Stress Management, 26*(2), 162–172. doi:10.1037tr0000096

Joshi, A. (2018, October 17). *Memes can help people cope.* The Daily Evergreen. https://dailyevergreen.com/38952/opinion/memes-can-help-people-cope/

Kabat-Zinn, J. (2015). *Wherever you go, there you are: mindfulness meditation in everyday life.* Hachette Books.

Kabat-Zinn, J. (2003). Mindfulness-based interventions in context: Past, present, and future. *Clinical Psychology: Science and Practice, 10*(2), 144–156. doi:10.1093/clipsy.bpg016

Kaden, U. (2020). Covid-19 school closure-related changes to the professional life of a k–12 teacher. *Education Sciences, 10*(6), 165. doi:10.3390/educsci10060165

Kamarudin, H. (2013). Work stress factors among Mains Holdings Sdn. Bhd. Research Project. Kuala Lumpur: Open University Malaysia.

Kamus Dewan. (Edisi Ke-4). (2005). Kuala Lumpur: Dewan Bahasa dan Pustaka.

Kanter, R. (1977). Some effects of proportions on group life: Skewed sex ratios and responses to token women. *American Journal of Sociology, 82*(5), 965–990. doi:10.1086/226425

Kassam-Adams, N. (1995). The risks of treating sexual trauma: Stress and secondary trauma in psychotherapists. In B. H. Stamm (Ed.), *Secondary traumatic stress: Self-care issues for clinicians, researchers, and educators* (pp. 37–48). Sidran Press.

Kassel, J. (2020). *6 Chiropractor-Approved Exercises to Fight Text Neck.* Healthline. https://www.healthline.com/health/fitness-exercise/text-neck-treatment#does-text-neck-really-cause-pain

Katella, K. (2020). *Quarantine 15? What to Do About Weight Gain During the Pandemic.* Yale Medicine. https://www.yalemedicine.org/news/quarantine-15-weight-gain-pandemic

Kaynak, N. E. (2020). A close look at teachers' lives: Caring for the well-being of elementary teachers in the US. *The International Journal of Emotional Education, 12*(1), 19–34.

Kekatos, M. (2017). *Work at home? Watch out! You're more likely to suffer insomnia, stress and depression.* Daily Mail. https://www.dailymail.co.uk/health/article-4227786/Work-home-likely-suffer-insomnia.html

Kelloway, E. K., & Day, A. (2005). Building healthy workplaces: Where we need to be. *Canadian Journal of Behavioural Science / Revue Canadienne Des Sciences Du Comportement, 37*(4), 309–312. https://doi-org.proxy-library.ashford.edu/10.1037/h0087265

Kelloway, E. K., Inness, M., Barling, J., Francis, L., & Turner, N. (2010). Loving one's job: Construct development and implications for individual well-being. In *New developments in theoretical and conceptual approaches to job stress*. Emerald Group Publishing Limited. doi:10.1108/S1479-3555(2010)0000008006

Kelly, J. (2020). *Q&A: Why people are 'stress eating' during the pandemic, and how to stop*. https://news.virginia.edu/content/qa-why-people-are-stress-eating-during-pandemic-and-how-stop

Kelly, L. (2021). Playing with the diary: how crafting a multimodal and sensory diary can have a positive impact on teacher wellbeing. *Reflective Practice, 23*(1), 1–16. . 2021.1973986 doi:10.1080/14623943

Kenny, N., & Berenson, K. (2014). *Creating a teaching dossier.* Taylor Institute for Teaching and Learning Educational Development Unit. Retrieved from http://ucalgary.ca/taylorinstitute/edu/sites/default/files/Teaching%20Dossier%20Handout_0.pdf

Kerekes, S., Ji, M., Shu-Fang, S., Hao-Yuan, C., Harapan, H., Rajamoorthy, Y., & Wagner, A. L. (2021). Differential effect of vaccine effectiveness and safety on COVID-19 vaccine acceptance across socioeconomic groups in an international sample. *Vaccines*, *9*(9), 1010. doi:10.3390/vaccines9091010 PMID:34579247

Kiger, P. J. (2020). *Pandemic Is Turning Some Older Telecommuters Into Insomniacs*. AARP. https://www.aarp.org/work/working-at-50-plus/info-2020/work-from-home-insomnia.html

Kiral, B. (2020). The relationship between the empowerment of teachers by school administrators and organizational commitments of teachers. *International Online Journal of Education & Teaching*, *7*(1), 248–265.

Kirk-Jenkins, A. J., & Hughey, A. W. (2021). Abrupt adaption: A review of the impact of the COVID-19 pandemic on faculty in higher education. *Journal of the Professoriate*, *12*(1), 104–121.

Klassen, R. M., & Tze, V. M. (2014). Teachers' self-efficacy, personality, and teaching effectiveness: A meta-analysis. *Educational Research Review*, *12*, 59–76. doi:10.1016/j.edurev.2014.06.001

Klepinger, D., Lundberg, S., & Plotnick, R. (1999). How does adolescent fertility affect the human capital and wages of young women? *The Journal of Human Resources*, *34*(3), 421–448. doi:10.2307/146375

Klocko, B., & Wells, C. (2015). Workload Pressures of Principals: A Focus on Renewal, Support, and Mindfulness. *NASSP Bulletin*, *99*(4), 332–355. Advance online publication. doi:10.1177/0192636515619727

Konradt, U., Schmook, R., Wilm, A., & Hertel, G. (2000). Health circles for teleworkers: Selective results on stress, strain and coping styles. *Health Education Research*, *15*(3), 327–338. doi:10.1093/her/15.3.327 PMID:10977380

Koole, S. L., & Rothermund, K. (2011). "I feel better but I don't know why" The psychology of implicit emotion regulation. *Cognition and Emotion*, *25*(3), 389–399. doi:10.1080/02699931.2010.550505 PMID:21432681

Krechevsky, M., Mardell, B., Filippini, T., & Tedeschi, M. (2016). Children are citizens: The everyday and the razzle-dazzle. *Innovations in Early Education: The International Reggio Emilia Exchange*, *23*(4), 4–15.

Krechevsky, M., Mardell, B., & Romans, A. N. (2014). Engaging city hall: Children as citizens. *New Educator*, *10*(1), 10–20. doi:10.1080/1547688X.2014.868212

Kuhfeld, Soland, Tarasawa, Johnson, Ruzek, & Liu. (2020, June 13). *Projecting the potential impacts of COVID-19 school closures on academic achievement*. . doi:10.26300/cdrv-yw05

Kuhnke, J. L., & Jack-Malik, S. (2021). Roofs, Nesting Instincts, and Student Evaluations of Teaching During a Pandemic. *Currere Exchange Journal*, *5*(2), 44–52.

LaBorde, S. (2020). *What is a vision board?* https://makeavisionboard.com/what-is-a-

Lackritz, J. R. (2004). Exploring burnout among university faculty: Incidence, performance, and demographic issues. *Teaching and Teacher Education, 20*(7), 713–729. doi:10.1016/j.tate.2004.07.002

Laghi, F., Lonigro, A., Levanto, S., Ferraro, M., Baumgartner, E., & Baiocco, R. (2016). The role of nice and nasty theory of mind in teacher-selected peer models for adolescents with autism spectrum disorders. *Measurement & Evaluation in Counseling & Development, 49*(3), 207–216. doi:10.1177/0748175615596784

Lane, L., Jones, D., & Penny, G. E. (2019). Qualitative case study of teachers' morale in a turnaround school. *Research in Higher Education, 37*(Nov), 1–12.

Langford, S., & Crawford, M. (2022). Walking with teachers: A study to explore the importance of teacher wellbeing and their careers. *Management in Education.* Advance online publication. doi:10.1177/08920206221075750

Larson, L. M., Seipel, M. T., Shelley, M. C., Gahn, S. W., Ko, S. Y., Schenkenfelder, M., Rover, D. T., Schmittmann, B., & Heitmann, M. M. (2019). The academic environment and faculty well-being: The role of psychological needs. *Journal of Career Assessment, 27*(1), 167–182. doi:10.1177/1069072717748667

Laschinger, H. K., Borgogni, L., Consiglio, C., & Read, E. (2015). The effects of authentic leadership, six areas of worklife, and occupational coping self-efficacy on new graduate nurses' burnout and mental health: A cross-sectional study. *International Journal of Nursing Studies, 52*(6), 1080–1089. doi:10.1016/j.ijnurstu.2015.03.002 PMID:25801311

Laschinger, H. K., Wong, C. A., & Grau, A. L. (2013). Authentic leadership, empowerment and burnout: A comparison in new graduates and experienced nurses. *Journal of Nursing Management, 21*(3), 541–552. doi:10.1111/j.1365-2834.2012.01375.x PMID:23405976

Lassonde, C. A., Galman, S., & Kosnik, C. M. (2019). *Self-study research methodologies for teacher educators.* Sense Publishers.

Lawler, E. E., & Mohrman, S. A. (1985). Quality circles after the fad. *Harvard Business Review, 63*(1), 65–71. PMID:10269357

Lawlor, K. B. (2012). Smart goals: How the application of smart goals can contribute to achievement of student learning outcomes. *Developments in Business Simulation and Experiential Learning, 39,* 259–267.

Lazarus, R. S. (1966). *Psychological stress and the coping process.* McGraw-Hill.

Lazarus, R. S. (2006). *Stress and emotion: A new synthesis.* Springer Publishing Company.

Lazarus, R. S., & Folkman, S. (1984). *Stress, Appraisal, and Coping.* Springer Publishing, Inc.

Leahy, J., & Wolfe, J. (2021). *Teacher Self-Care: A Guide for Educators* (Dissertation). Spiral.

Learning Policy Institute. (2021, March 4). *Covid-19 is worsening already critical teacher shortages, potentially jeopardizing school openings.* https://learningpolicyinstitute.org/press-release/covid-19-worsening-already-critical-teacher-shortages-potentially-jeopardizing-school

Lease, S. H. (1999). Occupational role stressors, coping, support, and hardiness as predictors of strain in academic faculty: An emphasis on female faculty. *Research in Higher Education, 40*(3), 285–307. doi:10.1023/A:1018747000082

Leckey, R. (2021). *A year of screens: How more remote work & virtual learning affects our eye health.* https://www.wnep.com/article/entertainment/television/leckey-live/computer-screens-remote-

Lee, J. J., & Miller, S. E. (2013). A self-care framework for social workers: Building a strong foundation for practice. *Families in Society, 94*(2), 96–103.

Lee, J. J., Miller, S. E., & Bride, B. (2020). Development and initial validation of the self-care practices scale. *Social Work*, *65*(1), 21–28. doi:10.1093wwz045 PMID:31846041

Leinbaugh, T., Hazler, R. J., Bradley, C., & Hill, N. R. (2003). Factors influencing counselor educators' subjective sense of well-being. *Counselor Education and Supervision*, *43*(1), 52–64. doi:10.1002/j.1556-6978.2003.tb01829.x

Leiter, M. P., & Maslach, C. (2004). *Areas of worklife: A structured approach to organizational predictors of job burnout. In Emotional and Physiological Processes and Positive Intervention Strategies* (Vol. 3). doi:10.1016/S1479-3555(03)03003-8

Lerner, R. M., & Overton, W. F. (2010). The Handbook of Life-Span Development: Vol. 1. *Cognition, Biology, and Methods*. John Wiley & Sons.

Levecque, K., Anseel, F., De, B. A., Van, H. J., & Gisle, L. (2017). Work organization and mental health problems in PhD students. *Research Policy*, *46*(4), 868–879. doi:10.1016/j.respol.2017.02.008

Lever, N., Mathis, E., & Mayworm, A. (2017). *School mental health is not just for students: Why teacher and school staff wellness matters*. Report on emotional & behavioral disorders in youth. https://www.ncbi.nlm.nih.gov/pmc/articles/PMC6350815/

Levin, S., Scott, C., Yang, M., Leung, M., & Bradley, K. (2020, June 13). *Supporting a Strong, Stable Principal Workforce: What Matters and What Can be Done*. Retrieved from: https://www.nassp.org/wordpress/wp-content/uploads/2020/04/LPI-and-NASSP-Research-Agenda-Final-Report.pdf

Levin, L. S., & Idler, E. L. (1983). Self-care in health. *Annual Review of Public Health*, *4*(1), 181–201.

Levin, S., & Bradley, K. (2019). *Understanding and Addressing Principal Turnover: A Review of the Research*. National Association of Secondary School Principals.

Lewin, K. (1936). *Principles of topological psychology*. McGraw-Hill. doi:10.1037/10019-000

Linley, A., & Joseph, S. (2007). Therapy work and therapists' positive and negative well-being. *Journal of Social and Clinical Psychology*, *26*(3), 385–403. doi:10.1521/jscp.2007.26.3.385

Linos, A., & Kirch, W. (Eds.). (2008). *Promoting health for working women*. Springer.

Lin, S.-H., & Huang, Y.-C. (2014). Life stress and academic burnout. *Active Learning in Higher Education*, *15*(1), 77–90. doi:10.1177/1469787413514651

Loewus, L. (2021, May 4). Why teachers leave—or don't: A look at the numbers. *Education Week*, *5*. https://www.edweek.org/teaching-learning/why-teachers-leave-or-dont-a-look-at-the-numbers/2021/05#:~:text=And%20yet%20about%208%20percent%20of%20teachers%20leave

Lorde, A. (2007). *Sister outsider*. Crossing Press.

Louis, K.S. & Murphy, J. (2017). Trust, caring, and organizational learning: the leader's role. *Journal of Educational Administration*, *55*(1), 103 – 126.

Love, B. (2019). *We want to do more than survive*. Beacon Press.

Loziak, A., Fedáková, D., & Čopková, R. (2020). Work-related Stressors of Female Teachers During Covid-19 School Closure. *Journal of Women's Entrepreneurship and Education*, *3-4*. Advance online publication. doi:10.28934/jwee20.34.pp59-78

Lupton, D. (2013). The digitally engaged patient: Self-monitoring and self-care in the digital health era. *Social Theory & Health*, *11*(3), 256–270.

Luster, J., & Luster, J. (2015). *Calm classroom: In thirty seconds to three minutes, help your students develop self awareness, mental focus, inner calm*. Luster Learning Institute.

Mabry, L., Elliot, D. L., MacKinnon, D. P., Thoemmes, F., & Kuehl, K. S. (2013). Understanding the durability of a fire department wellness program. *American Journal of Health Behavior, 37*(5), 693–702. doi:10.5993/AJHB.37.5.13 PMID:23985292

Madigan, D. J., & Kim, L. E. (2021). Towards an understanding of teacher attrition: A meta-analysis of burnout, job satisfaction, and teachers' intentions to quit. *Teaching and Teacher Education, 105*, 103425. doi:10.1016/j.tate.2021.103425

Magnuson, S., Norem, K., & Lonneman-Doroff, T. (2009). The 2000 cohort of new assistant professors of counselor education: Reflecting at the culmination of six years. *Counselor Education and Supervision, 49*(1), 54–71. doi:10.1002/j.1556-6978.2009.tb00086.x

Mahfouz, J. (2017). Mindfulness Training for School Administrators: effects on wellbeing and leadership. *Journal of Educational Administration, 56*(6), 602 –619.

Maizan Mat @ Muhammad. (2018). Profile of negative emotional levels among lecturers of Selangor International Islamic University College. *Proceeding International Research Management & Innovation Conference (5th IRMIC).*

Maloney, J. V. (2014). Nursing and philanthropy. *Nursing Administration Quarterly, 38*(4), 280–282. doi:10.1097/NAQ.0000000000000052 PMID:25208143

Mannila, L., Nordén, L., & Pears, A. (2018). Digital Competence, teacher self-efficacy and training needs. *Proceedings of the 2018 ACM Conference on International Computing Education Research*. 10.1145/3230977.3230993

Manturuk, K., & Reavis, G. (2022). Pedagogical implications of COVID-19: A case study of what faculty learned about teaching well by teaching remotely during the COVID-19 pandemic. In J. S. McKeown, K. Bista, & R. Y. Chan (Eds.), *Global higher education during COVID-19: Policy, society, and technology* (pp. 154–166). STAR Scholars. https://starscholars.org/product/global-education/

Mardell, B., & Carpenter, B. (2012). Places to Play in Providence Valuing Preschool Children as Citizens. *Young Children, 67*(5), 76–78.

Marimuthu, K. (2019). *Demographic factors and work stress of Kedah PDRM Traffic Investigating Officer* (Master Thesis). Sintok: Universiti Utara Malaysia.

Marino, G. D. (2020). *Ethics: The essential writings*. Modern Library.

Martin, E. M., Myers, K., & Brickman, K. (2020). Self-preservation in the workplace: The importance of well-being for social work practitioners and field supervisors. *Social Work, 65*(1), 74–81. doi:10.1093wwz040 PMID:31846026

Martínez-Mejía, E., Villa-George, F. I., & Martínez-Guerrero, J. I. (2020). Prevalence of Burnout Syndrome in Mexican Employees in Mexico City. *Journal of Basic and Applied Psychology Research, 2*(3), 23–33.

Martin, J. (2020). Teaching without fear: Psychology safety can alter the professional learning landscape. *The Learning Professional, 41*(2), 36–38.

Maruyama, T., Hopkinson, P. G., & James, P. W. (2009). A multivariate analysis of work– life balance outcomes from a large-scale telework programme. *New Technology, Work and Employment, 24*(1), 76–88.

Maslach, C. (1982). *Burnout: The cost of caring*. Malor Book Publisher, ISHK.

Maslach, C., & Jackson, S. E. (1981). The measurement of experienced burnout. *Journal of Organizational Behavior, 2*(2), 99–113. doi:10.1002/job.4030020205

Maslach, C., & Leiter, M. P. (1997). The truth about burnout. San Francisco, CA: Jossey-Bass. Maslach, C. & Leiter, M. P. (2008). Early predictors of job burnout and engagement. *The Journal of Applied Psychology*, *93*(3), 498–512. doi:10.1037/0021-9010.93.3.498 PMID:18457483

Maslach, C., Schaufeli, W. B., & Leiter, M. P. (2001). Job burnout. *Annual Review of Psychology*, *52*(1), 397–422. doi:10.1146/annurev.psych.52.1.397 PMID:11148311

Mason, M. A., Wolfinger, N. H., & Goulden, M. (2013). *Do babies matter: Gender and family in the ivory tower*. Rutgers University Press. doi:10.36019/9780813560823

Mason, M. A., Wolfinger, N. H., & Goulden, M. (2013). *Do babies matter? Gender and family in the ivory tower*. Rutgers University Press.

Masten, A. S., & Motti-Stefanidi, F. (2020). Multisystem resilience for children and youth in disaster: Reflections in the context of Covid-19. *Adv Res Sci, 1*, 95–106. doi:10.1007/s42844-020-00010-w

Matheson, J. L., & Rosen, K. H. (2012). Marriage and family therapy faculty members' balance of work and personal life. *Journal of Marital and Family Therapy*, *38*(2), 394–416. doi:10.1111/j.1752-0606.2009.00137.x PMID:22512300

Maxwell, J. (2016, August 30). *The 5 Levels of Leadership*. John Maxwell. https://www.johnmaxwell.com/blog/the-5-levels-of-leadership1/

Mayer, L. (2013). Empowerment zone: Coaching academy primes teachers to become instructional leaders. *Journal of Staff Development*, *34*(6), 30–33.

McCallum, K. (2020). *Is Excess Screen Time Causing Your Headaches?* Houston Methodist. https://www.houstonmethodist.org/blog/articles/2020/apr/is-extra-screen-time-causing-your-headaches/

McCann, I. L., & Pearlman, L. A. (1990). Vicarious traumatization: A framework for understanding the psychological effects of working with victims. *Journal of Traumatic Stress*, *3*(1), 131–149. doi:10.1007/BF00975140

McCarthy, W. C., & Frieze, I. H. (1999). Negative aspects of therapy: Client perceptions of therapists' social influence, burnout, and quality of care. *The Journal of Social Issues*, *55*(1), 33–50. doi:10.1111/0022-4537.00103

McFadden, P., Moriarty, J., Schröder, H., Gillen, P., Manthorpe, G., & Mallett, J. (2020). Growing older in social work: Perspective on systems of support to extend working lives -Findings from a UK survey. *British Journal of Social Work*, *50*(2), 405–426. doi:10.1093/bjsw/bcz165

McKee, A., Boyatzis, R., & Johnston, F. (2008). *Becoming a resonant leader: Develop your emotional intelligence, renew your relationships, sustain your effectiveness*. Harvard Business Press.

McKimmie, B. M., Butler, T., Chan, E., Rogers, A., & Jimmieson, N. L. (2019). Reducing stress: Social support and group identification. *Group Processes & Intergroup Relations*, *23*(2), 241–261. doi:10.1177/1368430218818733

McLean, L., Abry, T., Taylor, M., Jimenez, M., & Granger, K. (2017). Teachers' mental health and perceptions of school climate across the transition from training to teaching. *Teaching and Teacher Education*, *65*, 230–240. doi:10.1016/j.tate.2017.03.018

Meltzoff, A. N. (2011). Social cognition and the origins of imitation, empathy, and theory of mind. In U. Goswami (Ed.), *The Wiley-Blackwell handbook of childhood cognitive development* (Vol. 2, pp. 49–75). John Wiley & Sons.

Meng, Y., Tan, J., & Li, J. (2017). Abusive supervision by academic supervisors and postgraduate research students' creativity: The mediating role of leader-member exchange and intrinsic motivation. *International Journal of Leadership in Education*, *20*(5), 605–617. doi:10.1080/13603124.2017.1304576

Meng, Y., & Zhao, C. (2018). Academic supervisor leadership and its influencing mechanism on postgraduate creativity in China. *Thinking Skills and Creativity*, *29*, 32–44. doi:10.1016/j.tsc.2018.05.006

Mental Health America. (n.d.). *The state of mental health in America.* https://mhanational.org/issues/state-mental-health-america

MetLife. (2013). *The MetLife Survey of the American Teacher: Challenges for School Leadership.* https://www.metlife.com/content/dam/microsites/about/corporate-profile/MetLife-Teacher-Survey-2012.pdf

Mews, J. G. (2019). Effective leadership in higher education: A review of leadership style preferences among faculty and staff within the United States. *Open Journal of Leadership*, *8*(02), 58–74. doi:10.4236/ojl.2019.82004

Michael, J. (2021). *Remote Work And Mental Health: How To Maximize Your Time For Micro Self-Care.* https://www.forbes.com/sites/forbescoachescouncil/2021/07/19/remote-work-and-mental-health-how-to-maximize-your-time-for-micro-self-care/?sh=122430144a7b

Mielke, C. (2019). *The burnout cure: Learning to love teaching again.* ASCD.

Miller, L. (2020). *How bad is working from home making your tech neck?* EWIWORKS. https://www.ewiworks.com/blog/bad-text-neck/

Miller, M. N., & McGowen, R. (2020). Strategies to avoid burnout in professional practice: Some practical suggestions. *The Psychiatric Times*, *27*(2), 25–25.

Mills, J., Wand, T., & Fraser, J. A. (2018). Exploring the meaning and practice of self-care among palliative care nurses and doctors: A qualitative study. *BMC Palliative Care*, *17*(1), 63. Advance online publication. doi:10.118612904-018-0318-0 PMID:29669559

Minero, E. (2017, October 4). *When students are traumatized, teachers are too.* Edutopia. https://www.edutopia.org/article/when-students-are-traumatized-teachers-are-too

Mohamad, N. I., Ismail, A., Rozi, M. S. A. M., & Ahmad, S. (2015). Work stress and its relation to employee health: An empirical study of a police contingent in Peninsular Malaysia. *Malaysian Journal of Society and Space*, *11*(10), 63–75.

Mohd Akmal Firdaus Mohamad Hamim. (2017). *Kompetensi guru reka cipta dalam bidang elektrik di sekolah menengah harian di Johor (Disertasi Sarjana).* Universiti Tun Hussein Onn Malaysia.

Montaudon-Tomas, C., Pinto-López, C. M., Olivera-Pérez, E., & Amsler, A. (2021). *Informe: El Estado del Trabajo Remoto en México durante la Pandemia de COVID-19. Observatorio de Competitividad y Nuevas Formas de Trabajo.* UPAEP Universidad.

Moore, S. E., Bledsoe, L. K., Perry, A., & Robinson, M. A. (2011). Social work students and self-care: A model assignment for teaching. *Journal of Social Work Education*, *47*(3), 545–553. doi:10.5175/JSWE.2011.201000004

Morales-Cadena, G. M., Fonseca-Salazar, N. F., & Fonseca-Chávez, M. G. (2020). Prevalence of professional burnout syndrome in postgraduate residents of surgical and non-surgical specialties. *Anales de Otorrinolaringología Mexicana*, *65*(2), 64–70.

Moretti, A., Menna, F., Aulicino, M., Paoletta, M., Liguori, S., & Iolascon, G. (2020). Characterization of Home Working Population during COVID-19 Emergency: A Cross-Sectional Analysis. *International Journal of Environmental Research and Public Health*, *17*(17), 6284.

Morgan, G. A., Gliner, J. A., & Harmon, R. (1999). Definition, Purposes, and Dimensions of Research. *Journal of the American Academy of Child and Adolescent Psychiatry, 38*(2), 217–219. doi:10.1097/00004583-199902000-00023 PMID:9951223

Morris, M. (2019). Currere or the Erasure of the Author. *The Currere Exchange Journal, 3*(1), 5–17. https://cej.lib.miamioh.edu/index.php/ CEJ/article/view/10

Mostafa, B. A. (2021). The Effect of Remote Working on Employees Wellbeing and Work-Life Integration during Pandemic in Egypt. *International Business Research, 14*(3), 41–52.

Muhammad, F. M. R., & Abu Bakar, A. Y. (2020). Stress and Job Satisfaction Among Polytechnic Lecturers in Malaysia: A Need Analysis Study. *Bisma The Journal of Counseling, 4*(1), 1–6. doi:10.23887/bisma.v4i1.24708

Munn-Giddings, C., Hart, C., & Ramos, S. (2005). A participatory approach to the promotion of well-being in the workplace: Lessons from empirical research. *International Review of Psychiatry (Abingdon, England), 17*(5), 409–417.

Munroe, J. F. (1999). Ethical Issues associated with secondary trauma in therapists. In H. Stamm (Ed.), *Secondary Traumatic Stress: Self-care issues for clinicians, researchers and educators.* Sidran Press.

Murphey, D., & Sacks, V. (2020, September 10). *Supporting students with adverse childhood experiences.* American Federation of Teachers. https://www.aft.org/ae/summer2019/murphey_sacks

Murphy, J. T. (2011). Dancing in the rain: Tips of thriving as a leader in tough times. *Phi Delta Kappan, 93*, 36-41.

Murphy, J., Louis, K. S., & Smylie, M. (2017). Positive school leadership: How the Professional Standards for Educational Leaders can be brought to life. *Phi Delta Kappan, 99*(1), 21 – 24. . doi:10.1177/0031721717728273

Murphy, M. (2019, November 25). Does Anyone Actually Like Autocratic Leaders? New Data Says Yes. *Forbes.* https://www.forbes.com/sites/markmurphy/2019/11/24/does-anyone-actually-like-autocratic-leaders-new-data-says-yes/?sh=5697cbc610de

Musek, J., & Polic, M. (2014). Personal Well-Being. Encyclopedia of Quality of Life and Well-Being Research. doi:10.1007/978-94-007-0753-5_2148

Myers, J. E., Sweeney, T. J., & Witmer, J. M. (2000). The Wheel of Wellness counseling for wellness: A holistic model for treatment planning. *Journal of Counseling and Development, 78*(3), 251–266. doi:10.1002/j.1556-6676.2000.tb01906.x

NAESP Releases Results of Midyear National Principal Survey on COVID-19 in Schools. (2021, February 20). Retrieved from: https://www.naesp.org/news/naesp-releases-results-of-midyear-national-principal-survey-on-covid-19-in-schools/

Nagamine, M., Shigemura, J., Fujiwara, T., Waki, F., Tanichi, M., Saito, T., Toda, H., Yoshino, A., & Shimizu, K. (2018). The relationship between dispositional empathy, psychological distress, and posttraumatic stress responses among Japanese uniformed disaster workers: A cross-sectional study. *BMC Psychiatry, 18*(1), 328. doi:10.118612888-018-1915-4 PMID:30309334

National Association of Social Workers. (2021). https://www.socialworkers.org/about/ethics/code-of-ethics

National Sleep Foundation. (2006). *Sleep-wake cycle: Its physiology and impact on health.* Author.

Neale-McFall, C., Hermann, M. A., & Eckart, E. (2020). Predictive variables of faculty retention in the counselor education field: A gender perspective. *Journal of Education and Training Studies, 8*(10), 1–9. doi:10.11114/jets.v8i10.4989

Neff, K. D. (2003). Development and validation of a scale to measure self-compassion. *Self and Identity, 2*(3), 223–250. doi:10.1080/15298860309027

Neff, K. D., Kirkpatrick, K. L., & Rude, S. S. (2007). Self-compassion and adaptive psychological functioning. *Journal of Research in Personality, 41*(1), 139–154. doi:10.1016/j.jrp.2006.03.004

Neff, K. D., & Pommier, E. (2013). The relationship between self-compassion and other-focused concern among college undergraduates, community adults, and practicing meditators. *Self and Identity, 12*(2), 160–176. doi:10.1080/15298868.2011.649546

Negash, S., & Sahin, S. (2011). Compassion fatigue in marriage and family therapy: Implications for therapists and clients. *Journal of Marital and Family Therapy, 37*(1), 1–13. doi:10.1111/j.1752-0606.2009.00147.x PMID:21198684

Nelson-Gardell, D., & Harris, D. (2003). Childhood abuse history, secondary traumatic stress, and child welfare workers. *Child Welfare, 82*, 5–26. PMID:12641376

Neumann, A. (2016). Professing passion: Emotion in the scholarship of professors at research universities. *American Educational Research Journal, 43*(3), 381-421. Retrieved January from https://www.jstor.org/stable/4121764

Neuman, S. (1986). Religious observance within a human capital framework: Theory and application. *Applied Economics, 18*(11), 1193–1202. doi:10.1080/00036848600000072

News Center 1. (2020). *How to alleviate digital eye strain while working from home*. https://www.newscenter1.tv/how-to-alleviate-digital-eye-strain-while-working-from-home/

NIH. (2018). *The power of pets: Health benefits of human-animal interactions*. https://newsinhealth.nih.gov/sites/nihNIH/files/2018/February/NIHNiHFeb2018.pdf

Niles, S. G., Akos, P., & Cutler, H. (2001). Counselor educators' strategies for success. *Counselor Education and Supervision, 40*(4), 276–291. doi:10.1002/j.1556-6978.2001.tb01260.x

Nissen-Lie, H. A., Rønnestad, M. H., Høglend, P. A., Havik, O. E., Solbakken, O. A., Stiles, T. C., & Monsen, J. T. (2015). Love yourself as a person, doubt yourself as a therapist? *Clinical Psychology & Psychotherapy.*

Nor Azimah Chew Abdullah. (2016). Konflik Kerja-Keluarga Dalam Kalangan Pensyarah: Satu Tinjauan. *Sains Humanika, 8*(4-2), 131-135.

Norcross, J. C., & Barnett, J. E. (2017). *Self-care as ethical imperative. The Register Report: Spring 2008*. The Guilford Press.

Norcross, J. C., & Guy, J. D. (2007). *Leaving it at the office: A guide to psychotherapist self-care.*

Nugraheny, A. R. (2020). *Peran teknologi, guru dan orang tua dalam pembelajaran daring di masa pandemi*. https://osf.io/preprints/lissa/hz57r/

Nyunt, G., O'Meara, K., Bach, L., & LaFave, A. (2022). Tenure Undone: Faculty Experiences of Organizational Justice When Tenure Seems or Becomes Unattainable. *Equity & Excellence in Education*, 1–15. doi:10.1080/10665684.2021.2010013

Obama, M. (2021). *Becoming*. Crown.

Ohaeri, J. U. (2003). The burden of caregiving in families with a mental illness: A review of 2002. *Current Opinion in Psychiatry, 16*(4), 457–465. doi:10.1097/01.yco.0000079212.36371.c0

Okeke, C. I., & Mtyuda, P. N. (2017). Teacher Job Dissatisfaction: Implications for Teacher Sustainability and Social Transformation. *Journal of Teacher Education for Sustainability, 19*(1), 54–68. doi:10.1515/jtes-2017-0004

Okeke, M. N., Echo, O., & Oboreh, J. C. (2016). Effects of stress on employee productivity. *International Journal of Accounting Research, 42*(3495), 1–12.

Olivo, E. (2015). Two simple mindful meditation exercises for teachers. *The Guardian.* https://www.theguardian.com/teacher-network/2015/dec/06/two-simple-mindful-meditation-exercises-for-teachers

Omisakin, F. D., & Ncama, B. P. (2011). Self, self-care and self-management concepts: Implications for self-management education. *Educational Research, 2*(12), 1733–1737.

Oplatka, I. (2017). Principal workload: Components, determinants and coping strategies in an era of standardization and accountability. *Journal of Educational Administration, 55*(5), 552 – 68. . doi:10.1108/JEA-06-2016-0071

Orem, D. E. (1985). *Nursing: Concepts of practice. 3.* McGraw-Hill.

Ostovar-Nameghi, S. A., & Sheikhahmadi, M. (2016). From teacher isolation to teacher collaboration: Theoretical Perspectives and empirical findings. *English Language Teaching, 9*(5), 197. doi:10.5539/elt.v9n5p197

Panter-Brick, C., & Smith, M. T. (2000). *Abandoned children.* Cambridge University Press.

Parent-Lamarche, A., Marchand, A., & Saade, S. (2020). Does Depression Mediate the Effect of Work Organization Conditions on Job Performance? *Journal of Occupational and Environmental Medicine, 62*(4), 296–302. doi:10.1097/JOM.0000000000001822 PMID:31977926

Park, S. G., Min, K. B., Chang, S. J., Kim, H. C., & Min, J. Y. (2009). Job stress and depressive symptoms among Korean employees: The effects of culture on work. *International Archives of Occupational and Environmental Health, 82*(3), 397–405. doi:10.100700420-008-0347-8 PMID:18622624

Pascoe, M. C., Hetrick, S. E., & Parker, A. G. (2020). The impact of stress on students in secondary school and higher education. *International Journal of Adolescence and Youth, 25*(1), 104–112. doi:10.1080/02673843.2019.1596823

Pate, C. (2020, May). *Self-Care Strategies for Educators During the Coronavirus Crisis.* https://selcenter.wested.org/wp-content/uploads/sites/3/2020/05/Self_Care_Strategies_for_Educators_During_the_Coronavirus_Crisis.pdf

Pearlin, L. I. (1989). The sociological study of stress. *Journal of Health and Social Behavior, 30*(3), 241–256. doi:10.2307/2136956 PMID:2674272

Pearlman, L. A. (1995). Self-care for trauma therapists: Ameliorating vicarious traumatization. In B. H. Stamm (Ed.), *Secondary traumatic stress: Selfcare issues for clinicians, researchers, and educators* (pp. 51–64). Sidran Press.

Pearlman, L. A., & MacIan, P. J. (1995). Vicarious traumatization: An empirical study of the effects of trauma work on trauma therapists. *Professional Psychology, Research and Practice, 26*(6), 558–565. doi:10.1037/0735-7028.26.6.558

Pearlman, L. A., & Saakvitne, K. W. (1995). Treating therapists with vicarious traumatization and secondary traumatic stress disorders. In C. R. Figley (Ed.), *Compassion fatigue: Coping with secondary traumatic stress disorder in those who treat the traumatized* (pp. 150–177). Brunner/Maze.

Pearman, C., Bowles, F., & Polka, W. (2021). Teacher educator perceptions of characteristics of self-efficacy. *Critical Questions in Education, 12*(1), 81–99.

Pembroke, N. (2016). Contributions from Christian ethics and Buddhist philosophy to the management of compassion fatigue in nurses. *Nursing & Health Sciences, 18*(1), 120–124. doi:10.1111/nhs.12252 PMID:26694199

Penedo, F. J., & Dahn, J. R. (2005). Exercise and well-being: A review of mental and physical health benefits associated with physical activity. *Current Opinion in Psychiatry, 18*(2), 189–193. doi:10.1097/00001504-200503000-00013 PMID:16639173

Peters, R. M., & Templin, T. N. (2010). Theory of planned behavior, self-care motivation, and blood pressure self-care. *Research and Theory for Nursing Practice*, *24*(3), 172–186.

Petzko, V. (2008). The perceptions of new principals regarding the knowledge and skills important to their initial success. *NASSP Bulletin*, *92*(3), 242-250. . doi:10.1177/0192636508322824

Pffifferling, J. H., & Gilley, K. (2000). *Compassion fatigue self-assessment.* American Academy of Family Physicians. https://www.aafp.org/fpm/2000/0400/fpm20000400p39-rt1.pdf

Phipps, S. T. A., & Prieto, L.C. (2017). Why Emotional Intelligence Is Necessary For Effective Leadership: Know the four reasons! *Leadership Excellence*, *34*(6), 56 – 57.

Pijanowski, J.C., Hewitt, P.M. & Brady, K.P. (2009). Superintendents' perceptions of the principal shortage. *NASSP Bulletin*, *93*(2), 85 – 95.

Pinar, W. (1975). Currere: toward reconceptualization. In W. F. Pinar (Ed.), Curriculum theorizing: The reconceptualists (pp. 396–414). Academic Press.

Pinar, W. F. (2019). Currere. In Key Concepts in Curriculum Studies (pp. 50–52). Routledge.

Pinar, W. F. (2012). *What is curriculum theory?* Routledge.

Pliner, S. M., Iuzzini, J., & Banks, C. A. (2011). Using an intersectional approach to deepen collaborative teaching. *New Directions for Teaching and Learning*, *2011*(125), 43–51. doi:10.1002/tl.432

Poetter, T. S. (2020). The thicket. *Currere Exchange Journal*, *4*(2), 1–15. https://cej.lib.miamioh.edu/ index.php/CEJ/article/view/128

Poetter, T. S. (2012). *Teaching again: A professor's tale of returning to a ninth grade classroom*. Information Age Publishing.

Porter, R. (2021). *Is COVID-19 Causing Carpal Tunnel?* Korn Ferry. https://www.kornferry.com/insights/this-week-in-leadership/is-covid-19-causing-carpal-tunnel

Potratz, A. (2020). *Managing remote workers during the COVID-19 Pandemi*. https://ohsonline.com/Articles/2020/08/09/Managing-Remote-Workers-During-the-COVID-19-Pandemic.aspx?Page=7

Potratz, A. (2020). *Managing remote workers during the COVID-19 Pandemic*. https://ohsonline.com/Articles/2020/08/09/Managing-Remote-Workers-During-the-COVID-19-Pandemic.aspx?Page=7

Premack, D., & Woodruff, G. (1978). Does the chimpanzee have a theory of mind? *Behavioral and Brain Sciences*, *1*(4), 515–526. doi:10.1017/S0140525X00076512

Pressley, T. (2021). Factors contributing to teacher burnout during COVID-19. *Educational Researcher*, *50*(5), 325–327. Advance online publication. doi:10.3102/0013189X211004138

Previsor Insurance. (2020). *Tips to Avoid Work-Related Injuries While Working from Home*. https://previsorinsurance.com/blog/tips-to-avoid-work-related-injuries-while-working-from-home/

Price, D., & McCallum, F. (2015). Ecological influences on teachers' well-being and "fitness.". *Asia-Pacific Journal of Teacher Education*, *43*(3), 195–209. doi:10.1080/1359866X.2014.932329

Qi, C. (2019). A double-edged sword? Exploring the impact of students' academic usage of mobile devices on technostress and academic performance. *Behaviour & Information Technology*, *38*(12), 1337–1354. doi:10.1080/0144929X.2019.1585476

Radey, M., & Figley, C. R. (2007). The social psychology of compassion. *Clinical Social Work Journal, 35*(3), 207–214. doi:10.100710615-007-0087-3

Ragu-Nathan, T. S., Tarafdar, M., Ragu-Nathan, B. S., & Tu, Q. (2008). The consequences of technostress for end users in organizations: Conceptual Development and empirical validation. *Information Systems Research, 19*(4), 417–433. doi:10.1287/isre.1070.0165

Rahim, N. A., & Yatim, N. M. (2017). *Hubungan Kepuasan Kerja Terhadap Prestasi Kerja Dalam Kalangan Pensyarah: Satu Kajian Di Kolej Komuniti Bukit Beruang Melaka*. Academic Press.

Rai, S. (2021, April). *Teaching and the New Education Policy*. The Tribute. https://www.tribuneindia.com/news/schools/teaching-and-the-new-education-policy-240818

Ramachandran, V. (2005). Why School Teachers Are Demotivated and Disheartened. *Economic and Political Weekly*.

Ramlee, N. (2015). *Tahap Stress dalam Kalangan Pensyarah Kolej Vokasional di Johor*. Tesis Sarjana. Universiti Tun Husseion Onn Malaysia.

Rand, A., & Branden, N. (1970). *The virtue of selfishness: A new concept of egoism*. Signet/New American Library.

Ransdell, S. (2020). *Teacher Self-Care*. Cambridge Scholars Publishing. http://www.cambridgescholars.com/teacher-self-care

Rapanta, C., Botturi, L., Goodyear, P., Guàrdia, L., & Koole, M. (2020). Online university teaching during and after the COVID-19 crisis: Refocusing teacher presence and learning activity. *Postdigital Science and Education, 2*(3), 923–945. doi:10.100742438-020-00155-y

Rathakrishnan, M. (2020). Covid -19 Ubah Pengajaran dan Pembelajaran dari Rumah. *BH Online*. https://www.bharian.com.my/rencana/komentar/2020/07/710464/covid-19

Rauvola, R. S., Vega, D. M., & Lavigne, K. N. (2019). Compassion Fatigue, Secondary Traumatic Stress, and Vicarious Traumatization: A Qualitative Review and Research Agenda. Occupational Health Science, 3, 297–336. doi:10.100741542-019-00045-1

Reeves, D. B., & Allison, E. (2009). *Renewal coaching: Sustainable change for individuals and organizations*. Jossey-Bass.

Reeves, D. B., & Allison, E. (2010). *Renewal coaching workbook*. Jossey-Bass.

Reevy, G., & Deason, G. (2014). Predictors of depression, stress, and anxiety among non-tenure track faculty. *Frontiers in Psychology, 5*(701), 1–17. doi:10.3389/fpsyg.2014.00701 PMID:25071667

Regional Educational Laboratory at Mathematica Policy Research. (2019, March). *What are effective school leaders, and how can states and districts develop them?* REL Mid-Atlantic. https://ies.ed.gov/ncee/edlabs/regions/midatlantic/pdf/RELMA_Characteristics_effective_school_leaders_fact_sheet.pdf

Rego, A., Sousa, F., Marques, C., & Cunha, M. (2012). Authentic leadership promoting employees' psychological capital and creativity. *Journal of Business Research, 65*(3), 429–437. doi:10.1016/j.jbusres.2011.10.003

Richards, R. (2020, May 21). *Improve teacher wellbeing with self-care strategies and formalized peer connections*. EAB. https://eab.com/insights/blogs/district-leadership/improve-teacher-wellbeing/

Rietman, G. C., & Karge, B. D. (2019). Investing in teacher support leads to teacher retention: Six supports administrators should consider for new teachers. *School Administration, Multicultural Education, and Inclusion, 27*(1), 7–18.

Ringkasan Eksekutif Pelan Pembangunan Pendidikan Malaysia 2015-2025 (Pendidikan Tinggi). (n.d.). *Kementerian Pendidikan Malaysia*. Retrieved on 16 March 2022 https://www.mohe.gov.my/muat-turun/penerbitan-jurnal-dan-laporan/pppm-2015-2025pt/104-ringkasan-eksekutif-pppm-2015-2025/file

Roberts, A., & Kim, H. (2019, May 6). *To promote success in schools, focus on teacher well-being*. Education Plus Development. https://www.brookings.edu/blog/education-plus-development/2019/05/06/to-promote-success-in-schools-focus-on-teacher-well-being/

Robertson, D. A., Padesky, L. R., & Brock, C. H. (2020). Cultivating student agency through teachers' professional learning. *Theory into Practice*, *59*(2), 192–201. doi:10.1080/00405841.2019.1705090

Robinson, L., Smith, M., & Segal, J. (2021). *Laughter is the best medicine*. https://www.helpguide.org/articles/mental-health/laughter-is-the-best-medicine.htm?pdf=13511

Robinson, K. J., Mayer, S., Allen, A. B., Terry, M., Chilton, A., & Leary, M. R. (2016). Resisting self-compassion: Why are some people opposed to being kind to themselves? *Self and Identity*, *15*(5), 505–524. doi:10.1080/15298868.2016.1160952

Roeser, R., Skinner, E., Beers, J., & Jennings, P. (2012). Mindfulness Training and Teachers' Professional Development: An Emerging Area of Research and Practice Child Development Perspectives. *Child Development Perspectives, 6*(2), 167-173. doi:10.1111/j.1750-8606.2012.00238.x

Roos, B. H., & Borkoski, C. C. (2021). Attending to the teacher in teaching: Prioritizing faculty well-being. *Perspectives of the ASHA Special Interest Groups*, *6*(4), 831–840. doi:10.1044/2021_PERSP-21-00006

Ropers-Huilman, B. (2000). Are you satisfied yet? Women faculty members' interpretations of their academic work. *New Directions for Institutional Research*, *2000*(105), 21–32. doi:10.1002/ir.10502

Ross, K. T., & Squires, P. (2015). Tone at the top: Leadership as the foundation of organizational health and wellness. *People & Strategy*, *38*(1), 36–41.

Rudolph, J. M., Stamm, B. H., & Stamm, H. E. (1997). *Compassion fatigue: A concern for mental health policy, providers, & administration.* In Poster presentation at the Annual Meeting of the International Society for Traumatic Stress Studies, Montreal, Canada.

Sabin-Farrell, R., & Turpin, G. (2003). Vicarious traumatization: Implications for the mental health of health workers? *Clinical Psychology Review*, *23*(3), 449–480. doi:10.1016/S0272-7358(03)00030-8 PMID:12729680

Salston, M., & Figley, C. R. (2003). Secondary traumatic stress effects of working with survivors of criminal victimization. *Journal of Traumatic Stress*, *16*(2), 167–174. doi:10.1023/A:1022899207206 PMID:12699204

Sameroff, A. J., & Fiese, B. H. (2000). Transactional regulation: The developmental ecology of early intervention. In J. P. Shonkoff & S. J. Meisels (Eds.), *Handbook of early childhood intervention* (revised edition, Vol. 2, pp. 135–159). Cambridge University Press. doi:10.1017/CBO9780511529320.009

Sánchez, B. (2020). *Coronavirus and Sleep: How Work From Home Has Affected Americans' Bedtime Habits.* The Active Times. https://www.theactivetimes.com/coronavirus-work-from-home-sleep

Sandorf, B. (2019). *Home Accident Statistics: Is Your Home as Safe as You Think?* https://www.asecurelife.com/home-accident-statistics/

Santos, L. (n.d.). *The Science of Well-Being*. Dr. Laurie Santos. https://www.drlauriesantos.com/science-well-being

Schafer, W. (1996). *Stress management for wellness*. Harcourt Brace.

Schauben, L. J., & Frazier, P. A. (1995). Vicarious trauma: The effects on female counselors of working with sexual violence survivors. *Psychology of Women Quarterly*, *19*(1), 49–64. doi:10.1111/j.1471-6402.1995.tb00278.x

Scherer, R., & Teo, T. (2019). Unpacking teachers' intentions to integrate technology: A meta-analysis. *Educational Research Review*, *27*, 90–109. doi:10.1016/j.edurev.2019.03.001

Schimanski, L. A., & Alperin, J. P. (2018). The evaluation of scholarship in academic promotion and tenure processes: Past, present, and future. *F1000 Research*, *7*(1605), 1–20. doi:10.12688/f1000research.16493.1 PMID:30647909

Schmitz, T. (2016, October 28). *Empathy - empathetic listening*. The Conover Company. Retrieved from https://www.conovercompany.com/empathy-empathetic-listening/

Schuldt, B., & Totten, J. (2008). An exploratory study: Business faculty and the faculty stress index. *Proceedings of the Allied Academies*, *13*(2), 128–133.

Schultz, T. W. (1961). Investment in human capital. *The American Economic Review*, *51*(1), 1–17.

Schultz, T. W. (1971). *Investment in human capital. The role of education and of research.* The Free Press.

Schwartz, K. (2016). *I wish my teacher knew: How one question can change everything for our kids*. Da Capo Lifelong Books, a member of the Perseus Books Group.

Scott, E. (2020, August 3). *5 Self-Care Practices for Every Area of Your Life*. Verywell Mind. https://www.verywellmind.com/self-care-strategies-overall-stress-reduction-3144729

Scott, E. (2021). *8 Tips to Handle the Stress of Working From Home*. https://www.verywellmind.com/the-stress-of-working-from-home-4141174

Seipel, M. T., & Larson, L. M. (2018). Supporting non-tenure-track faculty well-being. *Journal of Career Assessment*, *26*(1), 154–171. doi:10.1177/1069072716680046

Selye, H. (1976a). The stress of life. McGraw-Hill.

Selye, H. (1976b). Stress without distress. In G. Serban (Ed.), *Psychopathology of human adaptation* (pp. 137–146). Springer. doi:10.1007/978-1-4684-2238-2_9

Shah, P. F. (2020). *Working Remotely? Here Are 21 Self-Care Tips For Remote Workers Thrive Gobal*. https://thriveglobal.com/stories/working-remotely-here-are-21-self-care-tips-for-remote-workers/

Shah, D. T., Williams, V. N., Thorndyke, L. E., Marsh, E. E., Sonnino, R. E., Block, S. M., & Viggiano, T. R. (2018). Restoring faculty vitality in academic medicine when burnout threatens. *Academic Medicine*, *93*(7), 979–984. doi:10.1097/ACM.0000000000002013 PMID:29166355

Sham, F. M. (2005). Tekanan emosi remaja Islam. *Jurnal Islamiyat*, *27*(1), 3–24.

Shanafelt, T., Trockel, M., Rodriguez, A., & Logan, D. (2021). Wellness-centered leadership: Equipping health care leaders to cultivate physician well-being and professional fulfillment. *Academic Medicine*, *96*(5), 641–651. doi:10.1097/ACM.0000000000003907 PMID:33394666

Shanker, S. (2020, June 20). *What is Shanker Self-Reg?* www.self-reg.ca/self-reg

Shanker, S. (2013). *Calm, alert and learning: Classroom strategies for self-regulation*. Pearson.

Sharmaa, U., Sokalb, L., Wangc, M., & Loreman, T. (2021). Measuring the use of inclusive practices among pre-service educators:A multi-national study. *Teaching and Teacher Education*, *107*, 2–9. doi:10.1016/j.tate.2021.103506

Sharrocks, L. (2014). School staff perceptions of well-being and experience of an intervention to promote well-being. *Educational Psychology in Practice, 30*(1), 19–36. doi:10.1080/02667363.2013.868787

Shepherd, M. A., & Newell, J. M. (2020). Stress and health in social workers: Implications for self-care practice. *Best Practices in Mental Health, 16*(1), 46–65.

Shirey, M. R. (2015). Enhance your self-awareness to be an authentic leader. *American Nurse Today, 10*(8). http://www.americannursetoday.com/enhance-self-awareness-authentic-leader/

Showalter, S. E. (2010). Compassion Fatigue: What Is It? Why Does It Matter? Recognizing the Symptoms, Acknowledging the Impact, Developing the Tools to Prevent Compassion Fatigue, and Strengthen the Professional Already Suffering From the Effects. *The American Journal of Hospice & Palliative Care, 27*(4), 239–242. doi:10.1177/1049909109354096 PMID:20075423

Siegel, D. J. (2015). *Brainstorm: The power and purpose of the teenage brain.* Penguin Books.

Siejka, A. (2016). Tail waggin' tutors. *Children & Libraries, 14*(2), 32–33.

Sinclair, S., Raffin-Bouchal, S., Venturato, L., Mijovic-Kondejewski, J., & Smith-MacDonald, L. (2017). Compassion fatigue: A meta-narrative review of the healthcare literature. *International Journal of Nursing Studies, 69*, 9–24. doi:10.1016/j.ijnurstu.2017.01.003 PMID:28119163

Singh, H. (2020, July 14). *Official languages in Indian Constitution.* https://www.jagranjosh.com/general-knowledge/official-language-in-indian-constitution-1438068790-1

Skorupa, J., & Agresti, A. A. (1993). Ethical beliefs about burnout and continued professional practice. *Professional Psychology, Research and Practice, 24*(3), 281–285. doi:10.1037/0735-7028.24.3.281

Skovholt, T. M., Morgan, J., & Cunningham, H. N. (1989). Mental imagery in career counseling and life planning: A review of research and intervention methods. *Journal of Counseling and Development, 67*(5), 287–291. doi:10.1002/j.1556-6676.1989.tb02604.x

Skovholt, T. M., Rønnestad, M. H., & Jennings, L. (1997). Searching for Expertise in Counseling, Psychotherapy, and Professional Psychology. *Educational Psychology Review, 9*(4), 361–369. doi:10.1023/A:1024798723295

Smiley, A. (2020, February 7). *Why School Wellness Isn't Just for Kids: Many Teachers are Stressed and Depressed.* Occupational Health & Safety. https://ohsonline.com/articles/2020/02/07/why-school-wellness-isnt-just-for-kids-many-teachers-are-stressed-and-depressed.aspx

Sogunro, O. A. (2012). Stress in school administration: Coping tips for principals. *Journal of School Leadership, 22*, 664 – 700.

Sood, S. (2020). Psychological effects of the Coronavirus disease-2019 pandemic. *RHiME., 7*, 23–26.

Sorenson, R. D. (2007). Stress management in education: Warning signs and coping mechanisms. *Management in Education, 21*(3), 10 – 13. doi:10.1177/089202607077985

Sorenson, C., Bolick, B., Wright, K., & Hamilton, R. (2016). Understanding compassion fatigue in healthcare providers: A review of current literature. *Journal of Nursing Scholarship, 48*(5), 456–465. doi:10.1111/jnu.12229 PMID:27351469

Soulen, R. R. (2020). The continuum of care: A model of collaboration with new teachers. *Knowledge Quest, 48*(4), 36–42.

Sowani, D. A., & Lavalekar, A. (2020). Exploring psychological well-being of college students in relation to college classroom environment. *International Journal of Education and Management Studies, 10*(4), 428–433.

Stamm, B. H. (1995). Preface. In B. H. Stamm (Ed.), *Secondary traumatic stress: Self-care issues for clinicians, researchers, and educators* (pp. ix–xii). Sidran Press.

Stamm, B. H. (1997). Work-related secondary traumatic stress. *PTSD Research Quarterly*, *8*(2).

Stange, J. (2021). *6 Ways to Support Remote Worker Wellbeing*. Quantum Workplace. https://www.quantumworkplace.com/future-of-work/remote-worker-wellbeing

Staniscia, B., Deravignone, L., González-Martín, B., & Pumares, P. (2021). Youth mobility and the development of human capital: Is there a Southern European model? *Journal of Ethnic and Migration Studies*, *47*(8), 1866–1882. doi:10.1080/1369183X.2019.1679417

Stapp, A. C., & Lambert, A. B. (2020). The impact of mindfulness-based yoga interventions on fifth-grade students' perceived anxiety and stress. *International Electronic Journal of Elementary Education*, *12*(5), 471–480. doi:10.26822/iejee.2020562137

Starr Commonwealth. (2020, February 13). *The national institute for trauma and loss in children (TLC)*. https://starr.org/programs/national-institute-for-trauma-and-loss-in-children-tlc/

Steele, D. (2018, May 24). *Teaching's far from a 9-to-3:30 job: Here's what our day really entails*. ABC News. https://www.abc.net.au/news/2018-05-24/teachers-pay-teaching-profession-hours-duties-education/9786176

Stevanovic, P., & Rupert, P. A. (2004). Career-sustaining behaviors, satisfactions, and stresses of professional psychologists. *Psychotherapy (Chicago, Ill.)*, *41*(3), 301–309. doi:10.1037/0033-3204.41.3.301

Stinchfield, T. A., & Trepal, H. (2010). Academic motherhood for counselor educators: Navigating through the academic pipeline. *International Journal for the Advancement of Counseling*, *32*(2), 91–100. doi:10.100710447-009-9086-0

Strauss, J. L., Hayes, A. M., Johnson, S. L., Newman, C. F., Brown, G. K., Barber, J. P., Laurenceau, J.-P., & Beck, A. T. (2006). Early alliance, alliance ruptures, and symptom change in a nonrandomized trial of cognitive therapy for avoidant and obsessive-compulsive personality disorders. *Journal of Consulting and Clinical Psychology*, *74*(2), 337–345. doi:10.1037/0022-006X.74.2.337 PMID:16649878

Stress and the Family. (2016). *Coping with Catastrophe* (C. R. Figley, Ed.). Academic Press.

Su, A. J. (2017). 6 Ways to Weave Self-Care into Your Workday. *Harvard Business Review*. https://hbr.org/2017/06/6-ways-to-weave-self-care-into-your-workday

Sunarsi, D. (2020). The Analysis of The Work Environmental and Organizational Cultural Impact on The Performance and Implication of The Work Satisfaction. *Jurnal Ilmiah Ilmu Administrasi Publik*, *9*(2), 237-246. doi:10.26858/jiap.v9i2.11761

Surcher, L., Darling-Hammond, L., & Carver-Thomas. (2016, September 15). *A Coming Crisis in Teaching? Teacher supply, demand, and shortages in the U.S.* Learning Policy Institute. https://learningpolicyinstitute.org/product/coming-crisis-teaching

Sutcher, L., Darling-Hammond, L., & Carver-Thomas, D. (2016). *A coming crisis in teaching? Teacher supply, demand, and shortages in the U.S. Learning Policy Institute*. Learning Policy Institute. https://learningpolicyinstitute.org/

Sweeney, T. J., & Witmer, J. M. (1991). Beyond social interest: Striving toward optimum health and wellness. *Individual Psychology: The Journal of Adlerian Theory. Research & Practice*, *47*(4), 527–540.

Sweeny, K., Howell, J. L., & Kwan, V. W. (2020). Losing control: Comparing the role of personality during two types of stressful life experiences. *Personality and Individual Differences*, *156*, 109771. doi:10.1016/j.paid.2019.109771

Syrek, C., Kühnel, J., Vahle-Hinz, T., & Bloom, J. (2021). Being an accountant, cook, entertainer and teacher—all at the same time: Changes in employees' work and work-related well-being during the coronavirus (COVID -19) pandemic. *International Journal of Psychology*. Advance online publication. doi:10.1002/ijop.12761 PMID:33826148

Sze, W. Y., Surat, S., & Amat, S. (2022). Teacher pressures and challenges towards new norms during the covid-19 pandemic in a Sarawak State District. *Malaysian Journal of Social Sciences and Humanities*, *7*(1), 230–239.

Tagurum, Y., Okonoda, K., Miner, C., Bello, D., & Tagurum, D. (2017). Effect of technostress on job performance and coping strategies among academic staff of a tertiary institution in north-central Nigeria. *International Journal of Biomedical Research*, *8*(6), 312–319.

Tajudeen, A. B. A. (2004). *Kepuasan kerja dan tekanan yang dihadapi oleh guru sekolah menengah.* Retrieved from http://psasir.upm.edu.my/6399/1/FPP_2004_20(1-%0A24).pdf%0A

Takamatsu, R. (2018). Turning off the empathy switch: Lower empathic concern for the victim leads to utilitarian choices of action. *PLoS One*, *13*(9), e0203826. doi:10.1371/journal.pone.0203826 PMID:30212541

Tambi & Awang. (2019). Hubungan Antara Tekanan Kerja Dan Kecerdasan Emosi Terhadap Kepuasan Kerja Dalam Kalangan Pensyarah Fakulti Sains Sosial Dan Kemanusiaan, Universiti Kebangsaan Malaysia. *Journal of Social Sciences and Humanities, 16*(5), 1-19.

Tan, S. Y., & Castillo, M. (2014). Self-care and beyond: A brief literature review from a Christian perspective. *Journal of Psychology and Christianity*, *33*(1), 90–95.

Taylor, S. G., & Renpenning, K. M. (2021). *Self-care science, nursing theory, and evidence-based practice.* Retrieved from http://lghttp.48653.nexcesscdn.net/80223CF/springer-

Taylor, M. (2018). Using CALMERSS to enhance teacher well-being: A pilot study. *International Journal of Disability Development and Education*, *65*(3), 243–261. doi:10.1080/1034912X.2017.1394985

Temple, J. (1999). A positive effect of human capital on growth. *Economics Letters*, *65*(1), 131–134. doi:10.1016/S0165-1765(99)00120-2

Tengku Sarina Aini Tengku Kasim & Fatimah Sahida AbduRajak. (2018). Pengalaman pengajaran guru novis Pendidikan Islam: Implikasi terhadap reka bentuk kurikulum latihan pendidikan guru. *Jurnal Pendidikan Malaysia*, *43*(1), 59–66.

The Center for Occupational Safety. (2020). *Mobile work and remote work.* Finlandia. https://ttk.fi/en/well-being_at_work_and_occupational_health_and_safety/the_basics_for_occupational_safety_and_health/work_environment/mobile_work_and_remote_work

The Chronicle of Higher Education. (2021). *"On the Verge of Burnout" Covid-19's impact on faculty well-being and career plans.* https://connect.chronicle.com/rs/931-EKA-218/images/Covid%26FacultyCareerPaths_Fidelity_ResearchBrief_v3%20%281%29.pdf

The Crisis Intervention and Suicide Prevention Centre of BC. (2013). *Coping & self-care.* Retrieved from https://crisiscentre.bc.ca/coping-and-self-care/

The Pennsylvania State University. (2016, September). *Teacher health and stress.* https://www.prevention.psu.edu/uploads/files/rwjf430428-TeacherStress.pdf

Thoits, P. A. (1986). Social support as coping assistance. *Journal of Consulting and Clinical Psychology*, *54*(4), 416–423. doi:10.1037/0022-006X.54.4.416 PMID:3745593

Thoits, P. A. (1995). Stress, coping, and social support processes: Where are we? What next? *Journal of Health and Social Behavior, 35*, 53–79. doi:10.2307/2626957 PMID:7560850

Thoits, P. A. (2011). Mechanisms linking social ties and support to physical and mental health. *Journal of Health and Social Behavior, 52*(2), 145–161. doi:10.1177/0022146510395592 PMID:21673143

Thomas, J. (2013). Association of personal distress with burnout, compassion fatigue, and compassion satisfaction among clinical social workers. *Journal of Social Service Research, 39*(3), 365–379. doi:10.1080/01488376.2013.771596

Tomlin, A. D. (2021). *When they see us: Narratives of black male teachers*. Dissertation. University of Maryland.

Tomlin, A. D. (2022b, January 12). 4 Strategies to Foster Equity and Inclusion in the Classroom. *Interfolio*. https://www.interfolio.com/resources/blog/four-strategies-to-foster-equity-and-inclusion-in-the-classroom/

Tomlin, A. D., & Hoey, D. M. (2021). *4 Tips for gaining/progressing in an administrative appointment*. Available online: https://www.interfolio.com/resources/blog/four-tips-for-progressing-in-an-administrative-appointment/

Tomlin, A. D. (2022c). I'm a black PhD, and I still have to fight! In A. Allen & J. Stewart (Eds.), *We are not okay: Black faculty experiences & higher education strategies*. Cambridge University Press. doi:10.1017/9781009064668.005

Tomlin, A. D. (Ed.). (2022a). *Working while black: The untold stories of student affairs practitioners*. Information Age Publishing.

Torres, M. (2020). *This Is What Happens To Your Body When You Work From Home*. Huffpost. https://www.huffpost.com/entry/what-happens-body-work-from-home_l_5e84bfb5c5b6a1bb765185df

Towbes, L. C., & Cohen, L. H. (1996). Chronic stress in the lives of college students: Scale development and prospective prediction of distress. *Journal of Youth and Adolescence, 25*(2), 199–217. doi:10.1007/BF01537344

Tschannen-Moran, M., & Gareis, C. R. (2004). Principals' Sense of Efficacy. *Journal of Educational Administration, 42*, 573 – 585. . doi:10.1108/09578230410554070

TTT4U. (n.d.). *How to create a teacher vision board to visualize your goals*. https://www.teachandtaketime4u.com/2018/03/08/create-teacher-vision-board/

Tutt, P. (2021, August 12). *You Can't Lead on Empty: Supporting School Staff with Vicarious Trauma*. Edutopia. https://www.edutopia.org/ article/ you – cant – lead – empty – supporting – staff – vicarious - trauma? Utm _ content = linkpos9 &utm _ source = edu – newsletter &utm _ medium = email &utm _ campaign = weekly – 2021 – 08 – 18 - A

Tzima, S., Styliaras, G., & Bassounas, A. (2019). Augmented reality applications in education: Teachers point of view. *Education Sciences, 9*(2), 99. doi:10.3390/educsci9020099

UC Davis Health. (2020). *COVID-19 is wrecking our sleep with coronasomnia – tips to fight back*. https://health.ucdavis.edu/health-news/newsroom/covid-19-is-wrecking-our-sleep-with-coronasomnia--tips-to-fight-back-/2020/09#:~:text=And%20a%20report%20from%20the,a%20surprise%20to%20no%20one

Udipi, S., Veach, P. M., Kao, J., & LeRoy, B. S. (2008). The psychic costs of empathic engagement: Personal and demographic predictors of genetic counselor compassion fatigue. *Journal of Genetic Counseling, 17*(5), 459–471. doi:10.100710897-008-9162-3 PMID:18704664

Unimap Academic Regulations for Postgraduate Research Programs. (2021). Retrieved on 14 March 2022. https://cgs.unimap.edu.my/images/REGULATIONS/R.pdf

University at Buffalo. (2017). *Introduction to self-care*. Retrieved from https://socialwork.buffalo.edu/resources/self-care-starter-kit/introduction-to-self-care.htm

University of Michigan. (2017). *Ten things you can do for your mental health* Retrieved from https://www.uhs.umich.edu/tenthings

UNUM. (2020). *Remote working and the risks to physical health.* https://www.unum.co.uk/resources/remote-working-and-the-risks-to-physical-health

Upham, B. (2021). *The Link Between Migraine Headache and Neck Pain.* Everyday Health. https://www.everydayhealth.com/migraine/the-link-between-migraine-headache-and-neck-pain/

Valcour, M. (2016). Beating Burnout. *Harvard Business Review.* https://hbr.org/2016/11/beating-burnout

Valente, V., & Marotta, A. (2015). The impact of yoga on the professional and personal life of the psychotherapist. *Contemporary Family Therapy, 27*(1), 65–80. doi:10.100710591- 004-1971-4

van der Kolk, B. A. (2014). *The body keeps the score: Brain, mind, and body in the healing of trauma.* Penguin Books.

Varanasi, R. A., Vashistha, A., Kizilcec, R. F., & Dell, N. (2021). Investigating technostress among teachers in low-income Indian Schools. *Proceedings of the ACM on Human-Computer Interaction, 5*(CSCW2), 1-29. 10.1145/3476081

Vekeman, E., Devos, G., Valcke, M., & Rosseel, Y. (2017). Do teachers leave the profession or move to another school when they don't fit? *Educational Review, 69*(4), 411–434. doi:10.1080/00131911.2016.1228610

VIA Institute on Character. (n.d.). *Bring Your Strengths to Life & Live More Fully.* https://www.viacharacter.org/

Viner, R. (1999). Putting stress in life: Hans Selye and the making of stress theory. *Social Studies of Science, 29*(3), 391–410. doi:10.1177/030631299029003003

Vision Health. (2020). *Tips to Reduce Eye Strain When Working From Home.* https://www.deltadentalia.com/a-healthy-life/vision-health/tips-to-reduce-eye-strain-when-working-from-home/

Vitello-Cicciu, J. M., Weatherford, B., Gemme, D., Glass, B., & Seymour-Route, P. (2014). The effectiveness of a leadership development program on self-awareness in practice. *The Journal of Nursing Administration, 44*(3), 170–174. doi:10.1097/nna.0000000000000046

Volberg, R. A., Gupta, R., Griffiths, M. D., Ólason, D. T., & Delfabbro, P. (2011). An international perspective on youth gambling prevalence studies. In Youth Gambling (pp. 21-56). De Gruyter. doi:10.1515/9783110255690.21

Wagoner, R. L., & Star, H. (2021). Confronting Ourselves: An Autoethnographic Approach to Whiteness in Higher Education. In K. R. Roth & Z. S. Ritter (Eds.), *Whiteness, Power, and Resisting Change in US Higher Education.* Palgrave Studies in Race, Inequality and Social Justice in Education. Palgrave Macmillan. doi:10.1007/978-3-030-57292-1_3

Waite, R., Mckinney, N., Smith-Glasgow, M., & Meloy, F. (2014). The embodiment of authentic leadership. *Journal of Professional Nursing, 30*(4), 282–291. doi:10.1016/j.profnurs.2013.11.004

Walker, T. (2021, June 17). *Educators ready for fall, but a teacher shortage looms.* NEA. https://www.nea.org/advocating-for-change/new-from-nea/educators-ready-fall-teacher-shortage-looms

Walters, R. (2021). *9 self-care strategies for remote workers.* https://www.robertwalters.com.br/en/hiring/hiring-advice/9-self-care-strategies-for-remote-workers.html

Walumbwa, F. O., Avolio, B. J., Gardner, W. L., Wernsing, T. S., & Peterson, S. J. (2018). Authentic leadership: Development and validation of a theory-based measure. *Journal of Management, 34*(1), 89–126. doi:10.1177/0149206307308913

Wang, J., Straubhaar, R., & Ong, C. (2020). Teacher and administrator experiences with teacher recruitment, retention, and support in a California charter-led turnaround school. *Inquiry in Education, 12*(1), 1–17.

Wang, X., Hegde, S., Son, C., Keller, B., Smith, A., & Sasangohar, F. (2020). Investigating mental health of US college students during the COVID-19 pandemic: Cross-sectional survey study. *Journal of Medical Internet Research, 22*(9), e22817. doi:10.2196/22817 PMID:32897868

Wang, X., & Li, B. (2019). Technostress among university teachers in Higher Education: A study using Multidimensional person-environment misfit theory. *Frontiers in Psychology, 10*, 1791. Advance online publication. doi:10.3389/fpsyg.2019.01791 PMID:31447734

Ward, K., & Wolf-Wendel, L. (2004). Academic motherhood: Managing complex roles in research universities. *Review of Higher Education, 27*(2), 233–257. doi:10.1353/rhe.2003.0079

Wearing, J., Ingersoll, M., DeLuca, C., Bolden, B., Ogden, H., & Christou, T. M. (Eds.). (2019). *Key Concepts in Curriculum Studies: Perspectives on the Fundamentals*. Routledge. doi:10.4324/9781351167086

Weber, M. (2001). *The Protestant Ethic Debate Max Weber's Replies to His Critics, 1907–1910*. Liverpool University Press.

Wells, C. M. (2013a). Educational leaders describe a job too big for one: Stress reduction in the midst of leading. *AASA Journal of Scholarship & Practice, 10*(3), 32 – 45.

Wells, C.M. (2015). Conceptualizing Mindful Leadership in Schools: How the Practice of Mindfulness Informs the Practice of Leading. *Education Leadership Review of Doctoral Research, 2*(1).

West, D. L., Peck, C. M., Reitzug, U. C., & Crane, E. A. (2014). Accountability, autonomy, and stress: Principal responses to superintendent change in a large U.S. urban school district. *School Leadership & Management, 34*, 372 – 39. doi:10.1080/136324.2014.928683

Wester, K. L., Trepal, H. C., & Myers, J. E. (2009). Wellness of counselor educators: An initial look. *Journal of Humanistic Counseling, Education, and Supervision, 48*(1), 91–109. doi:10.1002/j.2161-1939.2009.tb00070.x

What is Stress. (2021, September 18). *American Institute of Stress*. https://www.stress.org/

White, K. N. (2007). *The effects of background music in the classroom on the productivity, motivation, and behavior of fourth grade students*. https://files.eric.ed.gov/fulltext/ED522618.pdf

White, R. (2014). Foucault on the care of the self as an ethical project and a spiritual goal. *Human Studies: A Journal for Philosophy and the Social Sciences, 37*(4), 489-504. doi:10.1007/s10746-014-9331-3

White, R., & Wyn, J. (2004). *Youth and society*. Oxford University Press.

Wilcox, P., Winn, S., & Fyvie-Gauld, M. (2015). 'It was noting to do with the university, it was just the people': The role of social support in the first-year experience of higher education. *Studies in Higher Education, 30*(6), 707–722.

Williams, I. D., Richardson, T. A., Moore, D. D., Gambrel, L. E., & Keeling, M. L. (2020). Perspectives on self-care. *Journal of Creativity in Mental Health, 5*(3), 320–338. doi:10.1080/15401383.2010.507700

Williams, S. A. S., Conyers, A., & Garcia, F. (2018). Practical applications of ecological consultation in higher education: Diversity and inclusion initiatives. *Public Administration Quarterly, 42*(2), 183–212.

Wilshire, B. W. (1990). *The moral collapse of the university: Professionalism, purity, and alienation*. State University of New York Press.

Wilson, A.G. (2021). Emotionally Agile Leadership Amid COVID-19. *School Leadership Review, 15*(2).

Wilson, A. G., Almerico, G., Johnston, P., & Ensmann, S. (2020). Examining Educational Leadership Dispositions: A Valid and Reliable Assessment of Leadership Dispositions. *Journal of Educational Leadership Preparation, 15*(1).

Wilson, M. (2014). Critical reflection on authentic leadership and school leader development from a virtue ethical perspective. *Educational Review, 66*(4), 482–496. doi:10.1080/00131911.2013.812062

Wilton, T. (2021, October 26). *Facebook to Invest $10B this Year in VR and AR to Help Fuel the Metaverse*. Academic Press.

Wisconsin Initiative for Stigma Elimination. (2021, September 18). https://compassionresiliencetoolkit.org/schools/compassion-resilience/

Witters, D., & Agrawal, S. (2021, December 6). *Well-Being Enhances Benefits of Employee Engagement.* Gallup.com. https://www.gallup.com/workplace/236483/enhances-benefits-employee-engagement.aspx

Wood, A., & Thomas, N. (2021). *If you've gained weight during the pandemic, you're not alone. Here's what to do about it.* CNN. https://www.cnn.com/2021/03/24/health/weight-gain-during-covid-wellness/index.html

Woodhall, M. (1987). Human capital concepts. In G. psacharopoulos (Ed.), Economics of education (pp. 21-24). Elsevier. doi:10.1016/B978-0-08-033379-3.50011-5

Woodman, D. (2003). Responsibility and time for escape: The meaning of wellbeing to young Australians. *Melbourne Journal of Politics, 29*(2003-2004), 82–94.

Woods, C. (2019). Employee wellbeing in the higher education workplace: A role for emotion scholarship. *Higher Education, 60*(2), 171–185. doi:10.100710734-009-9293-y

Woodyard, C. (2011). Exploring the therapeutic effects of yoga and its ability to increase quality of life. *International Journal of Yoga, 4*(2), 49–54. doi:10.4103/0973-6131.85485

Woo, H., Kim, H., & Park, S. (2019). Burnout and turnover intentions among junior counseling faculty: Moderating role of mentoring. *Journal of Employment Counseling, 58*(2), 85–94. doi:10.1002/joec.12114

World Economic Forum. (2020). *The Future of Jobs Report 2020.* World Economic Forum. https://www.weforum.org/reports/the-future-of-jobs-report-2020

World Health Organization (WHO). (2021b). *What do we mean by self-care?* https://www.who.int/reproductivehealth/self-care-interventions/definitions/en/

World Health Organization. (2019). *Burn-out an "occupational phenomenon": International Classification of Diseases.* https://www.who.int/news/item/28-05-2019-burn-out-an-occupational-phenomenon-international-classification-of-diseases

World health Organization. (2020). *Pandemic fatigue. Reinvigorating the public to prevent COVID-19.* https://apps.who.int/iris/bitstream/handle/10665/335820/WHO-EURO-2020-1160-40906-55390-eng.pdf

World Health Organization. (2021). *What do we mean by self-care?* https://www.who.int/reproductivehealth/self-care-interventions/definitions/en/

World Health Organization. (2021a). *Occupational health.* https://www.who.int/health-topics/occupational-health

Wrzesniewski, A., McCauley, C., Rozin, P., & Schwartz, B. (1997). Jobs, careers, and callings: People's relations to their work. *Journal of Research in Personality, 31*(1), 21–33. doi:10.1006/jrpe.1997.2162

Yakaboski, T. (2019, November 13). *Making space under the weight of growing expectations.* Inside Higher Ed. https://www.insidehighered.com/advice/2019/11/13/how-set-boundaries-support-your-personal-life-and-career-opinion

Yan, Y.-W., Lin, R.-M., Su, Y.-K., & Liu, M.-Y. (2018). The relationship between adolescent academic stress and sleep quality: A multiple mediation model. *Social Behavior and Personality, 46*(1), 63–77. doi:10.2224bp.6530

Yoder, E. A. (2010). Compassion fatigue in nurses. *Applied Nursing Research, 23*(4), 191–197. doi:10.1016/j.apnr.2008.09.003

Ysseldyk, R., Greenaway, K. H., Hassinger, E., Zutrauen, S., Lintz, J., Bhatia, M. P., Frye, M., Starkenburg, E., & Tai, V. (2019). A leak in the academic pipeline: Identity and health among postdoctoral women. *Frontiers in Psychology, 10*(1297), 1–17. doi:10.3389/fpsyg.2019.01297 PMID:31231285

Yu, H., Jiang, A., & Shen, J. (2016). Prevalence and predictors of compassion fatigue, burnout and compassion satisfaction among oncology nurses: A cross-sectional survey. *International Journal of Nursing Studies, 57*, 28–38. doi:10.1016/j.ijnurstu.2016.01.012 PMID:27045562

Yurtkorub, S. (2013). Job stress and job performance among employees in public sector in Istanbul: Examining the moderating role of emotional intelligence. *Procedia: Social and Behavioral Sciences, 75*, 518–524. doi:10.1016/j.sbspro.2013.04.056

Zafir, M. M., & Fazilah, M. H. (2010). Stress at the Workplace: How the Ergonomic Factors Minimize it? *The 5th National Human Resource Management Conference 2010*, 642–657. 10.1080/00140130400029282

Zaini, U. (2012). *Akademia Baru: Memartabat UTM Berjenama Global 2012-2020*. Penerbit UTM Press.

Zalat, M. M., Hamed, M. S., & Bolbol, S. A. (2021). The experiences, challenges, and acceptance of e-learning as a tool for teaching during the COVID-19 pandemic among University Medical Staff. *PLoS One, 16*(3), e0248758. Advance online publication. doi:10.1371/journal.pone.0248758 PMID:33770079

Zambrana, R. E., Valdez, R. B., Pittman, C. T., Bartko, T., Weber, L., & Parra-Medina, D. (2021). Workplace stress and discrimination effects on the physical and depressive symptoms of underrepresented minority faculty. *Stress and Health, 37*(1), 175–185. doi:10.1002mi.2983 PMID:32926523

Zerbe, K. J. (2020). Pandemic fatigue: Facing the body's inexorable demands in the time of Covid-19. *Journal of the American Psychoanalytic Association, 68*(3), 475–478.

Zhao, C., Shi, C., Zhang, L., Zhai, Z., Ren, Z., Lin, X., & Jiang, G. (2020). Establishment of online platform for psychological assistance during a public health emergency. *International Journal of Mental Health Promotion, 22*(3), 123–132. doi:10.32604/IJMHP.2020.011077

Zielinska, M., & Kirtzman, F. (2021). *The Mental Health Toll of Working in Isolation*. Korn Ferry. https://www.kornferry.com/insights/this-week-in-leadership/mental-health-remote-work-coronavirus

About the Contributors

Karis L. Clarke is an Associate Professor and Department Chair of Educational Leadership at Clark Atlanta University who works with leaders in the Educational Leadership Department to prepare them to work in diverse schools locally, nationally, and internationally. Karis is a passionate educator cultivating the growth and development of educators. For 15 years, Karis Clarke has driven the development of teacher education with oversight of training programs, instructional strategies, curriculum planning, and accreditation. As a leader and mentor, she fosters dynamic and high performing instructional environments to enhance the student experience and sustain retention. She further encouraged growth by collaborating cross-functionally with internal and external constituencies to drive strategic direction while articulating the institutional mission. Dr. Clarke is a certified early childhood teacher, elementary supervisor, elementary principal and superintendent in South Carolina and holds Elementary Education (P-5) and Educational Leadership-Tier II certification in Georgia. She taught pre-kindergarten, second grade and third grade in the Beaufort County School District (Beaufort, South Carolina). She has served as an instructor and university supervisor at Winthrop University; Assistant Professor, Coordinator, Title III Activity Director, and Interim Director of Teacher Education at Morris College; Director of Teacher Education at Columbia College; Associate Professor, Department Head of Early Childhood Education and Elementary Education at Anderson University, and Education Consultant. Dr. Karis Clarke holds a B.A. in political science from Florida A&M University, M.A.T. in early childhood education from the College of Charleston, Ed.S. and Ed.D. in educational administration from South Carolina State University. She has also completed post bachelor's work at Florida State University.

* * *

Ansar Abbas received an Airlangga Development Scholarship to complete his doctoral degree at the University of Airlangga in Surabaya, Indonesia. During his studies, he wrote a number of journal articles, both qualitative and quantitative, as well as book chapters. Some papers are already published in prestigious journals while others are still under the peer-review process. Some of the key areas of research he developed his research in are leadership theories, leadership psychology, modern slavery, human capital value creation, positive and negative elements of psychology, spirituality, spiritual intelligence, research modeling and framework design, well-being, and positive psychology research. In addition, he is broadening his expertise in order to contribute to various worthwhile academic activities for research advancement, such as serving as a reviewer, editorial assistant, and editor for a number of national and international journals. He has a total of 15 years of diverse experience in a variety of fields, including management, administration, academia, and research.

Anna Amsler is an independent consultant and researcher affiliated to the Observatory of Competitiveness and New Ways of Working. She holds a Bachelor's Degree in International Relations and a Master's in Political Communication and Marketing, having worked in private and public institutions in areas related to public policy, strategic planning and project evaluation.

Jia Borror earned her doctoral degree in Educational Leadership in May of 2012 and currently serves as a faculty member at NSU's Abraham S. Fischler College of Education and School of Criminal Justice. Prior to that she served as a teacher in Broward County Public Schools. She has over 18 years of classroom teaching experience and holds National Board Certification. She teaches multiple courses in education at the Undergraduate, Master's, and Educational Specialist level in the areas of Curriculum and Instruction, Teacher and Educational Leadership, and Early Childhood Education. She is involved with educational research, presents at national conferences, writes for professional journals, and volunteers in the community as a member of the Junior League of Greater Fort Lauderdale.

Whitney Chick, M.Ed., holds a Masters of Education in Instructional Accommodations from Francis Marion University and a degree in Educational Curriculum and Leadership from Winthrop University. Mrs. Chick is an instructor in the Early Childhood Education program at Columbia College whose research interests include resiliency practices for beginning teachers and trauma-informed education.

Paul Collins received his Ph.D. in Educational Leadership from Miami University. He holds undergraduate degrees in Liberal Studies and Elementary Education from The University of Central Florida and Florida A&M University, respectively. Dr. Collins also holds an M.Ed. in Elementary Education from Florida A&M University. He was an Academic All-American and the Scholar-Athlete award recipient during his senior year on the FAMU baseball team. Dr. Collins brings over 20 years of experience in the field of education at the levels of traditional public, public charter, private/independent, international, and higher ed. He has served as an Assistant Professor in the Division of Education at Baldwin-Wallace University, as well as, a Teaching Associate at Miami University where he facilitated undergraduate and graduate level courses, served on university committees, and advised students. He has authored publications and has made many conference presentations. Additionally, Dr. Collins conducted research in Ghana, West Africa and spent a summer term as Visiting Lecturer at the University of South Africa. He has served many years as an elementary and middle school educator and transformational school administrator in Florida and Georgia public schools. Dr. Collins also worked in various teaching and leadership roles with the Marva Collins/Cleaster Mims College Preparatory School of Cincinnati, Ohio; which operated as an independent educational institution. He also garnered international educational leadership expertise while serving as Dean of Students at a school in the United Arab Emirates. Dr. Collins is currently a Visiting Associate Professor, Interim Chairperson, and Master's Degree Program Coordinator in the Educational Leadership and Counseling Dept. at Florida A&M University. His research interests are in the areas of Black male educator representation/retention and historiography & education.

Brennan Davis, Ph.D., is an Assistant Professor of Education at Columbia College, where she teaches literacy, writing, and English education courses. Dr. Davis holds a Ph.D. in Language and Literacy from the University of South Carolina and maintains research interests in two primary areas: effective professional development tools and processes for addressing issues of diversity in schools and innovative support systems for pre-service and beginning teachers.

Dian Ekowati is Head of Planning board Airlangga and senior lecturer at Faculty of Economics and Business. She is engaged in doing several social and academic research projects related to human development, organizational learning and change management.

Mochammad Fahlevi is Lecturer at Department of Management, BINUS Online Learning, Bina Nusantara University, Indonesia. Mochammad Fahlevi research has been published in several Scopus and WOS journals. Mochammad Fahlevi also serves as a Chief Editor of Journal of Research in Business, Economics, and Education, Journal of Business Management and Accounting, Journal of Economics and Business Letters, Priviet Multidisciplinary Journal, and Priviet Social Sciences Journal and also serves as an Associate Editor of Frontiers in Psychology, and is on the reviewer board of several leading journals.

Rakotoarisoa Fenitra is Graduated from the Faculty of Economics and Business, Department of Management, Universitas Airlangga, Surabaya Indonesia. He was granted an ADS by The Airlangga Global Engagement. His area of interest falls in Entrepreneurship, human behavior, tourism and marketing in particular, while general interests are related to human development approaches and empirical research.

Kavita Gupta is an Assistant Professor in the Department of Psychology, Faculty of Education and Psychology at The Maharaja Sayajirao University of Baroda, Vadodara (Gujarat). She is Pursuing her Ph.D. in Clinical Psychology from Sardar Patel University, Anand (Gujarat). Besides, she has her Doctoral thesis on 'Quality of Life in Cancer Patients undergoing Chemotherapy and Radiotherapy'. She is working with the university students targeting their Personal, Emotional, Psychological problems and enhancement of their mental health and well-being. Her area of interest includes Positive Psychology, Clinical Psychology, Social Psychology, Research Methodology, Educational Psychology. She is dedicating to serving undergraduate, postgraduate and PG Diploma students. She further hopes to apply the knowledge and skills garnered from her various disciplines towards improving the welfare and happiness of people of the world. Her research findings have been published as 20 research papers and 5 chapters in edited book in national and international referred/indexed journals and presented 6 research papers at National and International conferences.

Aida Shakila Ishak is a Senior Lecturer at the Faculty of Applied and Human Sciences, Universiti Malaysia Perlis. Her area of expertise is psychology counselling including drug abuse, adolescent and mental health issue. She has several years of experience in teaching and handling academic research. Aside from that, she also has participate in lots of event such as seminars and participating in the international conferences. She is currently active as a reviewer panel of proposals for postgraduate students in the faculty. Apart from academic activities, she is also heavily involved in community service engagement to help the local community, especially in providing counselling services and crisis intervention.

Fauziah Ismail is a lecturer at the Centre for Liberal Sciences, Faculty of Applied Sciences and Humanities, Universiti Malaysia Perlis. She holds a Bachelor Degree Human Development and Management (Universiti Putra Malaysia), Master of Arts Communication (Universiti Sains Malaysia). Areas of expertise are Human Communication, Human development and Health Communication. Started working at Universiti Malaysia Perlis on 17 March 2017. Before appointed as a lecturer, she worked as a Medical Social Worker at University Malaya Medical Center, Kuala Lumpur for 3 years. Apart from that, she has served in the Department of Statistics Malaysia, Penang and also in industry sector, Kasatani Advance Technology, Penang.

Nur Qurratul' Aini Ismail is a Lecturer at Centre for Liberal Sciences, Faculty of Applied & Human Sciences, UniMAP. Experienced as a social research assistant for over 10 years. B.Comm (Universiti Utara Malaysia), MA (Universiti Utara Malaysia) and PhD (Universiti Utara Malaysia). Areas of expertise are organizational communication, community policing and volunteerism.

Sarah Jarvie is an Associate Professor at Colorado Christian University. She has been a full-time counselor educator since 2014. She has a background in community mental health and private practice with clients of all ages from children to adults. Dr. Jarvie enjoys infusing connections between clinical practice and the classroom. Her research interests include person-centered education, teaching applications to counseling, and counselor and counselor educator wellness.

Anindita Majumdar has completed her PhD in Applied Psychology from University of Calcutta. She is an academician and a Rehabilitation Council of India registered psychologist. She has more than 10 years of work experience, both in education and corporate sectors. She is associated with Association of Rehabilitation Psychologist & Professionals India, International Benevolent Research Foundation, and Indian Psychoanalytic Society as Professional Life & Affiliated Member. She has extensive experience in practicing psychometric assessment, counselling, psychotherapy, skill training & development. Her expertise area includes child development related parenting psycho-educational training along with behavioural and educational management in special education field. Her areas of teaching and research interest include- Creativity, Expressive psychotherapy, Clinical & Rehabilitation Psychology, Developmental Psychology, Psychosocial & Personality research, and Qualitative Analysis. She has several papers published and presented in these domains. Her publication list includes- Indian Journal of Health & Wellbeing, International Law Research, International Journal of Advanced Research & Innovative Ideas in Education, IGI Global, Emerald, and many other platforms.

Cara Metz is an Associate Professor at University of Arizona Global Campus. She received a master's degree in clinical mental health counseling and a doctorate in counselor education and supervision from the University of Cincinnati. She also holds a bachelor's degree in psychology and economics from Ohio University. Dr. Metz has been licensed as a counselor since 2006 and has worked in an elementary school, community mental health, and a private practice, seeing clients from 6 to 80, favoring working with transitional aged youth from 14 to 22. In 2013, she moved into teaching full time, working with master's- and doctoral-level students studying counseling. Dr. Metz is currently serving as the faculty lead of the BA health and human services program at UAGC. Her research interests include counselor and counselor educator wellness, person-centered education, and best practices for online education.

Noran L. Moffett is a tenured Professor of Education in the Department of Educational Leadership of the College of Education at Fayetteville State University. He has formerly served in roles of Associate Dean at two Educator Preparation Programs (EPPs) during the reaffirmation of their NCATE Legacy Visits and as a professor who served as dissertation advisor concurrently. Noran is the son of a deceased World War II veteran, the late Rev. M.J. Moffett, and a mother, Alice E. Moffett, who retired as a school cafeteria manager. Noran was honorably discharged from the United States Army. He never loses sight of the purpose for which he came to the profession of teacher education- CHILDREN. Dr. Moffett's educational philosophy is as follows: "I am an educational evangelist and I believe that the purpose of educational preparation in higher education should be to ensure that we prepare future educators to serve as advocates for the children with the least opportunity, so they can compete with the children with the greatest opportunity as contributors to the global community."

Siti Norayu Mohd Basir works as Senior Lecturer at Universiti Malaysia Perlis. She gain her PhD in Political Science from Universiti Sains Malaysia in 2021. She is a fellow researcher at Center of Excellent for Social Innovation and Sustainability (COESIS) Universiti Malaysia Perlis.Her areas of expertise are patriotism, nationhood, Malaysian politics and ethnic relations. She is active in writing journals, articles in books and seminars presenter on national identity, ethnic relations in Malaysia and is often an interview panellist in Malaysia newspapers on issues of Malaysian statehood and politics. Expertise in the field of ethnic relations allows her to teach several related subjects namely Appreciation of Ethics and Civilization and Ethnic Relations.

Cynthia Montaudon is a full-time professor and a business consultant at the Business School at UPAEP. Since September 2018, she became head of the Observatory on Competitiveness and New Ways of Working, which deals with numerous issues related to social problems and creates awareness about current and future social needs. She has obtained a Post Doctorate Certificate In Organizational Leadership from Regent University in Virginia, USA; a Ph.D. in Strategic Planning and Technology Management from UPAEP, in Puebla, Mexico; a Ph.D. in Business from the University of Lincoln in Lincolnshire, UK, and three masters degrees: one in Quality Engineering from the Universidad Iberoamericana in Puebla, Mexico, another in Communication and media from the Jean Moulin, Lyon II University in Lyon, France, and the last one in Business Administration from the Tec de Monterrey in Mexico.

B. S. Parimal is Assistant Professor in the Department of Psychology, The Maharaja Sayajirao University of Baroda, Vadodara, Gujarat since 1997. His PhD thesis was on "Comparative study of Value, Personality and Mental Health among Scheduled-Caste and Non-Scheduled-Caste Students". He has presented 15 research papers at National and International Conferences. He has Published 07 research papers in National and 05 International reviewed/referred journals. His specialization is Clinical Psychology and areas of interest for teaching are Positive Psychology, Health Psychology, Educational Psychology and Counselling Psychology. His Research interests include Stress Management, Interpersonal Relationship Skills, Happiness and Mental Health Awareness Programmes in Community. He has been NSS Programme Officer at University level, Dean of students at Faculty level and UGC nominee at National level. He has been recognized as PhD guide. He has been felicitated recently for his contribution in teaching field by International Association of Lions Club. His Life motto is "Learn Psychology, Teach Psychology and Live Psychology".

Ingrid Pinto López is a university professor, researcher and consultor at Business School of UPAEP University, recognized by the National System of Researchers (SNI Conacyt). Ph.D. in Strategic Planning and Technology Management. Currently coordinator of the competitiveness observatory and new forms of work, coordinator of the international arbitration of the Latin American Association of Accounting and Administration Schools ALAFEC, member of Barcelona Economics Network and the Illustrious Latin American Academy of doctors.

Sarah Ransdell is currently a professor of Health Science at Nova Southeastern University. She received her PhD in Cognitive Psychology from the University of Florida in 1987. She teaches statistics, research methods, and telehealth. She recently published a book called Teacher Self-Care: A joyful ode to good health (Cambridge Scholars, 2020). She currently conducts research on self-reported resilience and cognitive skill among university students, staff, and faculty.

Nalanda Ray is currently pursuing her master's degree in psychology at Amity University, Kolkata. Her primary area of interest is in the regulation and development of emotions and empathy, and how they could cumulatively enhance social wellbeing. Additionally, she explores ways through which these qualities may be nurtured within people, as she believes that they could help promote functional adaptation in an increasingly hyper-digitized world. She has interned at Karma Center for Counselling & Wellbeing and at the Department of Mental Health and Behavioural Sciences at Fortis Healthcare. Her publications include a paper in the book Digitalization: The Global Force Breaking all the Trends, 2019, New Media and Language Learning, 2020 - for which she won the Outstanding Paper Award - and Moving to Know Boundaries, 2021. She has also been a passionate social service worker and strives to show the importance of empathy and action through helping others. Her volunteer work includes being a teaching assistant for underprivileged children at Jan Seva School, and being the President of the non-profit service organization Leo Club of Calcutta Vriddhi under Lions Club International.

Nurul Naimah Rose is a senior lecturer at Universiti Malaysia Perlis, Malaysia. She received her PhD in Counselling from University of Science Malaysia in 2017, M.ed Guidance and Counselling in 2009 and Bachelor of Human Sciences majoring in Sociology and Anthropology in 2006 from International Islamic University Malaysia. Her research work mostly about psychological distress, organizational stress, stress management, counselling stress intervention and stress coping strategy intervention.

Gagan Singh received his Graduation Degree in Electrical Engineering from Dayalbagh Organization, India, in 1998, M. Tech (Engineering Systems) from Dayalbagh Educational Institute, Agra, India in 1999, and Ph.D. in Electrical Engineering from Uttarakhand Technical University in 2011. He is currently working as Professor in the Electrical and Electronics & Communication Engineering Department, DIT University, Dehradun, India since March'2000. He has an overall experience of above twenty-three years. He served as Head of the Department of Electrical Engineering for over seventeen years and also served as Controller of Examination of DIT University for six years. He has authored a book on 'Electrical Measurement and Measuring Instruments' in 2004 and has published more than fifty papers in conference proceedings and international journals. His research interests include hydro-power plant instrumentation, control, modeling, and simulation. Two research scholars completed their Ph.D. under his guidance and he is currently guiding 4 Ph.D. scholars. He is the receiver of the Young Scientist Award in the first Uttaranchal State Science Congress by the Uttaranchal Council of Science and Technology, Government of Uttaranchal, in November 2006. The Academic Council of ULektz has awarded and recognized him as one of India's Top 20 Thought Leaders in Higher Education for 2021 on ULektz Wall of Fame.

Sonika Singh is currently working as Associate Professor in the Electrical and Electronics & Communication Engineering Department, DIT University, Dehradun, India since April'2000. Holding her Ph.D. in Electronics and Communication Engineering, she is mentoring the young minds at DIT University to leverage the most in this field. She proudly walks along with an exceptional experience of more than twenty-two years, rendering additional administrative responsibilities as well. Her research interests include Mobile Satellite Systems, Photonics, and Channel modeling in Wireless Communication Systems. She has guided one Ph.D. in EECE Department. She authored a book on 'Solid State Devices and Circuit' in 2004 and proudly owns more than forty papers in Conference Proceedings and International Journals. She is also the Chairperson of ICEIT DIT University Organisational Member. The Academic Council of ULektz has awarded her as one of India's Top 50 Women Leaders in the Education Industry for 2020.

Cris Slotoroff is a K–12 Humanities, World Languages, and Fine Arts Supervisor for a New Jersey school district. He taught AP Language & Composition to high school seniors in New Jersey for 12 years. His research primarily focuses on the changes to students' and teachers' regard for communication and socialization in the wake of mobile technology's ubiquity. Ultimately, Cris's research seeks to create a more informed teacher workforce that can help students to navigate these behavioral changes to live happier, more autonomous lives.

Fendy Suhariadi is Professor of Psychology Faculty in the field Industrial and Organizational Psychology, and Now as a Head of Human Resource Development program of Post Graduate School, Universitas Airlangga. His area falls into human behavior, industrial psychology and human development research.

Antione D. Tomlin, Ph.D., is an associate professor and department chair of Academic Literacies at Anne Arundel Community College. He earned his Ph.D. in Language, Literacy and Culture from the University of Maryland, Baltimore County, his M.A. in Higher Education Administration with a specialization in student affairs from Morgan State University, and his B.S. in Psychology from Stevenson University. Antione's current research interests focus on exploring the experiences of Black professionals in higher education.

Adrianne Wilson is an Associate Professor for Educational Leadership at the University of Tampa in Tampa, Florida. Dr. Wilson is also the director of the master's in educational leadership program at her institution as well as the chair of the education department. Dr. Wilson teaches numerous educational leadership courses; however, she is most notably known for her work in launching the educational leadership program six years ago at her institution. Dr. Wilson also serves on the board of directors for the Florida Association of Professors of Educational Leadership. Dr. Wilson is also the co-author and developer of three professional disposition assessments, which are currently under adoption by universities and colleges across the United States. With more than 20 years of experience in education, Dr. Wilson continues to build strong partnerships with local surrounding school district in her community. Lastly, Dr. Wilson conducts diversity, equity, and inclusion trainings as a consultant and her research agenda includes professional dispositions, mindfulness for school leadership, and mentorship.

Trudi Wolfe is in her first year as school social worker at Loper Elementary School in Shelbyville, IN. Prior to this school year, she had been the school counselor at Central Elementary in Beech Grove for 16 years. While at Central Elementary, Trudi led her school and district in implementing brain-aligned and trauma informed practices. Prior to becoming a school counselor, Trudi worked in mental health settings for over 20 years, working with children and adults who have experienced trauma. Trudi holds licenses in school social work, school counseling, clinical social work, and marriage and family therapy. Trudi also holds a Certificate in Applied Educational Neuroscience from Butler University.

Index

www.ingramcontent.com/pod-product-compliance
Lightning Source LLC
LaVergne TN
LVHW062144300926
849161LV00010B/2625